Evidence-based Healthcare and Public Health

Dedication

This book is dedicated to the memory of my mother who taught me, by example, the benefits of optimism and irony.

Commissioning Editor: Timothy Horne
Development Editor: Barbara Simmons
Project Manager: Anne Dickie
Text Design: Charlotte Murray
Cover Design: Stewart Larking
Illustrator: David Graham
Illustration Manager: Kirsteen Wright

Evidence-based Healthcare and Public Health

How to make decisions about health services and public health

Sir Muir Gray CBE MD

Director, National Knowledge Service, NHS;
NHS Chief Knowledge Officer;
Professor of Knowledge Management, Nuffield Department of Surgery,
University of Oxford, UK;
Director, Better Value Healthcare Ltd, UK

Chapter 9 co-written by **Sasha Shepperd** MSc DPhil

Research Scientist in Evidence Synthesis, Department of Public Health,

University of Oxford, UK

Editor: **Erica Ison**
Editorial Assistant: **Rosemary Lees**
Information Scientist: **Nicola Pearce-Smith**

THIRD EDITION

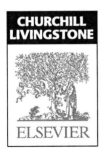

CHURCHILL
LIVINGSTONE

ELSEVIER

EDINBURGH LONDON NEW YORK OXFORD PHILADELPHIA ST LOUIS SYDNEY TORONTO 2009

CHURCHILL LIVINGSTONE
ELSEVIER

© Elsevier Limited 2001

© 2009, Elsevier Limited. All rights reserved.

No part of this publication may be reproduced or transmitted in any form or by any means, electronic or mechanical, including photocopying, recording, or any information storage and retrieval system, without permission in writing from the publisher. Permissions may be sought directly from Elsevier's Rights Department: phone: (+1) 215 239 3804 (US) or (+44) 1865 843830 (UK); fax: (+44) 1865 853333; e-mail: healthpermissions@elsevier.com. You may also complete your request on-line via the Elsevier website at http://www.elsevier .com/permissions.

First edition 1997

Second edition 2001

Third edition 2009

ISBN: 978 0 443 10123 6

British Library Cataloguing in Publication Data

A catalogue record for this book is available from the British Library

Library of Congress Cataloging in Publication Data

A catalog record for this book is available from the Library of Congress

Note

ELSEVIER your source for books, journals and multimedia in the health sciences

www.elsevierhealth.com

Working together to grow libraries in developing countries

www.elsevier.com | www.bookaid.org | www.sabre.org

 ELSEVIER   BOOK AID International   Sabre Foundation

Transferred to Digital Printing in 2010

The publisher's policy is to use paper manufactured from sustainable forests

Contents

Preface to third edition

I have written this book for those who make decisions about groups of patients or populations. My overall purpose is twofold:

1. to improve the competence of health service decision-makers
2. to strengthen the motivation of any health service decision-maker to use scientific methods when making a decision.

However, some opponents of this approach have characterised it as: 'Arrogant, seductive and controversial'.

It must be admitted that the terms 'evidence-based medicine' and 'evidence-based healthcare' were chosen partly for their provocative nature. However, those of us involved in developing these initiatives had evidence that:

- the findings from research were not being put into practice quickly and systematically because the process of decision-making was based on a random cocktail of drivers – values, resources, and evidence
- decision-makers were not aware which of these drivers were shaping their decisions, nor which of them was most important.

However, as proponents of an evidence-based approach, we may not have been as clear as we could have been in describing its development, partly because the ideas were continually evolving. This could provide an explanation of why one group of workers was critical.[1-3] Many other people have found the concepts useful.

The approach advocated in this book is one that emphasises the need to apply logic to:

- the analysis of healthcare problems
- the identification and appraisal of options for health improvement
- decision-making about the delivery of healthcare for groups of patients or populations.

This approach of evidence-based decision-making could be given one of several different generic terms; for example, it could be called reductionist or positivist. However, proponents regard it as an essential component of providing modern healthcare, in the same way that we regard evidence-based medicine as an essential approach to clinical practice in the 21st century.

The preoccupation with productivity and quality that dominated health service management towards the end of the twentieth century has not necessarily led to the development of evidence-based policies, nor to the implementation of knowledge derived from research for the improvement of the effectiveness, safety, acceptability and cost-effectiveness of healthcare. There is now a general appreciation that decisions made about health services and clinical practice must be based on evidence to a much greater degree than they have been in the past such that the knowledge derived from research can be used to improve the health of patients and the public.

References

1. Polychronis, A., Miles, A. and Bentley, P. (1996) *Evidence-based medicine: Reference? Dogma? Neologism? New orthodoxy?* J. Eval. Clin. Pract. 2: 1–5.
2. Polychronis, A., Miles, A. and Bentley, P. (1996) *The protagonists of 'evidence-based medicine' – arrogant, seductive and controversial.* J. Eval. Clin. Pract. 2: 9–13.
3. O'Neill, D., Miles, A. and Polychronis, A. (1996) *Central dimensions of clinical practice evaluation: efficiency, appropriateness and effectiveness – I.* J. Eval. Clin. Pract. 2: 13–29.

Confessions of an amanuensis

Although famous for his work on electromagnetism, it is far from common knowledge that the young Michael Faraday acted as an amanuensis to Sir Humphrey Davy, following an injury to Davy's eyes in a laboratory explosion.

The word 'amanuensis' was first recorded in 1619, derived from the Latin *manu* for hand and *-ensis*, a suffix meaning 'belonging to'. The definition in the *Shorter Oxford English Dictionary* is given as 'one who copies or writes from dictation'. This has been my main function in the preparation of this book, which takes as a starting point the work done during the 1990s, principally in Oxford, to promote 'evidence-based healthcare'.

The idea of commissioning a multi-author book was rejected because of the problems inherent in such a project, particularly on a topic like evidence-based healthcare in which there is so much cross-cutting from one approach to another. As it would have been difficult to fuse several different contributions into a coherent whole, the decision was taken for a small group to 'copy or write from dictation' from the work of many different people.

Many of the people whose work we have described worked in the four counties that comprised the old Oxford Regional Health Authority. This book also builds on the original ideas of the team at McMaster University, comprising Larry Chambers, Gordon Guyatt, Brian Haynes, Jonathan Lomas, Andy Oxman and Dave Sackett. Since then, Dave was a source of inspiration during the five years he spent in the UK, helping to change the culture and develop the skills of evidence-based decision-making.

Those whose work has been drawn upon for one or more of the three editions of this book are:

Clive Adams, Doug Altman, Chris Ball, Andrew Booth, Sandra Booth, Anne Brice, Catherine Brogan, Shaun Brogan, Chris Bulstrode, Iain Chalmers, Myles Chippendale, Andy Chivers, Martin Dawes, Anna Donald, Gordon Dooley, Martin Eccles, Adrian Edwards, Jayne Edwards, Jim Elliott, Katie Enock, John Fletcher, John Geddes, David Gill, Paul Glasziou, Michael Goldacre, Peter Gøtzsche, Sian Griffiths, Jeremy Grimshaw, Nick Hicks, Alison Hill, Richard Himsworth, Carol Lefebvre, Huw Llewelyn, Mark Lodge, Steve McDonald, Ian McKinnell, Henry McQuay, Theresa Marteau, Jill Meara, Ruairidh Milne, Andrew Moore, Al Mulley, David Naylor, Gill Needham, Ian Owens, Judy Palmer, David Pencheon, Bob Phillips, W. Scott Richardson, William Rosenberg, Jill

Sanders, Ken Schultz, Valerie Seagroatt, Sasha Shepperd, Mark Starr, Mike Stein, Barbara Stocking, Sharon Straus, Andre Tomlin, Ben Toth, Martin Vessey, and Chris Williams.

Many of these people have been supported by the UK National Health Service R&D programme, the initial leadership of which by Sir Michael Peckham was very important in the evolution of evidence-based healthcare.

I am also indebted to those people in various teams with whom I have worked on the development of these ideas: the GRiPP team, the CASP team, the R&D team, those in the Cochrane Collaboration, colleagues developing the National Library for Health, colleagues in the National Screening Programmes, and friends and colleagues at McMaster University (Canada) and at the National Library of Medicine (USA), who have continued to be inspirational and generous.

Simply stringing words together is only part of the preparation of a text like this; the final product, as I said, has been the combined work of a small team. The team is supported by Ann Southwell, who wields the business management skills underpinning the creation of many of the projects that contributed to the development of evidence-based healthcare. Karen McKendry, a wizard with PowerPoint, created some of the diagrams that punctuate and enliven the prose, and Nicola Pearce-Smith acted as the book's able information scientist. Without their contributions, the book would have been of much poorer quality.

The duo who shaped this book in its final form (for the third time of asking) – Rosemary Lees and Erica Ison – have continued to be endlessly good-humoured and hard-working and applied not only effort but also the highest level of skill to transforming base metal into gold, and transmuting discursive prose into a text that is much briefer, clearer, and more powerful than it was when it left the hand of the amanuensis.

Finally, like another Scottish amanuensis, James Boswell, I must acknowledge the burden borne by my family, Jackie, Em, and Tat, who have put up with it all three times over.

The production of all three editions of this book was supported by charitable trust funds. The objective in the disbursement of monies from these funds is the promotion of epidemiology as a practical tool for all healthcare decision-makers, working for what the president of the Royal Statistical Society in 1996 called the 'promotion of an evidence-based society'.[1]

Reference

1. Smith, A.F.M. (1996) Mad cows and Ecstasy: chance and choice in an evidence-based society. J. R. Statist. Soc. A. 159: 367–83.

How to use this book

As the main aim in writing this book is to help those people who have to make decisions about groups of patients or populations base those decisions on a careful appraisal of the best evidence available, it has been structured in such a way as to increase the level of evidence-based decision-making in the provision of health services. The scope of, and need for, evidence-based decision-making are described in Chapters 1 and 2.

The contents of the rest of the book cover four main topics:

- asking the right questions (Section 9.4.1)
- finding and appraising evidence (Chapters 4–6)
- developing the capacity of organisations and individuals to use evidence (Chapters 7 and 9)
- implementation – getting research into practice.

Finding and appraising evidence

The appraisal of evidence has three different dimensions:

- different types of healthcare decision, such as decisions about new treatment services or management changes (Chapter 3) and public health (Chapter 8)

- different types of outcome, such as effectiveness, safety or quality (Chapter 6)
- different types of research method, such as systematic reviews, randomised controlled trials, or cohort studies (Chapter 5).

For any problem, all three dimensions must be considered (Fig. 0.1).

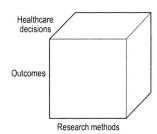

Fig. 0.1

Developing the capacity for evidence-based decision-making

In Chapter 7, the ways in which the level of evidence-based decision-making within an organisation can be increased are discussed. This is achieved by developing not only the skills of individuals (see Chapter 9) but also the culture, systems and bureaucratic structures within organisations (see Sections 7.1-7.4). These two facets of development are inter-related (Fig. 0.2).

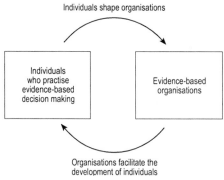

Fig. 0.2

Getting research into practice

Throughout the book, there is a focus on implementation, although it is recognised that it is often difficult to implement research evidence into clinical practice and health service management and policy.

The first step is to prepare a policy (Fig. 0.3), i.e. a statement of what should happen – for example, that all women aged over 50 years should undergo mammography, or that all people who have had a myocardial infarction should receive a treatment regimen of aspirin and beta-blockers.

Once a policy has been developed, systems must be designed to ensure that the policy is implemented. These systems must encompass organisational development (Chapter 7) and the education of both professionals and the public to improve not only healthcare but also the public health (Chapter 9).

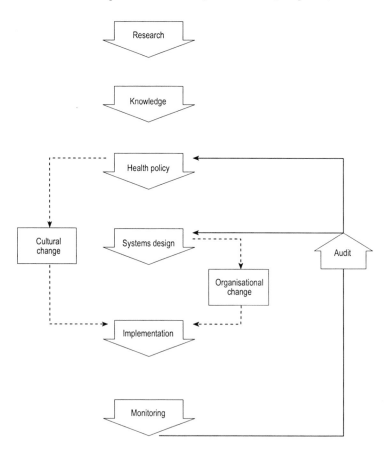

Fig. 0.3

Although a companion book on evidence-based medicine has been published, it is written primarily for clinicians.[1] The essence of this discipline has been distilled in Chapter 10 for the benefit of health service managers because decisions about individual patients and those about groups are inter-related. Clinicians who are also managers, or involved in managing, will benefit from developing the skills described in both books because, although concepts such as appropriateness or effectiveness are the same, a different perspective needs to be brought to bear in each sphere.

Reference

1. Straus, S. E., Richardson, W. S., Glasziou, P. and Haynes, R. B. (2005) *Evidence-based Medicine. How to Practice and Teach EBM*, 3rd edn. Churchill Livingstone, Edinburgh.

Defining our terms

A rose is a rose is a rose.

Gertrude Stein

What's in a name? That which we call a rose

By any other word would smell as sweet;

William Shakespeare, *Romeo and Juliet*, Act II, Scene ii

Gentle Reader,

Visualise, if you will, Newcastle General Hospital, the hub of hospital care in the north-east for many years – solid, Victorian and dependable. The hospital's honest, uncompromising and practical atmosphere might strike you as an unlikely setting for the 20th century's most influential philosopher, but Ludwig Wittgenstein was employed as a laboratory technician there during the Second World War. He showed such great promise as a laboratory investigator that attempts were made to persuade him to take up a scientific career. However, he chose to return to philosophy, linguistic philosophy in particular.

One of Wittgenstein's central tenets in linguistic philosophy was that differences of opinion or arguments between protagonists were often the result of a failure to recognise that both sides were using the same word but had a different understanding of its meaning when they used it.

Commentary

Throughout this book we have defined certain terms and attempted to use those definitions consistently. However, it is important to bear in mind, gentle reader, that our definitions may not be the same as yours.

Defining words with words

The definition of a word is the collation of its meanings by a lexicographer, preeminent among whom is Dr Johnson, some-time Fellow of Pembroke College, Oxford, and compiler of the first great English dictionary. It was another Fellow of an Oxford College, Dr James Murray, first editor of the *Oxford English Dictionary*, who decided that a dictionary should contain not only the definitions of words but also their meanings by providing examples of the word in use, and arranged chronologically so that the evolution of the word's meaning could be understood.[1]

Defining words by their usage

The meaning of a word is often different from its definitions, and meaning can best be appreciated by observing the way a word is used. At first, Murray's idea of illustrating meaning through usage was fiercely resisted by some delegates at the Oxford University Press, due to the effect this policy would have on the magnitude, and cost, of the exercise. Both sides were right: the delegates because the task took a long time – at Murray's death in 1915, 36 years after he took on the task, he had completed nearly half of the dictionary, having been responsible for words beginning with the letters A–D, H–K, O–P and T – and Murray, because the enduring success of the *Oxford English Dictionary* has changed for ever the way we think and find out about the meanings of words.

The principles of James Murray and the philosophy of Ludwig Wittgenstein are very similar. Wittgenstein's texts are difficult to read. His two great works, the *Tractatus Logico-Philosophicus* and *Philosophical Investigations*, consist of lean, numbered propositions, arranged hierarchically in the former and as a single sequence in the latter. Counter-intuitively, the absence of long paragraphs does not make them easy to understand. Access is facilitated by numerous books about, and commentaries on, Wittgenstein and his work, such as Anthony Kenny's book *Wittgenstein*.[2]

No single meaning of a word is always and indubitably right. There are only uses that are clear and those that are not clear, uses that are new and those that are not new. The need to observe how a word is used in order to understand its meaning is one of the principles of Wittgenstein's philosophy underpinning this book, and rather than expecting the reader to buy Last's *Dictionary of Epidemiology*,[3] excellent though it is, we have endeavoured to make it clear how we use particular terms.

Two other of Wittgenstein's principles are relevant to decision-makers:

- New words (e.g. Internet) or new uses of words (e.g. World Wide Web)

can clarify meaning and be useful or cause confusion. However, as any term becomes more widely used by more people, its use becomes increasingly diverse, and there may come a point at which the term causes more confusion than clarity and should no longer be used. Consider, for example, how often you have heard the term 'evidence' used when the way in which it was used indicated that it was being invested with a different meaning from that which you understood when using the word? (See also Casebook 1.)

- Many arguments – indeed, Wittgenstein believed all arguments – result from a failure to appreciate that the people involved do not agree on the meaning of the terms being used. Consider, for example, how often you have heard arguments about the proposition that 'evidence-based medicine destroys clinical freedom' without time being taken to reach agreement on the terms 'evidence-based medicine', 'destroys', and 'clinical freedom'.

Decision-making can be improved and arguments prevented, therefore, by prefacing the debate with statements such as:

When we use the word 'evidence' we mean 'knowledge derived from research'; when we use knowledge derived from our own experience, we shall make that clear.

Word euthanasia

Sometimes it is necessary to discontinue the use of a word or term that has become the cause of confusion and is preventing further understanding and progress. Active discontinuation of the use of a word may not be necessary in some disciplines, such

Casebook 1 The meanings of evidence

In the UK and other countries in which English is the first language, one of the connotations of the term 'evidence' is that the information used is the product of research; evidence-based propositions, therefore, are those that can be supported by good-quality research, and contrast with propositions that depend only on the experience of the person making the proposition. One implication of evidence-based decision-making is that the decision-maker is being scientific and orientated towards applying the findings from research.

In other languages, however, the word 'evidence' – *Evidenz* in German, *evidencia* in Spanish or Italian – has a different connotation. The use of the term implies what, in the UK, would be understood as 'self-evident'. It is self-evident that night follows the day; no research is needed, no critical appraisal is required. As such, the promotion of 'evidence'-based medicine would be interpreted as the promotion of the traditional style of decision-making in which a decision-maker assumes that the proposition on which a decision is based is true because it is self-evident, and does not invite or require critical appraisal and evaluation.

In Italy, therefore, 'evidence-based medicine' has been translated as 'medicine based on proof of efficacy'. In German, the closest translation of 'evidence-based medicine' would be *critische medizin* or 'critical medicine', but those who were involved in discussing the concept at the early workshops decided to adopt the term *Evidenz Basiert Medizin*, thereby boldly changing the German language.

as management, where many new terms are created and enter widespread use until they themselves become displaced by later fashions. 'Benchmarking' and 'modernising' are examples of such terms, and the same fate may, in time, befall 'evidence-based decision-making'. However, if any term causes more confusion than clarity, it should be dropped from decision-making discourse.

Even in clinical practice terms can cause confusion and may need to be deleted from debate. In his highly praised biography, Ray Monk[4] describes how Wittgenstein, when a technician in a research laboratory in Guy's Hospital in 1941, formed a Medical Research Council team, the leader of which, Dr Grant, observed that 'there is in practice a wide variation in the application of the diagnosis of "shock" without an agreed meaning of the term',

which was harmful to patients, and 'renders it impossible to assess the efficacy of the various methods of treatment adopted'. Grant argued that 'there is good ground, therefore' for the view that it is better to avoid the diagnosis of 'shock', and to replace it with an accurate and complete record of a patient's state and progress, together with the treatment given.

Wittgenstein was himself influenced by a physicist, Hertz, who had proposed dropping the use of the term 'force' from the debates of the time, accepting that if this were done 'the questions as to the nature of force will not have been answered but our minds, no longer vexed, will cease to ask illegitimate questions'.

Wittgenstein, in paying homage to this approach, said that 'in my way of doing philosophy, its whole aim is to give an expression to such a form that certain disquietudes disappear'. He also proposed that if Dr Grant was required to include the word 'shock' in his annual report, as some authorities wished, the word should be printed 'upside down to emphasize its unsuitability'.

Defining words by numbers

Vienna at the end of the Hapsburg Empire was in the final stages of its glory, already turning a little rotten on the bough. Although rottenness implies decay, decay is necessary for the renewal of life forms. Wittgenstein was a product of Vienna or, to be more precise, of the intellectual and wealthy Jewish community living in Vienna at the time; so, too, was Malinowski. Malinowski argued, contrary to Wittgenstein, that knowledge was created, not by the lonely intellectual sitting at his desk, as Wittgenstein did throughout the English winters, but by groups of people talking and using language to create new knowledge.

The Vienna school of philosophy was flourishing as Wittgenstein left the city, and it became very influential, particularly in Britain, where it gave rise to what is known as 'logical positivism', the leading figure and most eloquent reporter of which was A. J. Ayer. In *Language, Truth and Logic*,[5] Ayer took an approach to the definition of a term that did not rely on words at all.

He proposed that instead of trying to understand the meaning of a proposition by analysing the meaning of the individual terms within that proposition it was better to determine whether a proposition could be verified:

> *The criteria which we use to test the genuineness of apparent statements of fact is the criterion of verifiability. We say that a sentence is factually signifi-cant to any given person, if, and only if,*

> *he knows how to verify the propositions which it purports to express – that is, if he knows what observations would lead him, under certain conditions, to accept the proposition as being true, or reject it as being false. And with regard to questions the procedure is the same. We enquire in every case what observations would lead us to answer the question, one way or the other; and, if none can be discovered, we must conclude that the sentence under consideration does not, as far as we are concerned, express a genuine question, however strongly its grammatical appearance may suggest that it does.*

> A. J. Ayer[5]

The logical positivists believe that no term should be examined in isolation – a study of the term 'efficiency' would be pointless – but investigated in the context of propositions, such as 'this hospital is more efficient than that hospital'. To define the meaning of this proposition, a logical positivist would not have recourse to a dictionary, but instead seek to agree on the data that would need to be collected to confirm or refute the statement. Thus, for this particular proposition, the debate immediately becomes: 'How would you measure efficiency?'. Options include:

- cost per case
- throughput per bed
- percentage of costs spent on administration.

Meaning, reality and language

The traditional view of language was that it described reality. This is undoubtedly true for physical objects, such as 'a table' or 'a chair', unless one adheres to the more sceptical school of philosophy which holds that everything ceases to exist when one closes one's eyes. For social constructs, however, language does not simply describe reality; it creates it.

The clearest description of the relationship between language and reality comes from anthropologists, notably Benjamin Lee Whorf, who worked as a fire prevention engineer for the Hartford Fire Insurance Company and studied Native American languages, particularly the language of the Hopi people. He created a theory he called the principle of linguistic relativity,[6] in which he proposes that language creates social realities such as 'the future', 'the quality of evidence' or even 'evidence-based healthcare'. The Sapir–Whorf hypothesis of linguistic relativity is the best articulation of this concept: 'the fact of the matter is that the "real world" is to a large extent unconsciously built up on the language habits of the group'. Through the use and evolution of language comes social change and social reality. The work of anthropologists has since been developed by sociologists, the most accessible text being *The Social Construction of Reality* by Berger and Luckman.[7]

Words have meanings but the meanings create and change reality as well as expressing it.

Indefinite definitions

Throughout this book, we have tried to give a clear definition of a term without implying that our definition is *the* definition; *caveat lector*, 'let the reader beware'.

References

1. Winchester, S. (2003) *The Meaning of Everything: The Story of the Oxford English Dictionary.* Oxford University Press, Oxford.
2. Kenny, A. (1973) *Wittgenstein.* Penguin Books, London.
3. Last, J.M. (2000) *A Dictionary of Epidemiology.* Oxford University Press, Oxford.
4. Monk, R. (1991) *Wittgenstein.* Vintage Press, New York, pp. 445–7.
5. Ayer, A.J. (1936) *Language, Truth and Logic.* Penguin Books, London.
6. Carroll, J.B. (ed.) (1956) *Language, Thought, and Reality: Selected Writings of Benjamin Lee Whorf.* Technology Press of Massachusetts Institute of Technology, Cambridge, Massachusetts.
7. Berger, P.L. and Luckman, T. (1966) *The Social Construction of Reality. A Treatise in the Sociology of Knowledge.* Doubleday, Garden City, New York.

Despite the differences in the ways in which health services around the world are funded and organised, many of the major problems in the delivery of healthcare are similar:

- the increasing costs of healthcare (Fig. P.1)
- the lack of capacity in any country to pay for the totality of health services demanded by healthcare professionals and the general public.

In addition, in most countries, the inflation in healthcare costs is greater than the growth of the economy. This rate of inflation is related to inefficiencies in the delivery of healthcare arising from:

- the supply-led nature of healthcare in which the professional tells the patient what is needed, thereby creating demand, or develops and advocates the use of a new service
- the provision of inappropriate care.

Moreover, although the mode of health service provision appears to differ greatly from one country to another, there are certain common factors that are beginning to influence the evolution of systems of health service organisation and healthcare delivery in all countries irrespective of their geographical latitude:

- population ageing
- the advent of new technology and new knowledge
- rising patient and professional expectations
- new diseases, such as SARS.

In addition to these macro problems affecting healthcare as a whole, eight problems can be observed in every service:

1. errors and mistakes
2. poor-quality healthcare
3. waste of resources
4. variations in policy and practice

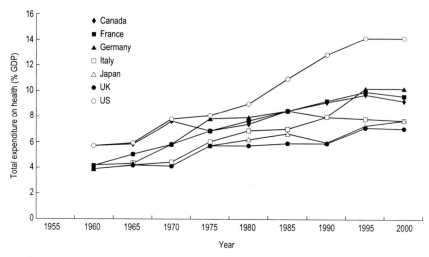

Fig. P.1
Expenditure on healthcare as a percentage of gross domestic product (GDP) in Canada, France, Germany, Italy, Japan, the UK and the USA from 1960 to 1996 (Source: Hicks and Gray, ref. 1, Section 2.3)

5. patient's poor experience of healthcare
6. over-enthusiastic adoption of interventions of low value
7. failure to get evidence and new interventions of high value into practice
8. failure to manage ignorance and uncertainty.

Common problems: common solutions

As the problems associated with the delivery of healthcare worldwide converge, the solutions being sought can be characterised by certain features that are not only evident in the health services of post-industrial nations but also important to the structural reforms of healthcare in developing economies:

- a preoccupation with cost control
- the development of systems to prevent the burden of cost falling on the individual
- an increasing authority being given to the function of paying for healthcare either for people who live within a particular area or for those who are members of a health plan or insurance fund
- a clearer definition and delineation of the function of paying for healthcare such that responsibility is being

shifted from the heartland of government to an agency or agencies, the primary responsibility of which is to pay for healthcare and obtain value for money; in Germany, for example, there is now an increased emphasis on the power of insurance schemes

- a growing appreciation of the need for those who pay for healthcare to manage the evolution and development of clinical practice in partnership with the clinical professions
- increasing public and political interest in the evidence on which decisions about the effectiveness and safety of healthcare are based.

As a result of these common problems, pressures and solutions, systems of health service organisation are also beginning to converge. In order to meet these powerful challenges, the principles of evidence-based healthcare can be applied to great effect, irrespective of whether a health service is organised nationally (as in the UK) or by province (as in Canada), whether it is tax-based or insurance-based (as in Japan), or whether the main source of funding is public or private (as in the USA).

Indeed, the teaching and learning of evidence-based practice can bring previously hidden elements of healthcare practice into sharp focus as assumptions and habits are challenged through the application of reliable knowledge. Healthcare professionals at all levels should know:

- how to convert an information need or healthcare problem into an answerable question
- where to find the best evidence to answer questions
- when to apply the evidence if found.

Against this background, it is important to recognise that healthcare information needs, and barriers to meeting those information needs, vary not only among countries but also among healthcare systems.

Margin Note P.1
Evidence-based practice

Learning and teaching evidence-based practice integrates principles from problem-based learning and reflective learning. By seeking the active engagement of the learner through focused learning in real work activity, the gap between what is known and what is practised diminishes (see Chapter 9).

Problems and solutions in poorer countries

The challenges to the provision of healthcare may be obvious in post-industrial nations, but these challenges also affect developing countries. Thus, a minister of health in a developing economy is responsible for providing appropriate services to meet not only the typical health problems of less developed countries, such as high infant mortality rates, and high mortality and morbidity rates resulting from the prevalence of infectious diseases – problems resolved in the 19th century in what were then industrial nations – but also the consequences of lifestyle habits, such as cigarette smoking, drug abuse and dangerous driving, which became predominant in the post-industrial societies of the late 20th century.

New healthcare technologies may be introduced into a developing country by practitioners, or developed in teaching hospitals that have been built in emulation of famous centres in the USA or Europe. These technological developments, however, will be relevant to only a small proportion of the population, although they can consume a large proportion of healthcare resources. Thus, it is vital that health services in a developing economy are managed using an evidence-based approach, although it may prove more difficult to implement in this context than in that of a developed economy. In countries that do have well-developed economies, private practice, which is much more difficult to influence, is relatively less important than care provided within formal managed systems. In developing countries, physicians can sometimes be so poorly paid that incentives other than conforming to the best evidence available may prevail.

There are interventions that have been shown to do more good than harm at reasonable cost but which are not yet widely adopted in countries with developing economies, such as the administration of aspirin, which reduces the health and economic burden resulting from stroke.

Conversely, there are other interventions that have not yet been shown to be effective but which are in routine use; these interventions of unproven effectiveness consume resources that could be expended on interventions that do more good than harm at reasonable cost. Evidence-based decision-making has a role in the provision of healthcare in all countries, irrespective of the stage of their economic development (see Section 7.8.5).

The absence of reliable information due to inadequate access to information systems is a particular challenge for those working in low- and middle-income countries. Open-access initiatives, such as Healthcare Information For All by 2015 (HIFA2015), have been set up to resolve this problem in low-income countries (Margin Note P.2) using advocacy and evidence to ensure the availability of reliable information for safe and effective healthcare.

Margin Note P.2

Healthcare Information for All

Healthcare Information for all 2015 (HIFA2015) is available online at: http://www.dgroups.org/groups/child2015

The aim of Health Information for All by 2015 is to identify evidence-based solutions to address the information and learning needs of healthcare providers. The objective is to create a web-based resource providing different ways of meeting information needs.

Pre-conditions for evidence-based healthcare

It has emerged that there are two necessary pre-conditions to foster the practice of evidence-based healthcare:

1. a commitment to cover the whole population – where no such commitment exists, it is still possible to introduce any intervention that shows some evidence of effectiveness no matter how small
2. a fixed budget for healthcare – as healthcare budgets were capped during the final years of the 20th century, there was a growing appreciation of the need for evidence-based decision-making as an essential element in the provision of healthcare for the 21st century (see Casebook P.1).

The USA and the rest of the developed world

The difference between healthcare decision-making in the USA and in other developed countries is that the two pre-conditions for evidence-based decision-making – a fixed budget and a commitment to cover the entire population – are not present.

Casebook P.1 Poacher turned gamekeeper

In 1997 in France, the minister of health, M. Jacques Richir, himself a doctor, challenged the medical profession when they were complaining about the introduction of tougher controls on healthcare spending.

Le docteur Richir, qui continue à exercer la médecine, se lance: 'Pouvez-vous me dire avec certitude que chaque acte que vous effectuez a toujours une justification médicale?'

'Oui!', s'écrient les internes en chœur, manifestement choqués qu'on puisse mettre en doute leur conscience professionnelle.

'Au moment de rédiger votre ordonnance', poursuit imperturbalement M. Richir, 'vous devez réfléchir quinze secondes et vous demander si votre acte est indispensable. C'est sur les actes redondants qu'on économisera un ou deux pour cents.'
Le Monde, 4 Avril 1997

This difference between healthcare decision-making in the USA and in other developed countries was highlighted by the decision about which age-groups of women should undergo breast cancer screening, a decision that was taken at the second attempt. The decision in question was a recommendation that breast cancer screening be undertaken in women *under* the age of 50 years, which was elegantly analysed in a paper by Tannenbaum[1] (a summary of this analysis is presented in Casebook P.2).

Casebook P.2 Summary of the paper by Tannenbaum (Source: *Evidence-Based Health Policy and Management* 1998; 2: 53)

The epidemiological approach to the assessment of effectiveness in Canada and the United States is similar, although research results in Canada are expressed more often in terms of the population benefits that are likely to result, but in the United States the results of research are seen as something not only for policy-makers and managers but also as a resource for consumers to make more informed decisions. Much of the debate in Canada takes place between the government and the organisations representing physicians who argue both that they should be involved in decision-making about resource allocation and that, having made broad decisions on the amount of resources available, individual clinicians should retain a high level of freedom in interpreting evidence and maximising effectiveness. The Canadian government, in paying and negotiating medical prices, represents not only Canadian patients but also population health interests, and effectiveness research is used to obtain the best value for the population as a whole.

In the USA this type of negotiation does not take place at government level but is much more decentralised and dispersed, being interpreted by insurance companies and provider organisations on the one hand, and individual patients on the other. An analysis of who actually makes choices in the American health care system reveals that individual consumers do have choice, but this is often determined, or constrained, by their employer.

Physicians have a different part to play in the interpretation of evidence about effectiveness or ineffectiveness in the two systems. In one system the physicians are very much involved in negotiation with the government about the total amount of resources available for health care, and therefore priorities, whereas in the USA, physicians have a number of different types of relationships with those who pay for healthcare, depending on the type of organisation they work for and the patients they serve.

Author's conclusions

Both the USA and Canada have an explicit commitment to promote effective, and to discourage ineffective, care. However, the different cultures and the different decision-making processes mean that the knowledge about effectiveness and ineffectiveness, which is usually expressed in terms of probabilities, has a different contribution in decisions in both countries. The author's conclusion is that: 'Canadian policy-makers overstate the societal applicability and the US policy-makers the individual applicability of outcomes research findings'. The result of this is that different decisions may result from the same evidence.

Tannenbaum suggested that the main reason why the USA and Canada took different approaches (although the same argument could apply to any other developed country) was that in the USA decisions about health are individualistic, whereas in other developed countries they are primarily collective. In the USA, it is felt that government should recommend action if there is a possibility that the individual might benefit; it is then up to the individual to take the appropriate step – provided, of course, that they can afford to do so. In those countries in which healthcare is provided to the entire population, all decisions about health and healthcare have to be made taking into account finite resources and opportunity costs. Thus, people in other countries would not deny the possibility of a small benefit from universal screening for the population of women under 50 years, although they could point out that there will be a large number of women who would be harmed by the process and might be mindful of the other uses to which those resources could be put.

In the absence of the pre-conditions for evidence-based healthcare, those who pay for healthcare in the USA, such as for-profit and not-for-profit health maintenance organisations and the insurance companies that back them, may seek to live within their resources, either by increasing productivity, or by excluding patients who are likely to be heavy users of the service, or both. Thus, decisions taken about healthcare, at a collective level, are different in the USA than in other countries.

However, it should be noted that the Department of Health and Human Services and its related agencies, notably the Agency for Healthcare Quality and Research (previously known as the Agency for Health Care Policy and Research), and the Veterans Administration, which has to cover a whole population on a fixed budget, do try to practise evidence-based healthcare irrespective of the fact that the majority of healthcare in the USA, which is paid for by insurance companies, is provided on a different set of principles.

This is not to say that the USA is an evidence-free zone. On the contrary, there are many excellent initiatives shared with the rest of the world:

- the network of evidence-based practice centres funded by the Agency for Healthcare Quality and Research
- the decision-making in organisations that have a fixed budget, such as Medicare
- the promotion of evidence-based patient choice by the Foundation for Informed Medical Decision Making.

Despite these initiatives, a significant difference does remain in the nature of decision-making between the USA and the rest of the world, although this difference is likely to diminish as every American, apart from the super-rich, becomes dependent on cost-conscious insurance companies.

Reference

1. Tannenbaum, S.J. (1996) 'Medical effectiveness' in Canadian and U.S. Health Policy: the comparative politics of inferential ambiguity. Health Serv. Res. 31: 517–32.

Gentle Reader,

Empathise with the walnut. You have placed it in one of those nutcrackers where the nut is held in a wooden cup and pressure exerted by means of a wooden screw. The screw can be turned in such a way that it will either crack the shell and release the nut whole or smash it to smithereens.

Commentary

Any health service is in the same situation as the walnut: it operates within a fixed resource envelope that is subjected to increasing pressure as a result of the population ageing, rising patient and professional expectations and the advent of new technology and new knowledge.

What do I mean when I refer to a health service? In this context, a health service can be represented by a decision-maker, that is, a person like you who feels the pressure as the screw tightens.

Although there are significant differences in decision-making between publicly funded and insurance-based health services, these differences are diminishing as medical insurance companies become increasingly cost conscious.

Evidence-based health services

1.1 Evidence-based healthcare: a scientific approach to health services management

Over the last two decades, tremendous advances have been made in the health sciences with the development of new technology and new knowledge. Hitherto these advances have principally been used to support clinical practice, with the result that clinical decision-making is now based on information derived from research to a much greater degree than it was. This approach is referred to as evidence-based medicine; a more generic term, evidence-based practice, can also be used.

In this book, readers will be shown how some of the scientific advances and methods that have underpinned the development of this approach to clinical practice can also underpin decision-making involving the care of groups of patients and populations.

> Evidence-based healthcare is a discipline in which decisions about groups of patients or populations are based on best current evidence but also take into account the needs and values of those groups or populations. It may be manifest as evidence-based policy-making, evidence-based paying for or commissioning of health services, or evidence-based management.

The science of most relevance to this approach to healthcare decision-making is epidemiology, that is, the study of disease in groups of patients and in populations. Although other sciences, such as occupational psychology, can be a source of information, epidemiology is the foundation of evidence-based healthcare.

In this chapter, the process and parameters of evidence-based decision-making in the provision of healthcare will be described; in Chapter 2, the evolution of an evidence-based approach will be discussed in relation to increasing constraints on the availability of resources for healthcare.

1.2   Why focus on decision-making?

There are two main reasons why it is important to focus on decision-making:

1. In the provision of healthcare, an enormous number of decisions is made. In the UK each year, for every million population, 40–50 million decisions are made about individual patients by clinicians, and thousands of decisions are made about groups of patients or populations by managers.
2. Decision-making in the provision of healthcare has a direct influence on the cost of delivering a health service. Changes in the volume and intensity of clinical practice constitute the major factor driving the increase in those healthcare costs that it is possible to control.[1]

Although the changes in clinical practice that tend to receive prominence involve the introduction of a new treatment that is very expensive, it is the cumulative effect of small changes to clinical practice – such as the introduction of a new diagnostic test or an increase in the number of treatments for particular patients – across the service throughout the financial year (i.e. very large numbers of events) that substantially increases costs and has a massive impact on the healthcare budget.

Moreover, many of these small changes to clinical practice are those that have no good evidence of:

- doing more good than harm
- doing more good than harm at reasonable cost.

Furthermore, for some of these new interventions and procedures, there may be evidence of:

- doing more harm than good
- doing more good than harm but at unreasonable cost.

Although in many countries systems for technology assessment have been set up, innovations may bypass those systems (see Fig. 7.4).

Reference

1. Eddy, D.M. (1993) *Three battles to watch in the 1990s.* JAMA 270: 520–6.

1.3   The drivers of decision-making: evidence, values, and resources and needs

*Now according to Dionysius, between man and angel
there is this difference, that an angel perceives the truth by
simple apprehension, whereas man becomes acquainted
with a simple truth by a process from manifold data.*

Thomas Aquinas

In the past, it was not unusual for decisions about what
was effective to be based on opinion – opinion-based
decision-making. In more recent history, however, decisions
about groups of patients or populations tend to be based on
a combination of three factors (Margin Fig. 1.1):

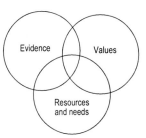

Margin Fig. 1.1

1. evidence
2. values
3. resources and needs.

At present, many healthcare decisions are still driven
principally by values and resources and needs – values-based
decision-making. Little attention has been given, or is paid,
to applying any evidence derived from research. However,
as the pressure on the resources available for healthcare
increases, decisions will have to be made explicitly and
openly, a process that will be accelerated by demands from
consumer groups, the media, and government for openness
and accountability. Those who take decisions will be expected
to present the evidence on which each decision was based.
Even in cases for which the evidence is difficult to find or
poor in quality, and the decision taken may ultimately be
driven by values and resources and needs, the decision-
maker must search for, appraise and present the evidence.

As the pressure on resources increases, opinion-based
decision-making will be eradicated, and there will be a
transition from opinion-based decision-making to evidence-
based decision-making (Margin Fig. 1.2).

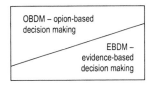

Increasing pressure ⟶

Margin Fig. 1.2

1.4   Evidence-based decision-making

*… policy makers and practitioners who intervene in other
people's lives should acknowledge that although they act with
the best of intentions, they may sometimes do more harm than
good. That possibility should be sufficient motivation for
them to ensure their prescriptions and proscriptions are
informed – even if not dictated – by reliable research evidence.*

Iain Chalmers[1]

During the 21st century, the healthcare decision-maker – that is, anyone who makes decisions about groups of patients or populations – will have to adopt an evidence-based approach. Indeed, to assume that healthcare decision-makers can operate in any other way in the hard times ahead is unrealistic. Every decision will have to be based on a systematic appraisal of the best evidence available in the context of the prevailing values and the resources available. To accomplish this, the best available evidence relating to a particular decision must be found and applied (Fig. 1.1). This requires the development of evidence management skills, the promotion of circumstances conducive to the use of an evidence-based approach, and a recognition of the need to renew decisions in the light of new evidence.

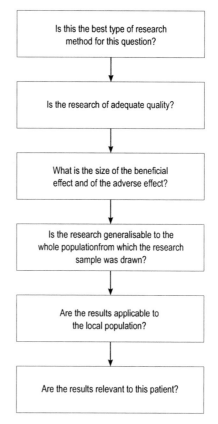

Fig. 1.1
The critical pathway of questions to help you find and apply the best evidence available

1.4.1 Skills for healthcare decision-makers

The skills necessary to practise evidence-based decision-making include being able to:

- ask the 'right' questions, i.e. converting a problem or information need into an answerable question (see Section 9.4.1)
- define criteria such as 'effectiveness', 'safety' and 'acceptability'
- find evidence about the effectiveness, safety and acceptability of a new test or treatment (see Section 9.4.2)
- assess the quality of evidence from research findings (see Section 9.4.3)
- assess whether the results of research are generalisable to the whole population from which the study sample was drawn
- assess whether the results of the research are applicable to the local context, setting and population (see Section 9.4.4)
- implement the changes indicated by the evidence.

The development of such skills may seem ambitious, but there is evidence that it can be done. Everyone involved in healthcare decision-making must have the skills to enable them to make decisions about 'doing the right things'.

- All chief executives should be able to discriminate between a good and a bad systematic review.
- All directors of finance should be able to find and appraise studies on health service cost-effectiveness.
- Every medical director should be able to determine whether a randomised controlled trial (RCT) in a specialty other than their own is biased.
- The board member who has responsibility to act as the chief knowledge officer (see Sections 2.5.1.1 and 7.4, and Box 2.4) should be able to appraise evidence about any innovation to ascertain whether it should be introduced.

These are the management skills necessary for the provision of healthcare in the 21st century.

1.4.2 Pre-requisites for good decision-making

The performance (**P**) of an individual or team is a function of (i.e. determined by) three variables:

1. the level of motivation (**M**) of the individual/team (a direct relation)

2. the level of competency (**C**) of the individual/team (a direct relation)
3. the barriers (**B**) the individual/team has to overcome in order to perform well (an inverse relation).

$$P = \frac{(M \times C)}{B}$$

The resources every decision-maker requires in order to be able to overcome any barriers and practise evidence-based decision-making are shown in Box 1.1.

It is also vital for any decision-maker intent upon using the evidence to be working in an environment in which appropriate and effective decision-making is encouraged, that is, an organisation committed to evidence-based decision-making (see Sections 7.1–7.4).

1.4.3   Reviewing decisions in the light of new evidence

Having made a decision on the basis of evidence (Margin Fig. 1.3), it is essential to keep that decision under review as new evidence becomes available (Margin Fig. 1.4). To illustrate this point, a list of screening programmes that the National Screening Committee of the UK had deemed inappropriate for introduction in 1997 is shown in Table 1.1, together with the status of these screening programmes up to the end of 2006. From this table, it can be seen how the publication of new evidence has altered the decisions being made about policy.

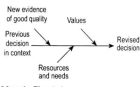

Margin Fig. 1.3

Margin Fig. 1.4

Box 1.1 Resources necessary to every decision-maker

- The support of a librarian or information scientist
- Access to electronic databases, most importantly the Cochrane Library, PubMED (or Medline) and EMBASE; these are accessible via the Internet
- Access to evidence-based resources or information gateways via the Internet, e.g. National Library for Health, available at: http://www.library.nhs.uk – it is advisable to set up a list of 'Favourites'
- Access to bibliographic management software so that any relevant citations can be stored systematically and easily retrieved

Table 1.1   The effect of publication of new evidence on evidence-based policy-making about screening in the UK (for reference, see specific conditions at http://www.screening.nhs.uk)

Screening programme	Status in 1997	Status in 2006
Prostate cancer	Inappropriate for introduction	Routine prostate cancer screening should not be introduced. Prostate cancer screening can be provided on request only if the man fully understands the lack of good-quality evidence about the benefits and risks of testing (provided by the Prostate Cancer Risk Management Programme)
Ovarian cancer	Inappropriate for introduction	No screening should be offered except in the context of the Medical Research Council RCT of ovarian cancer screening
Colorectal cancer	Inappropriate for introduction	Two RCTs were published in which there was a reduction in mortality, and a pilot of colorectal cancer screening was undertaken to see if the quality of service in a research setting could be reproduced in an ordinary service setting. Results from the pilot were reassuring and screening will be introduced in phases. The first phase commenced in July 2006
Chlamydia	Inappropriate for introduction	Further research published, including a Health Development Agency briefing in 2004; pilot of chlamydia screening was undertaken to see if the quality of service in a research setting could be reproduced in an ordinary service setting. Results from the pilot were reassuring and the National Chlamydia Screening Programme was rolled out in 2005
Human papilloma virus (HPV) testing as primary cervical screening test for cervical cancer	Inappropriate for introduction	More research available raising the possibility of using HPV tests during cervical screening to speed up and improve management of some types of positive smear results but the costs and benefits are evenly balanced. The National Screening Committee (NSC) has been piloting the use of a test for cervical cancer — liquid-based cytology (LBC) with triage of borderline and mildly dyskaryotic cytology specimens — at three sites in England
Congenital biliary atresia for neonates	Inappropriate for introduction	Screening for biliary atresia should not be offered. Research published in the British Medical Journal (1999) showed that screening the bloodspot sample using tandem mass spectrometry alone yielded a high false-positive rate, which would be financially and emotionally unacceptable
Cholesterol screening for whole population	Inappropriate for introduction	As a result of the Diabetes, Heart Disease and Stroke (DHDS) prevention project (October 2003 to September 2005), the NSC recommended the introduction of a vascular risk management programme, in which the whole population would be offered risk assessment that could include measurement of risk factors such as blood pressure, cholesterol and glucose

Reference

1. Chalmers, I. (2003) *Trying to do more good than harm in policy and practice: the role of rigorous, transparent, up-to-date evaluations.* Ann. Am. Acad. Pol. Soc. Sci. 589: 22–40.

1.5   Defining the scope of evidence-based healthcare

Evidence-based healthcare consists of three main stages (Fig. 1.2):

1. producing evidence
2. making evidence available
3. using evidence.

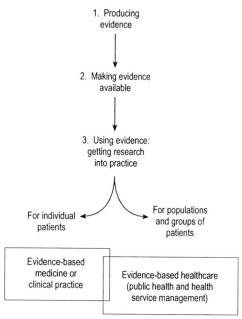

Fig. 1.2
The three main stages of evidence-based healthcare

1.5.1   Stage 1: Producing evidence

Producing evidence is the responsibility of research workers. In general, there are two main contexts in which research is conducted:

- a framework set by policy-makers, in which research is commissioned by governments or research councils
- a subject area or topic that has been determined by the researcher(s), who actively seeks funding from a charity or other body; the funding body will provide support if the research project is of good quality – this is known as responsive funding.

In every country, the trend is to reduce the amount of funding available to respond to the priorities of research workers and to transfer these funds into commissioning research to answer questions of importance to clinicians and patients, and to managers and policy-makers. Indeed, in recent years there has been the origination and initial development of an evidence base for involving consumers in setting the research and development agenda for the NHS.[1]

1.5.1.1 Ignorance is a type of evidence

The clever men at Oxford
Know all that there is to be knowed.
But they know none of them half as much
As intelligent Mr Toad.
　　　　　Kenneth Grahame, *The Wind in the Willows*

The development of systematic reviews gives us confidence about what is known and, conversely, about what is not known. It is now possible to classify what is not known – i.e. uncertainty – into two categories:

- uncertain uncertainty – we don't know if anyone knows
- certain uncertainty – we know that nobody knows, i.e. ignorance.

The James Lind Initiative, which produces the James Lind Library, has the aim of compiling a database of certain uncertainties or ignorance, known as the Database of Uncertainties about the Effectiveness of Treatments (DUETs). There are plans to make ignorance about treatments as readily available to patients as the knowledge contained in systematic reviews.

However, Iain Chalmers, coordinator of the James Lind Initiative, has pointed out that in order to hold a constructive debate about uncertainties and the effects of treatments we must find ways to engage patients in the discussion despite the challenges this will present.[2] Challenges posed by the explicit admission of uncertainty by clinicians include the potential to:

- undermine patients' confidence in the clinician
- reduce the therapeutic effectiveness of confidence in the clinician.

Chalmers suggests that an alliance of clinicians, patients, researchers and managers is needed for this discussion, and such a development would certainly be welcomed by some patients and their families. In a review of her experience of being the parent of a child with a complex health problem, Sandra Dunkelberg, who also happens to be a researcher in general practice, wrote that one of the things that was important to her family was: 'to be protected from specialists who propose more and more tests but cannot admit they do not know what is wrong'.[3]

For a discussion of the clinician's role with respect to uncertainty, see Chapter 10 and the Epilogue.

1.5.2   Stage 2: Making evidence available

Making the evidence derived from research available is vital, otherwise the potential value of new knowledge will never be realised. If research evidence is made available, is it possible to gain easy access to it? In this book, examples are given of ways in which healthcare professionals can access information in libraries and from databases such as Medline or PubMED. However, better systems for gaining access to information at the time it is needed, for example, on a ward round, in a surgery or in a patient's home, are now available using a tablet, PDA or mobile phone (especially as the evidence that mobile phones do not cause harm to patients is now clear if sensible precautions regarding their proximity to medical equipment are taken).[4]

For patients and carers, who can be 'locked out' of medical libraries, the development of the Internet has provided unparalleled access to medical information.

1.5.3   Stage 3: Using evidence

There are three main ways in which research evidence can be used:

- to improve patient choice (see Section 1.5.3.1)
- to improve clinical practice (see Section 1.5.3.2)
- to improve the value of the health service (see Section 1.5.3.3).

1.5.3.1 Evidence-based patient choice

If they wish, patients should have a choice of treatment options presented on the basis of best current knowledge.

1.5.3.2 Evidence-based clinical practice

Evidence-based clinical practice is:

> ... the conscientious, explicit and judicious use of current best evidence in making decisions about the care of individual patients. The practice of evidence-based medicine means integrating individual clinical expertise with the best available external clinical evidence from systematic research. By individual clinical expertise we mean the proficiency and judgement that individual clinicians acquire through clinical experience and clinical practice.[5]

In brief, evidence-based clinical practice is an approach to decision-making in which the clinician uses the best evidence available, in consultation with the patient, to decide upon the option that best suits the patient. In Chapter 10, evidence-based clinical practice is described in greater detail, partly as a resource for health service managers, who can do much to promote both evidence-based clinical practice and evidence-based patient choice.

1.5.3.3 Evidence-based policy-making, and paying for and managing health services on the basis of evidence

Managers who are responsible for health services for groups of patients or populations have to make many decisions, all of which fall into one of three main categories:

1. decisions about policy
2. decisions about paying for or commissioning healthcare
3. decisions about management.

As the number of constraints around decision-making increases, all three categories of decision will need to be based on evidence. The contents of this book will help health service personnel who make decisions about healthcare policy or when those paying for or managing healthcare develop the skills necessary to base those decisions on the best evidence available.

1. Policy decisions

Policy-making is a political process: it is based not only on the evidence but also on the value politicians place upon different types of decision-making, for example, centralised as opposed to decentralised decision-making.

There are two main types of policy concerning health:

- public health policy – concerning public health (see Chapter 8)
- healthcare policy – concerning health service financing and the way in which a health service is organised to account for the resources used.

In 1991, what was known as the purchaser/provider split was introduced into the UK. The aim of this policy was to alter the financial responsibility and the authority of those who pay for and those who provide healthcare. Although this particular UK healthcare policy decision was superseded over a decade ago, in almost every country, including the UK, a clear distinction has been drawn between those who pay for or commission healthcare for populations or groups of patients and those who provide that care, i.e. a distinction between the assessment of need together with the allocation of resources and the delivery of health services.

2. Decisions about paying for or commissioning healthcare

> Paying for or commissioning healthcare is a process by which those responsible for expenditure on health services for a population or group of patients first allocate resources to different patient groups and then enter into a set of contracts with the providers of those health services to obtain particular services at a specified level of quality and at an agreed cost to maximise the value derived from the resources invested.

The people who pay for healthcare can be public bodies, as is the case in the UK, or private organisations such as insurance companies, as is the case in the Netherlands. (It should be noted that insurance companies in many countries are supported by the state, provided certain requirements have been met.) If finance is limited, paying for healthcare is often linked to prioritisation (see Section 2.3).

For a discussion of the differences in roles between paying for and commissioning healthcare, see Section 7.6. For a discussion of evidence-based insurance, see Section 7.6.5.

3. Management decisions

> Management is the process whereby resources allocated to healthcare expenditure for a particular population or group of patients are utilised to best effect.

People who manage healthcare have to take many decisions, some of which can be evidence-based, for example, the decision whether to manage stroke patients in a stroke unit. Many decisions, however, have a weak or non-existent evidence base, such as a decision about whether to introduce a bonus scheme.

References

1. Oliver, S., Clarke-Jones, L., Rees, R. et al. (2004) *Involving consumers in research and development agenda setting for the NHS: developing an evidence-based approach.* Health Technol. Assess. 8(15): iii–iv, 1–148.
2. Chalmers, I. (2004) *Well informed uncertainties about the effects of treatment. How should patients and clinicians respond? [Editorial]* Br. Med. J. 328: 475–6.
3. Dunkelberg, S. (2006) *A patient's journey: our special girl.* Br. Med. J. 333: 430–1.
4. Derbyshire, S.W.G. and Burgess, A. (2006) *Use of mobile phones in hospitals. [Editorial]* Br. Med. J. 333: 767–8.
5. Sackett, D.L., Rosenberg, W.M.C., Gray, J.A.M. et al. (1996) *Evidence-based medicine: what it is and what it isn't. [Editorial]* Br. Med. J. 312: 71–2.

1.6   Realising the potential of evidence-based healthcare

The practice of evidence-based healthcare enables those managing a health service to determine the mix of services and procedures that will give the greatest benefit to the population served by that health service. However, there is no guarantee that any potential benefits identified within a research setting will be realised in practice, because one of the determinants of outcome is the quality of management. To ensure that a population/group of patients receives the maximum health benefit at the lowest possible risk and cost from the resources available, both evidence-based healthcare and quality management are essential practices (Table 1.2).

> Evidence-based healthcare + quality management
> = maximum health benefit at lowest risk and cost

1.7   Strategic approaches to implementing evidence-based decision-making in healthcare systems

Several strategic approaches have been taken towards implementing evidence-based decision-making in healthcare systems (Margin Fig. 1.5), including:

- the introduction of managed care – a high-level approach, which includes issues such as payment incentives and disincentives

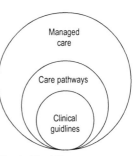

Margin Fig. 1.5

Table 1.2 The responsibilities and concomitant skills necessary for healthcare managers to realise the potential of research findings

Managerial responsibility	Skills necessary
Offering only valuable services: ensure that all the services and procedures are supported by good-quality evidence that they do more good than harm	Technology assessment Critical appraisal
Getting the mix right: ensure that the mix of services and procedures provided is that which will give the greatest benefit for the population served	Needs assessment Priority setting Evidence-based decision-making
Getting quality right: ensure that services and clinical practice are of sufficiently high quality to realise the potential for health improvement demonstrated in research settings	Professional education Public education Paying for or commissioning health services Quality management Clinical audit

- the production of care pathways
- the development of clinical guidelines.

1.7.1   Managed care

The physician has moved from Pegasus, soaring aloft on the heady excitement of biomedical science, to Sisyphus, condemned forever to push a boulder up a hill.

Lipkin[1]

In the past, it was possible to distinguish between two types of healthcare: clinical practice and public health (for the dichotomies between the two, see Table 1.3).

Nowadays, however, this sharp distinction no longer obtains, as increasing effort is being invested in standardising care for patients who suffer from the same condition; this is known as managed care. Managed care lies between clinical practice and public health on the spectrum of healthcare (Fig. 1.3).

In managed care, a systematic approach is taken to care management, whereby a pre-determined care package is delivered to groups of patients who have certain common conditions for which it is possible to define a core set of interventions and services those suffering from the condition should receive. The application of managed care has sometimes resulted in a greater involvement of nurses in clinical decision-making, for example, when offering a point of primary contact or ensuring that a proposed referral to a specialist service is appropriate. This development has

Table 1.3 The dichotomies between clinical practice and public health

Clinical practice	Public health
For individuals: Treatment for those who feel ill	For populations: Treatment of those who feel well
Low number needed to treat (NNT)	High number needed to treat (NNT)
Decisions unique to the individual	Decisions common to populations
Difficult to produce systems and guidelines	Easy to produce systems and guidelines
Paradigm problem: a patient who is feeling weak and tired	Paradigm problem: a population at risk of polio

Clinical practice	Managed care	Public health

Fig. 1.3
The spectrum of healthcare provided to a population

increased the need for care pathways in which the decision points are based on algorithms.

Clinicians in the UK have worked within a form of managed care since the inception of the NHS in 1948. In contrast, the development of a system of managed care has occurred rapidly in the USA where the trend towards its introduction has been most marked.[2] There is now a range of different approaches to regulating care in the USA, and here managed care has implications for:

- the sources of funding for healthcare
- the control of individual physicians (who in less than two decades were taken from a tradition of working as they chose to a system of strict controls)
- in cases where managed care is paid for by 'for-profit' health maintenance organisations, the amount of money made by those individuals who run such organisations at the expense of patients whose care is being limited to provide those profits.

Kassirer, in his review of managed care and the morality of the market place, pointed out that transformation of the US healthcare system 'is producing corporate conglomerates with billions of dollars in assets that compensate their executives as grandly as basketball players'.[3] Patients and those who pay for healthcare are increasingly in direct conflict in the courts as patients challenge the right of payers to deny them treatment. These conflicts become highly charged when insurance companies or 'for-profit' health maintenance organisations are making very large profits.

At first sight, it may seem as if the introduction of managed care would counteract some of the vagaries in clinical practice and facilitate the introduction of evidence-based healthcare. However, although managed care has an important contribution to make – for instance, by reducing the duration of hospital stay or increasing the proportion of heart attack patients who are prescribed beta-blocker drugs – it should not be regarded as a universal panacea for healthcare problems for the following reasons:

- Some patients may present with conditions that will not allow them to be slotted into a managed care system.
- Patients whom it is theoretically possible to treat within a managed care system, because they are suffering from a disease such as diabetes or asthma, may have individual characteristics that make it difficult to apply the guidelines to all aspects of their care.

- The rigorous control of decision-making inherent in a managed care system may cause clinicians to become disaffected; as a consequence, they may perform less well in another sphere of clinical practice, such as communication with the patient.

The development of managed care, however, does offer important opportunities for the introduction of evidence-based healthcare because it allows those who pay for healthcare to be explicit about the interventions that should and should not be offered to patients.

Margin Note 1.1
Care pathways

For more information about care pathways, access: http://www.library.nhs.uk/pathways/
An excellent common software platform, *Map of Medicine*, enables national guidelines to be converted into templates for pathways that can then be adapted to take account of local constraints and opportunities. Available online at:
http://www.mapofmedicine.com/

1.7.2   Care pathways

Care pathways 'define the expected course of events in the care of a patient with a particular condition, within a set time-scale'.[4] Care pathways are structured according to time intervals during which specific goals and the progress expected are indicated, together with guidance on the optimal timing of appropriate investigations and treatment.[5]

Pathways are developed by members of a team involved in patient care. Multidisciplinary guidelines are used to develop and implement clinical plans that represent current local best practice for specific conditions.[6] Care pathways are a tool that can be used to facilitate the introduction of an evidence-based approach into routine clinical practice.

Although generic pathways can be constructed, any care pathway is usually unique to the particular institution in which it is developed because it will reflect details of care, which vary among institutions, and current practice.

There is evidence that the use of care pathways can improve outcome and thereby reduce the cost of healthcare. Holtzman et al.[7] investigated the effect of the introduction of care pathways on the length of stay and patient outcomes for two cohorts of patients undergoing renal transplantation, one of which received organs from cadavers ($n = 170$), the other from living donors ($n = 178$). After the development and implementation of a care pathway for those undergoing transplantation with organs from cadavers, it was found that:

- mean length of stay declined from 17.5 to 11.8 days ($P = 0.008$)
- the rate of complications fell from 38.1% to 14.8% ($P = 0.002$)
- the incidence of infection was reduced from 33.3% to 7.4% ($P < 0.001$).

However, the implementation of a care pathway for those undergoing transplantation with organs from living donors did not affect any of the outcomes or length of stay.

1.7.3   Clinical guidelines

Clinical guidelines can be defined as systematically developed statements to support healthcare professionals and patients when making decisions about the most appropriate healthcare in particular circumstances.

In the NHS, the use of an evidence-based approach in general, and of clinical guidelines in particular, is viewed as a way to promote best practice. Between 2004 and the end of 2006, the National Institute of Health and Clinical Excellence had produced guidelines covering over 250 healthcare topics, and by 2010 the aim is to have produced guidelines covering all the major healthcare topics. In the independent sector, guidelines are being used increasingly to authorise the type of care a patient should receive before it is given, or to contract with preferred providers.[8] The latter approach is a springboard for the introduction of managed care, as practised in the USA.

Guidelines can be produced nationally or locally. The production of a set of guidelines should follow the well-established evidence about the factors determining success in development and implementation.[9] It is vital to obtain the best available evidence on which to develop clinical policy as expressed within guidelines or protocols (see Fig. 1.4) as opposed to justifying current practice *post hoc*. Recently, Oxman et al. have prepared a series of reviews on improving the use of research evidence in guideline development (Box 1.2).[10–26]

It is also important to ensure ownership of the guidelines by those professionals whom it is sought to influence.[27] Guidelines will be more effective on implementation if their development has involved all the relevant disciplines engaged in the care of a particular group of patients, including 'frontline staff' and the relevant managers. McDonald et al.[28] undertook qualitative research to explore the attitudes towards guidelines of doctors and nurses working together in surgical teams:

- nurses viewed guidelines as one key to providing safe good-quality care
- doctors perceived guidelines as unnecessary and potentially harmful.

Margin Note 1.2
The AGREE collaboration

The AGREE (Appraisal of Guidelines Research and Evaluation) Collaboration started as a research project in 1998. The aim was to develop an appraisal instrument to assess clinical guidelines. In 2002, the Collaboration received additional funding to disseminate further, and implement, the AGREE instrument as a way of enhancing effective healthcare policy in Europe. The objective was to promote the diffusion of a comprehensive approach to the production, dissemination and evaluation of high-quality clinical guidelines through established networks. Available online at: http://www.agreecollaboration.org/

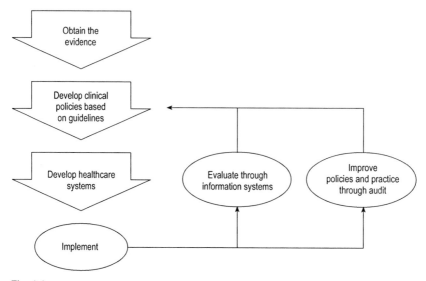

Fig. 1.4
From research to implementation and audit

Box 1.2 Improving the use of research evidence in guideline development

The Advisory Committee on Health Research (ACHR) of the World Health
Organization (WHO) set up a Subcommittee on the Use of Research Evidence (SURE)
to collect information relevant to giving WHO advice on how to improve the use of
research evidence in the development of recommendations, including guidelines and
policy. A series of reviews of methods used in the development of guidelines was
prepared, as follows:

Improving the use of research evidence in guideline development

Introduction[10]

1. Guidelines for guidelines[11]
2. Priority setting[12]
3. Group composition and consultation process[13]
4. Managing conflicts of interests[14]
5. Group processes[15]
6. Determining which outcomes are important[16]
7. Deciding what evidence to include[17]
8. Synthesis and presentation of evidence[18]
9. Grading evidence and recommendations[19]
10. Integrating values and consumer involvement[20]
11. Incorporating considerations of cost-effectiveness, affordability and resource
    implications[21]
12. Incorporating considerations of equity[22]
13. Applicability, transferability and adaptation[23]
14. Reporting guidelines[24]
15. Disseminating and implementing guidelines[25]
16. Evaluation[26]

Thus, different views exist about the value of guidelines. From this research, it would appear that doctors and nurses as professional groups each hold different but collective views about what constitutes safe clinical practice. Nurses may perceive doctors as rule-breakers, whereas doctors do not necessarily see certain rules as legitimate or indeed identify with rules written for them by other social groups. McDonald et al. suggest that, in future, safety research could have as a focus understanding the unwritten rules governing clinical behaviour and the way such rules are produced, maintained and accepted as legitimate.

Guidelines are more likely to be used if:

- a topic is chosen that clinicians believe to be important, as opposed to well-researched areas of practice
- acceptance is gained of the research evidence on which the guidelines are based
- the implementation of the guidelines is linked to established audit groups (Fig. 1.4).

Hutchings et al.[29] suggest that it may be important when publishing clinical guidelines to present group judgements separately, and the extent of agreement around those judgements. For instance, knowing that a recommendation is supported by a high level of agreement within the guideline development group might encourage higher levels of adherence by clinicians than one for which there is less agreement. Of further interest is the finding that formal consensus development was a robust method for guideline development in that the levels of agreement/disagreement were not dependent on the way the technique was conducted.[29]

In an observational study to determine which attributes of nationally produced clinical guidelines ($n = 10$) influence the use of guidelines during decision-making in general practice in the Netherlands, Grol et al.[30] found that overall guideline recommendations were followed in 61% of decisions (7915/12 880). However, when the decisions were analysed in relation to specific guideline attributes, they found the following types of recommendation to be influential:

- those that were non-controversial (followed in 68% of decisions)
- those that were clear (followed in 67% decisions)
- those that did not require a change in existing practice routines (followed in 67% of decisions)
- those that were based on research evidence (followed in 71% of decisions).

From these results, it would appear that evidence-based clinical guidelines are more likely to be used in clinical decision-making. However, the cost consequences for the health service of any of the recommendations made in a set of guidelines are also important, and should be borne in mind by those who produce and disseminate them.

1.7.3.1 Who is accountable for guidelines?

Gentle Reader,

Empathise with the relatives of people who were consumed by the Ravenous Bugblatter Beast of Traal. They tried to sue the publishers of the Hitch-Hiker's Guide to the Galaxy, *which claimed to be the definitive guide to the galaxy, because it contained a sentence that read 'The Ravenous Bugblatter Beast of Traal makes a good meal for visiting tourists', when the intention had been for it to read 'The Ravenous Bugblatter Beast of Traal makes a good meal of visiting tourists'.*

Commentary
In their defence, the publishers summoned a philosopher who claimed that the sentence as published was more beautiful than that originally intended and as beauty is truth, then it was also true. The relatives' case collapsed.

When a clinician makes a decision, he or she is accountable for that decision, but when a doctor follows a guideline who is responsible when something goes wrong? At one point, it was thought that the introduction of guidelines would be followed by a wave of litigation directed at those who developed them, but this fear has never materialised. There is evidence, however, that guidelines can be used as evidence to defend clinicians in court, as well as to bring a case against them (see Section 7.9.3).

1.7.3.2 Clinical guidelines and the law

Ms Baxendale QC: *Some of the witnesses we have had have described these guidelines as a framework, within which to work ... Does that fit in with how you saw the guidelines?*

Lady Thatcher: *They are exactly what they say, guidelines, they are not the law. They are guidelines.*

Ms Baxendale QC: *Did they have to be followed?*

Lady Thatcher: *Of course they have to be followed, but they are not strict law. That is why they are guidelines and not law and, of course, they have to be applied according to the relevant circumstances.*

Ms Baxendale QC: *They are expected to be followed?*

Lady Thatcher: *Of course they have to be followed. They need to be followed for what they are, guidelines.*

Cross-examination of Lady Thatcher during the Scott Enquiry into the 'Arms for Iraq' affair quoted in Hurwitz.[31]

In a very important book, Brian Hurwitz reviewed the evidence available in 1998 about the relationship between clinical guidelines and the law, [31] and considered the legal status of clinical guidelines in negligence case law. The main principle Hurwitz defined is that any doctor acting *outside* the guideline could expose him- or herself to the possibility of being found negligent unless able to provide a specific justification why they had done so. Hurwitz's opinion is that 'In the UK, it is unlikely that authors or sponsors of faulty guidelines would be held liable for patient injury', principally because the court would expect the treating clinician to use appropriate discretion and judgement. This conclusion, however, emphasises the importance of developing good-quality guidelines.

References

1. Lipkin, M. Jr. (1996) *Sisyphus or Pegasus? The physician interviewer in the era of corporatization of care.* Ann. Intern. Med. 124: 511–12.
2. Swartz, K. and Brennan, T.A. (1996) *Integrated health care, capitated payment, and quality: the role of regulation.* Ann. Intern. Med. 124: 442–8.
3. Kassirer, J.P. (1995) *Managed care and the morality of the marketplace.* [Editorial] N. Engl. J. Med. 333: 50–2.
4. Kitchiner, D., Davidson, D. and Bundred, P. (1996) *Integrated Care Pathways: effective tools for continuous evaluation of clinical practice.* J. Eval. Clin. Pract. 2: 65–9.
5. Coffey, R.J., Richards, J.S., Remmert, C.S. et al (1992) *An introduction to critical paths.* Qual. Manag. Health Care 1: 45–54.
6. Kitchiner, D. and Bundred, P. (1996) *Integrated care pathways.* Arch. Dis. Child. 75: 166–8.
7. Holtzman, J., Bjerke, T. and Kane, R. (1998) *The effects of clinical pathways for renal transplantation on patient outcomes and length of stay.* Med. Care 36: 826–34.
8. Fairfield, G. and Williams, R. (1996) *Clinical guidelines in the independent health care sector: an opportunity for the NHS to observe managed care in action.* [Editorial] Br. Med. J. 312: 1554–5.
9. NHS Centre for Reviews and Dissemination and Nuffield Institute For Health (1995) *Implementing clinical practice guidelines.* Effective Health Care Bulletin No. 8, University of Leeds, Leeds.
10. Oxman, A.D., Fretheim, A. and Schünemann, H.J. (2006) *Improving the use of research evidence in guideline development: introduction.* Health Res. Policy Syst. 4: 12.
11 Schünemann, H.J., Fretheim, A. and Oxman, A.D. (2006) *Improving the use of research evidence in guideline development: 1. Guidelines for guidelines.* Health Res. Policy Syst. 4: 13.

12. Oxman, A.D., Schünemann, H.J. and Fretheim, A. (2006) *Improving the use of research evidence in guideline development: 2. Priority setting.* Health Res. Policy Syst. 4: 14.

13. Fretheim, A., Schünemann, H.J. and Oxman, A.D. (2006) *Improving the use of research evidence in guideline development: 3. Group composition and consultation process.* Health Res. Policy Syst. 4: 15.

14. Boyd, E.A. and Bero, L.A. (2006) *Improving the use of research evidence in guideline development: 4. Managing conflicts of interests.* Health Res. Policy Syst. 4: 16.

15. Fretheim, A., Schünemann, H.J. and Oxman, A.D. (2006) *Improving the use of research evidence in guideline development: 5. Group processes.* Health Res. Policy Syst. 4: 17.

16. Schünemann, H.J., Oxman, A.D. and Fretheim, A. (2006) *Improving the use of research evidence in guideline development: 6. Determining which outcomes are important.* Health Res. Policy Syst. 4: 18.

17. Oxman, A.D., Schünemann, H.J. and Fretheim, A. (2006) *Improving the use of research evidence in guideline development: 7. Deciding what evidence to include.* Health Res. Policy Syst. 4: 19.

18. Oxman, A.D., Schünemann, H.J. and Fretheim, A. (2006) *Improving the use of research evidence in guideline development: 8. Synthesis and presentation of evidence.* Health Res. Policy Syst. 4: 20.

19. Schünemann, H.J., Fretheim, A. and Oxman, A.D. (2006) *Improving the use of research evidence in guideline development: 9. Grading evidence and recommendations.* Health Res. Policy Syst. 4: 21.

20. Schünemann, H.J., Fretheim, A. and Oxman, A.D. (2006) *Improving the use of research evidence in guideline development: 10. Integrating values and consumer involvement.* Health Res. Policy Syst. 4: 22.

21. Edejer, T.T. (2006) *Improving the use of research evidence in guideline development: 11. Incorporating considerations of cost-effectiveness, affordability and cost implications.* Health Res. Policy Syst. 4: 23.

22. Oxman, A.D., Schünemann, H.J. and Fretheim, A. *Improving the use of research evidence in guideline development: 12. Incorporating considerations of equity.* Health Res. Policy Syst. 4: 24.

23. Schünemann, H.J., Fretheim, A. and Oxman, A.D. (2006) *Improving the use of research evidence in guideline development: 13. Applicability, transferability and adaptation.* Health Res. Policy Syst. 4: 25.

24. Oxman, A.D., Schünemann, H.J. and Fretheim, A. (2006) *Improving the use of research evidence in guideline development: 14. Reporting guidelines.* Health Res. Policy Syst. 4: 26.

25. Fretheim, A., Schünemann, H.J. and Oxman, A.D. (2006) *Improving the use of research evidence in guideline development: 15. Disseminating and implementing guidelines.* Health Res. Policy Syst. 4: 27.

26. Oxman, A.D., Schünemann, H.J. and Fretheim, A. (2006) *Improving the use of research evidence in guideline development: 16 Evaluation.* Health Res. Policy Syst. 4: 28.

27. Grimshaw, J.M. and Russell, I.T. (1993) *Effect of clinical guidelines on medical practice: a systematic review of rigorous evaluations.* Lancet 342: 1317–22.

28. McDonald, R., Waring, J., Harrison, S. et al. (2005) *Rules and guidelines in clinical practice: a qualitative study in operating theatres of doctors' and nurses' views.* Qual. Saf. Health Care 14: 290–4.

29. Hutchings, A., Raine, R., Sanderson, C. et al. (2005) *An experimental study of the extent of disagreement within clinical guideline development groups.* Qual. Saf. Health Care 14: 240–5.

30. Grol, R., Dalhuijsen, J., Thomas, S. et al. (1998) *Attributes of clinical practice guidelines that influence use of guidelines in general practice: observational study.* Br. Med. J. 317: 858–61.

31. Hurwitz, B. (1998) *Clinical Guidelines and the Law: Negligence, Discretion and Judgement.* Radcliffe Medical Press, Abingdon, UK.

1.8   The limitations of healthcare in improving health

... three of the seven years' increase in life-expectancy since 1950 can be attributed to medical care. Medical care is also estimated to provide on average five years of partial or complete relief from the poor quality of life associated with chronic disease.

Bunker[1]

1.8.1   Improving the health of populations

The best healthcare can be defined as that:

- from which all ineffective interventions have been eliminated
- in which effective interventions are offered to those patients within the population most likely to benefit
- in which all services are delivered at the highest possible quality.

However, the health of a population is determined by five factors (Margin Fig. 1.6), only one of which is healthcare. The other four are:

- lifestyle
- socio-economic environment
- physical and biological environment
- genetics – an individual's genotype may confer a degree of protection or susceptibility to factors in the environment, whether physical or socio-economic, that trigger disease.

Thus, even the provision of the best healthcare will not necessarily ensure optimum levels of health in a population.

Margin Fig. 1.6

1.8.2   Improving the health of individual patients

Sick individuals present to clinicians with complicated problems which require an appreciation of the relationship between 'disease' and 'illness', terms which are sometimes used interchangeably but which have distinct meanings, as the definitions in the *Shorter Oxford English Dictionary* demonstrate:

- '**Disease:** a condition of the body, or of some part or organ of the body, in which its functions are disturbed or deranged.'
- '**Illness:** bad or unhealthy condition of the body (or, formerly, of a part); the condition of being ill.'

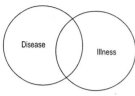

Margin Fig. 1.7

A disease is a condition from which an individual suffers, such as tuberculosis; an illness is a state of being, in which the individual enjoys the privileges of illness but must obey certain rules (Table 1.4).

The relationship between disease and illness is best shown in a Venn diagram (Margin Fig. 1.7). Most people who have a disease are also ill, although the degree to which any individual claims the privileges of illness varies considerably from one person to another.

1.8.2.1 Disease without illness

Some people have a disease but are not ill: an individual with undiagnosed diabetes has a disease but is unaware of the change in social status that will pertain when the diagnosis is known. Some people who have a disease do not wish to be ill or to be treated in a special way; for example, people who have disabilities do not wish to be discriminated against simply because of a disability resulting from disease.

1.8.2.2 Illness without disease

Some people feel ill but no causal disease can be found to explain their symptoms. This type of disorder has two common manifestations:

1. medically unexplained physical symptoms (MUPS), sometimes called somatoform disorders or somatisation, usually manifest as pain of various types
2. hypochondriasis or excessive anxiety about a disease, usually cancer.

These disorders are very common. One estimate is that about half of all new referrals attending a general medical outpatient clinic have MUPS.[2] MUPS are reactions to various forms of external strain which may occur:

- as an alternative to constructive adaptive behaviour that will remove or reduce the causal strain
- as an unproductive substitute for effective coping, as shown in Fig. 1.5.

Table 1.4   The privileges and rules of illness

Privileges	Rules
Being excused normal social duties	The patient must be seen to be trying to get better
Extra sympathy and attention	The patient must give up many social pleasures, e.g. going out to parties

There is, however, important evidence that MUPS can be treated effectively with cognitive therapy.[3] Indeed, as the pressure on resources increases, it will be necessary to treat this large group of patients in a more systematic manner. At present, a woman who presents with pelvic pain may be referred to as many as three different clinics and be subject to various investigations on separate occasions by doctors in training in different specialties in an attempt to cure the pain. In an RCT, Speckens et al.[3] evaluated the effect of additional cognitive behavioural therapy for patients with MUPS over optimised medical care. They found that the intervention group experienced a higher recovery rate at 6 months than the control subjects. This research is important: it shows that it is possible to apply the methodology of an RCT to such subtle and complex problems as MUPS.

Barsky and Borus, authors of a paper on somatisation and medicalisation in the era of managed care,[4] argue that the rate of presentation of MUPS in the USA will increase as managed care becomes more widespread. It is encouraging to note that some of the factors these authors identified as leading to increased referral rates are not relevant in the UK, where there has been a form of managed care, namely,

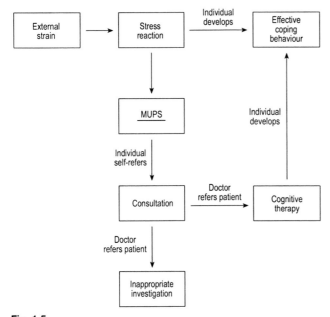

Fig. 1.5
Reactions to external strain

capitation-based general practice, since the inception of the NHS. Nonetheless, MUPS is a common problem in primary care, and its prevalence may increase as society enters the post-modern era (see Epilogue).

The application of knowledge alone cannot solve all health problems, but without knowledge subtle disorders such as MUPS and subtle concepts such as the distinction between disease and illness will be overlooked in the drive towards increasing investment in medical technology to produce, at best, progressively less benefit or, at worst, more harm than good.

References

1. Bunker, J.P. (1995) *Medicine matters after all*. J. Roy. Coll. Phys. Lond. 29: 105–12.
2. van Hemert, A.M., Hengeveld, M.W., Bolk, J.H. et al. (1993) *Psychiatric disorders in relation to medical illness among patients of a general medical out-patient clinic*. Psychol. Med. 23: 167–73.
3. Speckens, A.E.M., van Hemert, A.M., Spinhoven, P. et al. (1995) *Cognitive behavioural therapy for medically unexplained physical symptoms: a randomised controlled trial*. Br. Med. J. 311: 1328–32.
4. Barsky, A.J. and Borus, J.F. (1995) *Somatization and medicalization in the era of managed care*. JAMA 274: 1931–4.

1.9   Evidence and other types of knowledge

Evidence is one type of generalisable knowledge. There are other types of generalisable knowledge that are often of use to decision-makers, particularly when dealing with complex issues such as the reconfiguration of healthcare or social care.[1] For example, there is knowledge derived from:

- the analysis of routinely collected or audit data, sometimes called statistics
- the experience of clinicians or patients; this knowledge is often tacit and needs to be made explicit.

Any type of generalisable knowledge needs to be related to a specific context or situation, i.e.:

- to a particular patient
- to a particular health service.

In using other types of generalisable knowledge, it is important to be aware of the 'power of stories over statistics', especially in determining practice.[2] The power of story-telling rests in four main characteristics:

1. The human brain appears to be constructed in a way that processes stories better than other forms of input.
2. The storyteller, as the person who experienced an event, enables a connection to be made with the listener beyond that which is possible if the story were told by an observer.
3. The tendency to use the availability heuristic to estimate probabilities, i.e. basing an estimate on how well we can recall (or imagine) a case and in what level of detail – this leads to an over-estimation of events.
4. The apparent capacity to offer a solution to tragic outcomes, thereby giving meaning to the potentially unbearable.

However, a consideration of stories as the sole determinant of practice can lead to the neglect of a more complicated consideration of what else could be done with those resources and the most appropriate way of making those decisions.

Newman[2] offers four suggestions about ways to harness the power of stories more appropriately within the paradigm of evidence-based policy and practice (Box 1.3).

References

1. Pawson, R., Boaz, A., Grayson, L. et al. (2003) *Types and quality of knowledge in social care*. Knowledge Review 3. Social Care Institute for Excellence, and The Policy Press.
2. Newman, T.B. (2003) *The power of stories over statistics*. Br. Med. J. 327: 1424–7.

Box 1.3 Harnessing the power of stories within an evidence-based paradigm (Adapted from Newman[2])

1. Take care when experts in particular diseases write guidelines for the prevention of those diseases – it is important to have a widened perspective, including an awareness of the other ways in which resources could be spent
2. Raise awareness of the power of stories over statistics, and the availability heuristic
3. Tell stories about the suffering caused by misappropriation of resources, e.g. of children who suffer through lack of access to basic healthcare, or families traumatised by excessive medical intervention
4. Discuss how decisions should be made (as separate from making particular decisions)

1.10   Thinking and feeling

Every step in decision-making should be rational but, as Herbert Simon described in his monumental book *Administrative Behaviour* (the fourth edition of which was published 50 years after the first), irrational as well as rational actions play a part in decision-making.[1]

How people feel influences how they think. Since the publication of the second edition of this book, several important texts have been published on how clinicians think: *Complications*[2] by Atul Gawande, and books by Jerome Groopman, notably *Second Opinions*[3] and *How Doctors Think*[4] (which should really have been called 'How Doctors Think and Feel'). Indeed, two books entitled *How Doctors Think* have been published in recent years, the one by Groopman noted previously and another by Kathryn Montgomery,[5] a professor in humanities at Northwestern University, USA.

It is interesting to note that the way healthcare managers and public health practitioners feel has not been written about as clearly, partly because the decisions involved in health service delivery affect the lives (and deaths) of thousands of people, and telling the story of such decisions does not have the same impact as telling stories about the life and death of individual patients (see Section 1.9). However, two books related to this subject are of particular note. The first is by Sir Richard Packer, who wrote about the BSE crisis in the UK, based on his diaries at the time, and disclosed his feelings as a result of the political decision-making process, and also gave some account of his feelings during the crisis.[6] Mark Moore, in *In Creating Public Value*,[7] provides well-written studies of the process of decision-making in both the public sector and the public eye but without any individual testimony.

1.10.1   The need for bounded rationality

Even if public servants manage to keep emotions completely out of the process of decision-making, they, like clinicians, often have to use 'bounded rationality', a term introduced by Herbert Simon.[8] Bounded rationality is rationality employed in a situation in which:

- all the data are not available
- time is limited
- computers cannot solve the problem.

In such circumstances, decision-makers have to use what Gerd Gigerenzer has called 'fast and frugal heuristics',[9] rules of thumb based on their experience. In summary, therefore, it is possible to represent the process of good decision-making in the following equation:

Good decision-making = good use of evidence + good use of rules of thumb − emotion

References

1. Simon, H. (1997) *Administrative Behaviour: A Study of Decision-Making Processes in Administrative Organisations*, 4th edn. The Free Press, New York.
2. Gawande, A. (2002) *Complications: A Surgeon's Notes on an Imperfect Science*. Profile Books, London.
3. Groopman, J. (2001) *Second Opinions. Eight Clinical Dramas of Decision Making on the Front Lines of Medicine*. Penguin, New York.
4. Groopman, J. (2007) *How Doctors Think*. Houghton Mifflin, Boston.
5. Montgomery, K. (2005) *How Doctors Think: Clinical Judgement and the Practice of Medicine*. Oxford University Press, New York.
6. Packer, R. (2006) *The Politics of BSE*. Palgrave, Basingstoke.
7. Moore, M.H. (1997) *Creating Public Value. Strategic Management in Government*. Harvard University Press, Cambridge, Massachusetts.
8. Simon, H. (1957) *A Behavioural Model of Rational Choice*. In: *Models of Man, Social and Rational: Mathematical Essays on Rational Human Behaviour in a Social Setting*. Wiley, New York.
9. Gigerenzer, G. and Todd, P.M. and the ABC Research Group (1999) *Simple Heuristics That Make Us Smart*. Oxford University Press, New York.

Gentle Reader,

Empathise with the commissioner. He felt gutted. He had read with dismay the business case that the acute hospital Trust had put together to support the acquisition of spiral computed tomography (CT) which had revenue consequences of about £1 000 000 a year for several years. How could they? They knew their main commissioner faced a financial problem – a matter of a few millions. The Trust itself had a financial gap to close between their prices and the commissioner's position. Commissioner and provider had been discussing this gap 'maturely' for weeks, or so the commissioner thought, but of spiral CT nary a mention. Now it pops up like a jack-in-a-bloody-box.

Gentle Reader,

Empathise with the provider. She felt gutted. The commissioner had said they couldn't support the acquisition of new spiral CT kit. It was standard now; every NHS Trust had it. They would be virtually the only Trust without it, and the business case was good. When compared with ordinary CT, the images are more accurate, disease can be diagnosed earlier and the scanning time is much faster, which makes it more acceptable to patients. It would increase the productivity of the Trust, and reduce waiting times; surely the commissioner had been demanding all these things from them for months. Now they turn round and say it's no go.

Commentary

The prologue presents a seemingly intractable situation of irreconcilable differences. To resolve the conflict, both parties need to find and appraise the evidence on which claim and counter-claim are based and then discuss the quality of the evidence, the size of the effect suggested by that evidence, and the applicability of those research findings to the population being served. This approach will be increasingly required as those who make decisions are subject to increasing pressure to 'do the right things right'.

'Doing the right things right'

CHAPTER

2

2.1 The growing need for evidence-based healthcare

The need and the demand for healthcare are increasing. In almost every country, the rate of growth of both the need and the demand for healthcare is faster than the rate of increase in the resources available for providing it. There are three main reasons for this:

- population ageing
- new technology and new knowledge
- rising expectations for both patients and professionals.

The interaction of these factors is shown in Fig. 2.1.

2.1.1 Population ageing

Population ageing is the single most important factor increasing the need for healthcare. As the number of older people increases, so does the need for healthcare.

In addition, the interaction of an ageing population and rising patient expectations is significant. Cohorts of individuals currently approaching old age will have different expectations from those who are already old. In future, older people will be better organised, more assertive and have higher expectations of the quality of life that they wish to enjoy and of the quality and volume of health services to which they feel entitled.

2.1.2 New technology and new knowledge

The healthcare industry and those researchers working in health, health services and related disciplines will continue to develop new technologies. The nature of the technology may be 'high' – for instance, the development of biomaterials, sophisticated fundamental research on the human genome and the development of computer systems, or a combination of all three – or 'low' – for example, effective simple interventions to prevent postnatal depression. Such research

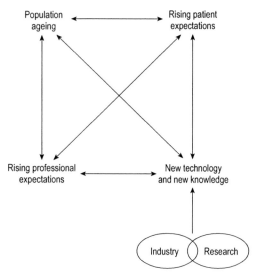

Fig. 2.1
The interaction of the three main factors that increase the need and demand for healthcare

indicates what it is possible to achieve, which then influences both patient and professional expectations.

Moreover, *effective* new technology increases the need for healthcare, if 'need' is defined as a health problem for which there is an effective intervention. Once an effective intervention has been developed, a previously insoluble problem becomes transformed into a health need for which there is a consequent claim on resources. The knowledge that such an effective intervention exists leads to public and professional demand for that service to be provided. If a misleading impression of effectiveness is given, this may precipitate inappropriate demand.

Sometimes, the application of a new technology will result in lower healthcare costs, or lower costs elsewhere in the economy, but even if healthcare costs are ultimately reduced by the use of a new technology there is often an increase in cost in the short term.

There is now evidence to show that new knowledge, i.e. research, obtained from clinical trials can be beneficial to the public health.[1] In a review of 28 trials costing $US355 million, it was found that 21% resulted in measurable improvements in health and 14% resulted in cost savings to society. Although the research results or new knowledge led to increases in healthcare expenditure, the health gains were large and valuable. However, long-term benefits may be of little comfort to the healthcare manager under immediate pressure.

2.1.3 Expectations about healthcare

Janzen et al.[2] found little good-quality research on expectations about healthcare or 'health expectations'. In response to their paper, Coulter[3] outlined nine questions that needed investigation if we were to gain a greater understanding of patient and public expectations (Box 2.1).

2.1.3.1 Rising patient expectations

Patient expectations of healthcare are rising, reflecting a societal change in attitude towards the provision of goods and services, a trend usually called 'consumerism'.

In most developed countries, the trend towards consumerism includes rising expectations of:

- the accessibility of health services
- the quality of health services
- the accountability of service providers, should there be any failure or perceived failure in the quality of healthcare.

There is general acceptance that the enjoyment of good health is a desirable and achievable objective; thus, if people have an expectation that their health should be better than it is, they will seek out services they believe will improve their health.

Changing attitudes in those approaching old age will mean that the sector of society which has the greatest need for healthcare will also make more demands in the future than it has in the past.

Box 2.1 Coulter's nine 'Great expectations': gaining a greater understanding of health expectations or expectancies (Source: Coulter[3])

1. How often are expectations unrealistic?
2. If unrealistic expectations are a real problem, how can they be modified?
3. What is the relationship between expectations and preferences?
4. Could measurement of patient satisfaction be improved by paying greater attention to prior expectations?
5. To what extent is there concordance, or dissonance, between patients' expectations and those of health professionals?
6. Do health professionals understand patients' expectations and in what ways do their perceptions of these influence their behaviour?
7. Are public expectations really rising, and if so, what problems does this cause?
8. Could high expectations act as a catalyst for quality improvement?
9. If so, should we be encouraging patients to have even higher expectations and to express these more forcefully?

Rising patient expectations are also fuelled by the development of new technology.

2.1.3.2 Rising professional expectations

Professional expectations are influenced by developments in technology in that any new developments serve as a stimulus to increase expectations. Two important managerial challenges for the future are:

- to help professionals be more critical in their appraisal of new technology
- to change the paradigm of healthcare such that a large proportion of the interventions offered to the population are those that have been shown to be effective through the performance of good-quality research.

Professional expectations and attitudes are also influenced by patient expectations. If patients who are 90 years old seek hip replacements, this will affect professional attitudes and expectations about the services that should be offered. Changing patient expectations about healthcare and the quality of healthcare can also influence professional attitudes and behaviour in a negative way: the threat of litigation may precipitate an increase in the practise of 'defensive medicine'.

References

1. Claibourne, S., Rootenberg, J.D., Katrak, S. et al. (2006) *Effect of a US National Institutes of Health programme of clinical trials on public health and costs.* Lancet 367: 1319–27.
2. Janzen, J.A., Silvius, J., Jacobs, S. et al. (2005) *What is a health expectation? Developing a pragmatic conceptual model from psychological theory.* Health Expect. 9: 37–48.
3. Coulter, A. (2005) *Examining health expectations.* Health Expect. 9: 1–2.

2.2   The evolution of evidence-based healthcare

The stages in the evolution of evidence-based healthcare from the early 1970s to the present day are described below and shown schematically in Fig. 2.2. During the 1970s and 1980s, the emphasis in the reform of health services or healthcare systems was on making structural changes or changes to the ways in which the systems were financed – 'doing things cheaper' (Section 2.2.1), 'doing things better' (Section 2.2.2) and 'doing things right'

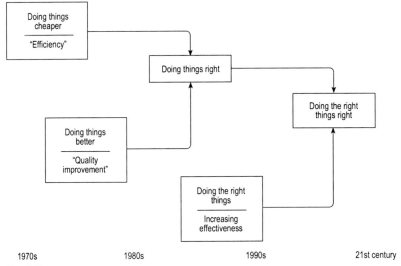

Fig. 2.2
The evolution of evidence-based healthcare from the 1970s to the 21st century

(Section 2.2.3). However, although structural reform is necessary, the impact it has is limited to:

- controlling the rate of cost increase
- increasing productivity
- increasing the quality of healthcare.

In order to gain the maximum value from the resources allocated to healthcare, it is necessary to 'do the right things' (Section 2.2.4), which requires a change in the way decisions within the health service are made.

2.2.1 Doing things cheaper

During the 1970s, financial pressure began to mount in the NHS after two decades during which investment in healthcare had increased steadily. The OPEC crisis and its financial consequences initiated an era in which healthcare decision-makers became more cost conscious. They were exhorted to increase efficiency, although this was actually manifest as an increase in productivity:

- **Productivity** is the relationship between inputs and outputs: number of bed days (therefore, the money necessary) per operation.
- **Efficiency** is the relationship between inputs and outcomes: number of bed days (therefore the money necessary) to obtain one extra year of life.

Unfortunately, these two words are often used as if they were synonymous (see Section 6.7.1.1).

The impetus to increase efficiency was to reduce cost per case by ensuring that healthcare was delivered:

- for the shortest time
- in the least expensive place
- by the least expensive professional
- using the cheapest possible drugs or equipment to provide an acceptable level of effectiveness and of safety.

2.2.2   Doing things better

During the 1980s, although the demand for increased efficiency was maintained, there was a new imperative, that of delivering quality improvement. As patients became better informed, more assertive and better organised, their expectations increased. Patients expected:

- easier access to services
- more effective healthcare
- safer care
- more information
- better communication.

These expectations for the provision of better healthcare reflected the general societal trend towards 'consumerism' (Section 2.1.3.1). The response within health services was 'to do things better' using the tools of quality assurance and clinical audit.

2.2.3   Doing things right

> Doing things cheaper + Doing things better
> = Doing things right

During the 1970s and 1980s, health service managers concentrated on 'doing things right', a combination of focusing on cost (i.e. 'doing things cheaper') and quality (i.e. 'doing things better'). Indeed, a great deal of attention and money was invested to ensure that clinicians 'do things right', by encouraging the performance of clinical audit, for instance. Unfortunately, 'doing things right' is only one side of the old management adage; the other is 'doing the right things'.

2.2.4   Doing the right things

In the past, healthcare managers tended to leave 'doing the right things' to other forces such as commercial pressure and chance. During the 1990s, this position was no longer tenable, especially as clinicians do not necessarily always 'do the right things'. In the provision of healthcare, the overall objective is to do more good than harm. However, it is important to be mindful in this situation that virtually all interventions have the potential to do harm, especially when those who champion the introduction of an innovation tend to emphasise the probability of benefit rather than that of harm occurring.

The interventions delivered within a health service can be categorised into three types according to their effect on patients:

1. doing more good than harm
2. doing more harm than good
3. of unknown effect or unproven efficacy.

The phrase 'more good than harm' encompasses four important concepts, three of which are embodied in the individual words whereas the fourth is unwritten:
'**Good**' – in this context, the word implies effectiveness but also includes safety and acceptability (see Sections 6.5 and 6.6.1.1, respectively).
'**Harm**' – the potential for this outcome of care should always be sought by decision-makers. The champions of a new service or intervention usually focus on the good the innovation will do, rather than the harm. Even when the possibility of harm is acknowledged, healthcare professionals may place a lower value on harm than the potential recipients of an intervention (see Section 10.3.1.2).
'**More**' – although the definition of 'more' may be self-evident, the *magnitude* of any difference described by the term is as important as the existence of a difference. The magnitude of any difference between the balance of good and harm observed in a research setting and the balance of good and harm in an ordinary service setting is determined by two main factors:

- the efficacy of the intervention as administered by the best hands in a research setting
- the quality of the service in which the intervention is actually delivered (Table 2.1 and Margin Fig. 2.1).

The degree of efficacy achieved in a research setting may not necessarily be reproducible in an ordinary service setting because the skills of the local healthcare professionals may not be of the same order as those of the researchers.

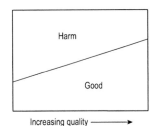

Margin Fig. 2.1

Table 2.1 The relationship between quality of service and the balance of good and harm conferred by an intervention

Quality of service	Balance
Very high	Good much greater than harm
Average	Good greater than harm
Below average	Good and harm equally balanced
Very low	Harm greater than good

The unwritten factor in this phrase is the **strength of the evidence**, which is determined by the quality of the research on which the evidence is based. The proposition that a therapy or test does more good than harm should be discarded if it is only an expression of personal opinion, but it should be used as evidence if it is a conclusion drawn from the conduct of high-quality research, the results of which showed that the intervention made a substantial difference with a low probability that the results were due to chance or biased findings.

Once the balance of good to harm has been established, decision-makers then need information on the costs of different options. This is because those interventions that do more good than harm can be subdivided into:

- those that do so at an affordable cost
- those that do so at an unaffordable cost.

2.2.5 Doing the right things right

For all healthcare professionals, but particularly clinicians, the important question to address at the beginning of the 21st century is not simply 'Are we doing things right?' or 'Are we doing the right things?' but:

'**Are we doing the right things right?'**

The need to do the right things right sets a new management agenda (see Section 2.5).

2.3 Decision rules for resource allocation in healthcare

In tandem with the evolution of evidence-based healthcare and the development of a new management agenda, the parameters used as a basis for decision-making about resource allocation have changed. A set of four decision rules for resource allocation[1] have been developed to illustrate the new paradigm.

Decision Rule I: The era of medical primacy
If resources are available, a healthcare intervention is provided (and thereby resources allocated) when a doctor is of the opinion that a particular intervention should be undertaken (Margin Fig. 2.2).

Decision Rule II: The era of effectiveness
If resources are available, a healthcare intervention is provided (and thereby resources allocated) if there is valid relevant evidence that a particular intervention will do more good than harm to a particular patient (Margin Fig. 2.3).

Decision Rule III: The era of cost-effectiveness
If resources are available, a healthcare intervention is provided (and thereby resources allocated) if there is valid relevant evidence that a particular intervention will do more good than harm to a particular patient *and* represents good value for money for the population (Margin Fig. 2.4).

Decision Rule IV: The era of best value healthcare
If resources are available, a healthcare intervention is provided (and thereby resources allocated) if there is valid relevant evidence that a particular intervention will do more good than harm to a particular patient *and* represents value for money for the whole population in relation to all other interventions (Margin Fig. 2.5).

Each of these decision rules can be described by a formula, all of which are given in Box 2.2.[1]

Decision Rule I describes the situation that pertained 20–30 years ago in the health services of most countries when a healthcare intervention was provided on the basis of unsubstantiated opinion. Decision Rule II describes the situation that developed during the last decade when it was recognised that not all healthcare interventions confer a net benefit. Decision Rule III describes the situation that pertains at the beginning of the 21st century when it has been acknowledged that the resources for healthcare are finite and that cost and value for money must be considered in any system of resource allocation. Decision Rule IV describes the situation that is set to become the prevailing system of resource allocation in which those who pay for healthcare will require that interventions are provided only when their outcomes give greater benefits than any of the alternative uses of equivalent resources. The application of Decision Rule IV maximises value across a health service and provides a net benefit to the population as a whole, as opposed to maximising the benefit for each individual irrespective of cost (Decision Rule II).

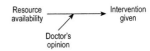

Margin Fig. 2.2

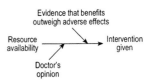

Margin Fig. 2.3

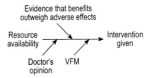

Margin Fig. 2.4

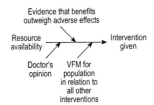

Margin Fig. 2.5

Box 2.2 Formulae for describing the decision rules for resource allocation (Source: Hicks and Gray[1])

For all decision rules (I–IV):

$Ralloc = \Sigma Iu + OH$

 where $Ralloc$ = resources allocated

   Iu = cost of intervention undertaken

   OH = cost of overheads

Decision Rule I:

$\Sigma Iu = \Sigma f(O.Ib > h) = Ravail$

 where O = doctor's opinion

   b = benefit

   h = harm

   $Ib > h$ = intervention confers net benefit

   $Ravail$ = resources available

Decision Rule II:

$\Sigma Iu = \Sigma f(E.Ib > h) = Ravail$

 where E = evidence

Decision Rule III:

$\Sigma Iu = \Sigma f(E.Ib > h.Ivfm) = Ravail$

 where vfm = value for money

   $Ivfm$ = intervention represents value for money

Decision Rule IV:

$\Sigma Iu = \Sigma f(E.Ispecb > h > E.Iotherb > h) = Ravail$

 where $Ispec$ = a specific intervention

   $Iother$ = all other interventions that could be undertaken in that clinical situation

---

Reference

1. Hicks, N.R. and Gray, J.A.M. (1998) *Evidence-based Medicine*. Financial Times Healthcare, London.

2.4 Value for money in healthcare

The value for money (VFM) of a health service can be measured directly by assessing the number of beneficial outcomes for the resources invested. In practice, value for money can be assessed by looking at the mix of services provided.

The factors that increase or decrease value for money are shown in Fig. 2.3.

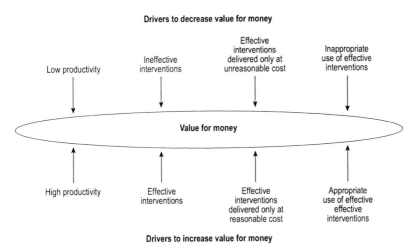

Drivers to decrease value for money

Fig. 2.3
Factors influencing value for money

In relation to cost, the concept of reasonableness is subtle, and its application poses difficulties because it involves value judgement. QALYs (Quality-adjusted Life Years) have been used to assess reasonableness of cost, and are a measure of length of life and quality of life. When QALYs are used to assess a range of new interventions, those interventions can usually be classified into one of three groups, as follows:

1. ridiculously cheap, a 'no-brainer decision' that should be implemented immediately, e.g. health workers giving brief advice to smokers to stop smoking at every consultation – excellent VFM
2. unreasonable cost, i.e. ridiculously expensive and irresponsible to fund, e.g. annual cervical screening – poor VFM
3. reasonable cost, i.e. gives a return on investment similar to that obtained for other interventions that are regarded as routine treatments, e.g. hip replacement or coronary artery bypass grafting – good VFM.

2.4.1 Better value healthcare

Decision-making in any health service is difficult. For almost every decision taken, there are some patients who will do better, and others who will do worse. However difficult such decision-taking may be, it is possible to get better value healthcare through evidence-based decision-making.[1] A toolkit for better value healthcare has been developed (Box 2.3).

Box 2.3 The Better Value Healthcare Toolkit (Source: Gray[1])

- How to respond to a bid for a new treatment or service
- How to conduct an annual value population review
- How to conduct a review of expenditure on a disease
- How to manage knowledge
- How to manage innovation
- How to carry out a systematic review
- How to reduce the number of errors
- How to engage patients and improve their experience
- How to improve productivity
- How to increase effectiveness
- How to get to the root of problems
- How to transform healthcare using information technology

Reference

1. Gray, J.A.M. (2007) *How to get Better Value Healthcare*. Offox Press, Oxford.

2.5 The new management agenda for health services

The need to 'do the right things right' generates a new management agenda for those in any health service, the implementation of which requires an evidence-based approach, the focus of this book. However, few health service management texts or courses appear to address the specific context that exists with respect to the delivery of a health service, namely, the nature of the provision of healthcare is driven not only by central policy-making but also by decentralised decision-making. Clinicians make many of the decisions, thereby determining not only service provision but also resource expenditure (see Section 1.2). Given this context, it is of paramount importance that those who make decisions about healthcare provision base those decisions on good evidence, using as a framework the classification of healthcare interventions set out in Section 2.2.4 (see also Table 2.2).

The new management agenda for the delivery of health services comprises four main strategies:

- the initiation of strategies to increase the good-to-harm ratio (Table 2.2)

Table 2.2 Strategies to increase the good-to-harm ratio in relation to the various types of intervention

Type of intervention	Strategies
Does more good than harm	• Promote use if it is affordable – starting starting right • Take steps to increase good and decrease harm to make ratio more favourable – quality improvement
Does more harm than good	• Stop them starting • Slow them starting • Start to stop them if it is not possible to increase good and decrease harm sufficiently to convert them into interventions that do more good than harm
Of unknown effect	• Stop them starting • Promote the conduct of RCTs both for new interventions and for interventions already in practice

- the promotion of relevant research
- the management of change in clinical practice
- minimising health inequalities.

In most health services being delivered, the distribution of the various types of interventions administered probably follows the pattern shown in Fig. 2.4.

The *optimal* distribution of interventions administered is represented in Fig. 2.5.

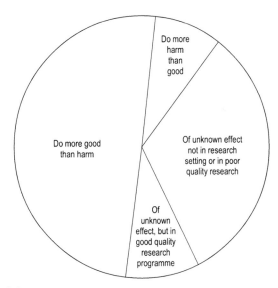

Fig. 2.4
Present distribution of various types of intervention

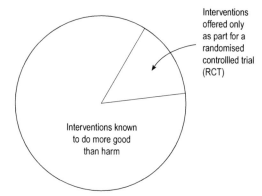

Fig. 2.5
Optimal distribution of interventions

Although quality improvement and cost reduction have been the imperatives in health service management since the 1980s, the other activities shown in Table 2.2, which will have an influence on not only *how* clinicians practise but *what* they practise, are new items on the management agenda.

2.5.1   Strategies to increase the good-to-harm ratio

It may take years for an effective intervention to be described, much less promoted, in a textbook. The classic study of this phenomenon was conducted by Antman et al.[1] into the delay in recommending thrombolysis as an effective intervention following myocardial infarction. In this study, it was demonstrated that even when information is available, implementation is often slow and sporadic, a finding as relevant today as it was in 1992.

A more pro-active approach to implementation is required to ensure that:

- patients are offered only those interventions that do more good than harm at reasonable cost
- the right patients are offered those interventions
- the interventions are delivered at a high standard.

As some of these management activities are new, managers need to combine several different approaches to ensure change takes place.

Although some clinicians believe delay in implementation to be advantageous, often citing, as justification for their stance, the consequences of the administration of thalidomide as a hypnotic to pregnant women, the keys to control lie not in delaying the implementation of research findings but in the critical appraisal of the best research evidence available and sound decision-making based on that appraisal. In fact, the use of thalidomide is an example of the failure to base decisions on good evidence.

In a review of the historical recommendations made about the sleeping position of infants, Gilbert et al.[2] concluded that the advice to put infants to sleep on their front, advice that was given for nearly 50 years, was contrary to evidence available from the year 1970, which showed that this position was likely to be harmful. Had a systematic review of preventable risk factors for sudden infant death syndrome (SIDS) from 1970 been conducted, Gilbert et al. estimated that over 10 000 infant deaths in the UK and at least 50 000 infant deaths in Europe, the USA and Australasia might have been prevented. Although the authors point out that it is unusual for health advice to have such a 'profound effect' on mortality, the results of this study underline the vital importance of developing pro-active mechanisms for the implementation of effective interventions.

2.5.1.1 Starting starting right

If there is evidence that an intervention does more good than harm, and it is affordable, decision-makers must manage its introduction within the health service (see Section 7.6.3.1). This will require appropriate professional training, including communication skills, patient education to promote good decision-making, and the development of systems of care supported by quality standards and mechanisms for the detection and correction of quality failures. All these steps are necessary to ensure good clinical outcomes.

> Good clinical decision-making + good systems
> = good clinical outcomes

For example, to promote the use of aspirin as a treatment after acute myocardial infarction (AMI) the following approaches are required:

- public education about the benefits of aspirin after AMI
- professional training, for instance, to promote the benefits of thrombolysis
- changes in purchasing requirements, for instance, to specify in contracts the standard of delivery of

thrombolysis treatment expected for patients with AMI (door-to-needle time)

- audit, in which performance is measured against a specified standard.

However, the problem of getting knowledge into practice, which has long been the preoccupation of policy-makers and managers, is twofold, comprising:

- the rapid adoption of some interventions
- the slow adoption of other interventions.

The speed and fact of adoption is not always proportionate to the value of interventions.

Although attention has been paid to the work of Everett Rogers, whose book *The Diffusion of Innovation* is a classic in the field, an outstanding systematic review of evidence by Greenhalgh and colleagues[3] suggests that there is no simple effective means for the diffusion of knowledge. While it is appropriate for people who wish to promote a new perfume, novel or fashion to rely on mechanisms such as word of mouth, television appearances and similar opportunities to change public consciousness, a powerful implication of Greenhalgh et al.'s work is that in a health service it is inappropriate to rely on diffusion (for greater detail, see Section 7.6.3.1).

For instance, if it is known – which it is – that pulmonary artery catheters do more harm than good,[4] then it is essential that action be taken both urgently and systematically to implement this knowledge. For such knowledge to be implemented, it requires that knowledge itself is perceived as a line-management responsibility and that every healthcare organisation should have a Chief Knowledge Officer (CKO). The CKO should be held to account for the following:

- allowing wrong information to seep into the organisation
- failing to ensure that high-quality and important information is implemented and delivered where and when it is needed in the organisation.

For further details of 'How to be a Chief Knowledge Officer', see Box 2.4. For further information about how the CKO can be integrated into an organisation, see Section 7.4.

2.5.1.2 Stopping starting and starting stopping

If interventions are doing more harm than good, decision-makers must ensure that either they are not introduced – 'stop them starting' – or, if they have already been

---

Box 2.4 How to be a Chief Knowledge Officer

What Chief Knowledge Officer (CKO)

When All the time

Who The CKO is a responsibility not a job. It is a responsibility that should be allocated to someone serving on the board or management team with direct accountability to the chief executive

Why To ensure that best use is made of knowledge to help the organisation achieve its objectives

How Ensure that the chief executive provides the support of a librarian to act as knowledge manager

Prepare a checklist of the groups of staff who need knowledge

Conduct a user needs review (a lunchtime meeting is better than nothing), and ascertain what each group needs

Ascertain what knowledge each group produces

With the librarian, set up a system for monitoring the knowledge that comes in to the organisation from:

- research outputs
- government agencies and other organisations who pay for healthcare, i.e. 'payers'
- statistical sources

Decide which sources of information are relevant to which group or groups of staff

Start a monthly 'New knowledge news' briefing for key contacts in every department

Identify the types of knowledge being produced by the organisation as a result of:

- research
- the production of patient leaflets
- central returns

Ask each producer of knowledge how they assess the quality of what they produce, and what steps they take to improve its quality; offer advice on how the quality of knowledge can be improved, e.g. encouraging those producing patient leaflets to use DISCERN (see Section 9.7.3)

At the end of each year, produce an annual knowledge report documenting developments in the use and production of knowledge in your organisation

---

introduced, that they are no longer practised – 'start stopping them'. However, starting stopping is much more difficult than stopping starting.

It is possible to stop an innovation completely and absolutely. For example, after consideration of the evidence on population screening for prostate cancer, the Department of Health in the UK issued guidance in 1997 that screening should *not* be introduced;[5] the guidance is shown in Box 2.5.

Box 2.5 Population screening for prostate cancer (Source: EL(97)12[5])

Summary

1. Population screening for prostate cancer, including the use of prostate specific antigen (PSA) as a screening test, should not be provided by the NHS or offered to the public until there is new evidence of an effective screening technology for prostate cancer. Screening, for the purposes of this Executive Letter, is defined as the application of a test or inquiry to identify individuals at sufficient risk of a specific disorder to warrant medical attention on account of symptoms of that disorder.[1]

Background

2. Two systematic reviews commissioned by the NHS Research and Development Health Technology Assessment Programme[2,3] have concluded that current evidence does not support a national screening programme for prostate cancer in the United Kingdom.

3. Current screening technologies (including the PSA test) have a limited accuracy that could lead to a positive result for those without the disease. Follow-up procedures could thus cause unnecessary harm to healthy individuals. The introduction of a prostatic cancer screening programme *at present* carries an unacceptable risk of more harm resulting than good.

4. The National Screening Committee has considered the evidence for introducing screening for prostate cancer and concluded that at this time and with current technology, there is no evidence of benefit resulting from population screening. This recommendation has been accepted by Department of Health Ministers.

5. Health Authority and General Practitioner Fund Holders are asked not to introduce or plan the purchase of population screening for prostate cancer until the National Screening Committee recommends an effective and reliable procedure.

6. This Executive Letter does not affect the clinical management of men presenting with symptoms of prostatic disease.

References

1. Adapted from: Wald, N.J. (1994) *Guidance on terminology.* J. Med. Screen. 1: 76.
2. Selley, S., Donovan, J., Faulkner, A. et al. (1997) *Diagnosis, management and screening of early localised prostate cancer.* Health Technol. Assess. 1(2): i, 1–96.
3. Chamberlain, J., Melia, J., Moss, S. et al. (1997) *The diagnosis, management, treatment and costs of prostate cancer in England and Wales.* Health Technol. Assess. 1(3): i–vi, 1–53.

The importance of stopping starting is heightened by the difficulty of starting stopping. Once an intervention is in routine use it can be very difficult to discontinue its use as demonstrated by the example shown in Casebook 2.1.[6,7]

Casebook 2.1 Albumin administration in the critically ill

The Cochrane Collaboration conducted a review of the effect of human albumin in critically ill patients.[6] The conclusion drawn was that:

there is no evidence that albumin administration reduces mortality in critically ill patients with hypovolaemia, burns or hypoalbuminaemia, and a strong suggestion that it may increase mortality.[6]

This review was published in the *British Medical Journal* of 25 July 1998. On 18 August that year, the Food and Drug Administration of the Department of Health and Human Services, USA, sent a letter to all doctors to draw their attention to the paper, to state that further research was needed, but:

the FDA urges treating physicians to exercise discretion in the use of albumin and plasma protein fraction based on their own assessment of these data.

The response in the UK to the findings of the review was slower and more hostile than that in the USA.

Since the initial review was conducted, the Albumin Reviewers have performed updates, the last substantive one dated 20 August 2004.[7] The message, however, remains the same.

2.5.1.3 Slowing starting

Slowing starting may be a more readily achievable objective than starting stopping. For instance, the use of printed educational material may help to modify the prescribing habits of GPs. The results of a study in England showed that the distribution to all GPs in 1993 (at a total cost of £25 000) of an *Effective Health Care* bulletin in which the cost-effectiveness of prescribing selective serotonin re-uptake inhibitors (SSRIs) for the treatment of depression was questioned, potentially avoided about 138 000 person-years of SSRI treatment.[8] The acquisition cost of this SSRI treatment, which is more expensive than the conventional therapy of tricyclic antidepressants, would have been nearly £40 million. Although the prescribing rate for SSRIs did continue to increase, the rate of increase was less than that which would have occurred had the bulletin not been sent out.

2.5.2 Promoting relevant research

If an intervention is of unknown effect, it should not be introduced; if it is already in service, it should be withdrawn until its effects have been investigated within an RCT to determine the beneficial effects (Section 5.4) and within a case-control or cohort study to identify any adverse effects (Sections 5.5 and 5.6, respectively).

It is possible to promote the performance of trials by:

- creating a culture in which interventions of unknown effect have to be evaluated scientifically from the first patient
- ensuring that those responsible for any health service invest in research and development, while recognising that there are two aspects to investing in research: the investment required for the research itself; and the health service costs of the research, because clinical care often takes longer, and therefore is more expensive, if patients and clinicians are involved in research.

2.5.2.1 Preventing unnecessary research

It is important to ensure that only *relevant* research is promoted. Young and Horton[9] have pointed out four main dangers of bad research practice (Margin Note 2.1), including unnecessary research. An example of unnecessary research is the investigation of the use of aprotinin to reduce peri-operative blood loss. Fergusson et al.[10] conducted a cumulative meta-analysis to show that although 64 trials were published between 1987 and 2002, the effectiveness and effect size of the intervention had been clearly established after the 12th trial in 1992. Thus, the subsequent 52 trials were unnecessary (see Margin Fig. 2.6 for an illustration of this). Unnecessary research raises many ethical questions, including the waste of resources and the opportunity costs of resources that could have been invested in relevant and necessary research.

Margin Note 2.1
Bad research practice

(Source: Young and Horton[9])

- Research conducted inappropriately
- Unnecessary research
- Research which is done but remains unpublished
- Research which is published but not in a way that justifies its existence or its relevance

2.5.3   Managing change in clinical practice

It is important to manage the introduction of any change in clinical practice; it is no longer sustainable to allow clinicians to make decisions about such changes in isolation. Although clinicians do implement changes in clinical practice that improve health, some of which will be achievable at a reasonable or reduced cost, they do not invariably choose 'the right things to do'. For example, during the 1980s, the surgical intervention laparoscopic cholecystectomy underwent rapid and widespread introduction in health services world-wide at the instigation of clinicians in the absence of good-quality evidence of its efficacy and despite concerns about its safety. The subsequent publication of the results of an RCT in which laparoscopic cholecystectomy was compared with conventional cholecystectomy showed there was no significant difference between the two study groups for hospital stay, time back to work for those employed, and time to full recovery, although laparoscopic cholecystectomy took significantly longer to perform.[11]

Sometimes changes to clinical practice can worsen outcomes overall; for instance, changes in the prescription of antibiotics have contributed to the genesis of a modern epidemic, the evolution of antibiotic-resistant bacteria, which has resulted not only in an increase in health service costs but also in mortality.

Until now, the evolution of clinical practice has been piecemeal, uncoordinated, and driven by individual clinicians. This situation is no longer acceptable and those responsible for the management and funding of health services must develop a new relationship in which clinicians (collectively) and managers can work together to guide the course of the evolution of clinical practice. In the UK, this approach is being promoted with the introduction of clinical governance (see Section 10.4.2.3). Managing the evolution of clinical practice is probably the most challenging item on the new management agenda.

2.5.4   Minimising health inequalities

In many countries, including the UK, the health inequalities gap is widening, i.e. the difference between the health of the poorest people in the population and that of the wealthiest people in the population is becoming greater. Furthermore, as medical care becomes more complicated and requires a greater level of contribution from the patient, the use of health services, and their degree of effectiveness, could begin to differ further between the poorest and the wealthiest in society, thereby exacerbating the underlying trend in increasing inequalities. For these reasons, those who manage health services must take steps to ensure that people with the least social and educational skills have access to healthcare that is appropriate to their needs.

References

1. Antman, E.M., Lau, J., Kupelnick, B. et al. (1992) *A comparison of results of meta-analysis of randomized control trials and recommendations of clinical experts.* JAMA 268: 240–8.
2. Gilbert, R., Salanti, G., Harden, M. et al. (2005) *Infant sleeping position and the sudden infant death syndrome: systematic review of observational studies and historical review of recommendations from 1940 to 2002.* Int. J. Epidemiol. 34: 874–87.
3. Greenhalgh, T., Robert, G., Bate, P. et al. (2005) *Diffusion of Innovations in Health Service Organisations. A systematic literature review.* BMJ Books and Blackwell Publishing, London.

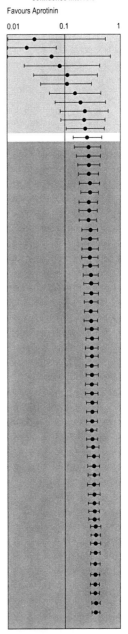

Odds ratio with 95% confidence intervals

Favours Aprotinin

0.01   0.1   1

Margin Fig. 2.6
Diagram to show that the conduct of 52 trials investigating the effectiveness of aprotinin in reducing peri-operative blood loss was unnecessary (Source: Fergusson et al.[10])

4. NHLBI ARDS Clinical Trials Network (2006) *Pulmonary artery catheters versus central venous catheters to guide the treatment of acute lung injury.* N. Engl. J. Med. 354: 2213–24.

5. Department of Health (1997) *Population Screening for Prostate Cancer.* EL (97)12.

6. Cochrane Injuries Group Albumin Reviewers (1998) *Human albumin administration in critically ill patients: systematic review of randomised controlled trials.* Br. Med. J. 317: 235–40.

7. The Albumin Reviewers (2007) *Human albumin solution for resuscitation and volume expansion in critically ill patients.* The Cochrane Database of Systematic Reviews, 2007, Issue 2. John Wiley and Sons Ltd. Abstract available online at: http://www.cochrane.org/reviews/en/ab001208.html

8. Mason, J., Freemantle, N. and Young, P. (1998/9) *The effect of the distribution of Effective Health Care Bulletins on prescribing selective serotonin reuptake inhibitors in primary care.* Health Trends 30: 120–2.

9. Young, C. and Horton, R. (2005) *Putting clinical trials into context.* [Comment] Lancet 366: 107–8.

10. Fergusson, D., Glass, K., Hutton, B. et al. (2005) *Randomized controlled trials of aprotinin in cardiac surgery: could clinical equipoise have stopped the bleeding?* Clin. Trials 2: 218–32.

11. Majeed, A.W., Troy, G., Nicholl, J.P. et al. (1996) *Randomised, prospective, single-blind comparison of laparoscopic versus small-incision cholecystectomy.* Lancet 347: 989–94.

2.6   The impact of science on clinical practice and healthcare costs

As a scientific approach to healthcare decision-making is championed in this book, it is appropriate to describe the impact that science – i.e. new technology and new knowledge – is having on clinical practice.

Sometimes, science may be put into practice by a well-considered national policy decision, for example, the introduction in the UK of breast cancer screening. However, most science is introduced into clinical practice by clinicians, who then seek the resources to fund the innovation from those who pay for the service to be delivered. The ways in which changes or innovations in clinical practice increase the cost of care are manifold (Box 2.6).

A study by Eddy in the USA showed that, in a healthcare system in which expenditure is not finite, changes in the 'volume and intensity' of clinical practice are the main factors driving increases in the cost of care that can be controlled by health service managers;[1] the other causes of increasing costs, population ageing and medical and general price inflation, are beyond the power of health service managers to control (Fig. 2.6). In other healthcare systems in which decisions are made within a context of finite resources, although expenditure does not

Box 2.6 The ways in which innovations in clinical practice increase costs

- Treating conditions that were previously untreatable
- Treating people who would previously have been untreated because of changing professional perceptions of need and appropriateness and changing public expectations. These may result from:
  - increasing safety of intervention
  - more acceptable, less invasive, less painful interventions
  - changing attitudes to chronological age as a reason for refusing treatment
  - changing expectations about health and disease
- Providing more expensive types of treatment:
  - more expensive drugs
  - more expensive imaging
  - more expensive tests
  - more expensive staff
- More intensive clinical practice:
  - longer duration of stay
  - more tests per patient
  - more professional interventions per patient
  - more treatments per patient

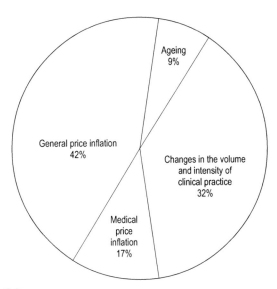

Fig. 2.6
Factors contributing to the increase in healthcare costs

spiral out of control, changes in the volume and intensity of clinical practice *will* generate financial and service pressures and can also drive the service in directions other than those that have been identified as priorities, such as those on the new management agenda.

Reference

1. Eddy, D.M. (1993) *Three battles to watch in the 1990s.* JAMA 270: 520–6.

2.7   Who 'carries the can'?

As need and demand for healthcare outstrip resources, and patient expectations rise, an increase in the number of complaints about the limitations of healthcare is to be anticipated. At present, much of the opprobrium falls on clinicians; in future, it may be appropriate to give guidance to disaffected people about who should receive complaints concerning particular aspects of the provision of health services in the UK, that is, who should 'carry the can' (Box 2.7).

Box 2.7 Checklist of who should 'carry the can' in the UK

If concerned about a shortage of resources affecting either yourself or a member of your family, work through the questions below to identify who should 'carry the can'.

*   Has the government decided to limit the amount of resources available for public services? *Write to the Chancellor of the Exchequer.*
*   Of the money allocated to public services, is insufficient going to health? *Write to the Prime Minister.*
*   Of the money allocated to health, is insufficient allocated to the population in which you live? *Write to the minister responsible for health services and ask that the formula used to distribute money geographically be reviewed.*
*   Of the money allocated to your population, is insufficient allocated to people with your type of health problem? *Write to the payer, such as the insurance company or primary care trust, responsible for allocating resources for the population in which you live.*
*   Of the money allocated to people with your type of health problem, is insufficient being allocated to people with your particular diagnosis? *Write to the chief executive of the hospital responsible for your service.*
*   Is the clinician giving you insufficient time and resources? *Write to the clinician.*

2.8   Industry and evidence-based decision-making

Industry has often found it difficult to come to terms with the shifting definition of evidence. In the early days, after Archie Cochrane's pioneering work, effectiveness was all that mattered. Then, cost-effectiveness became important, and in different countries the approach to defining and interpreting cost-effectiveness is different. In Australia, for example, there is a major programme reviewing drug cost-effectiveness; in England, Wales and Northern Ireland, the National Institute of Health and Clinical Excellence (NICE) gives guidance on cost-effectiveness of interventions. However, if an intervention is cost-effective that does not mean that it is affordable. Those working in industry have sometimes been disappointed that a new drug or new technology is not immediately taken up by a health service. The reasons for this are:

- It is often difficult for health services to identify cash in the short term for savings that will undoubtedly accrue in the long term
- Those who pay for or manage healthcare think of innovation not only in terms of cost-effectiveness expressed as cost per QALY, for example, but also as an intervention that can be funded only if less money is spent on another aspect of care, either for that particular group of patients or for different groups of patients.

Gentle Reader,

Empathise with the young public health physician. He was walking past the Radcliffe Camera which stands in the middle of one of Oxford's most beautiful squares. As he passed by, he caught a whiff of musty paper. It came from the ventilation shafts of the government paper rooms that lie under the green sward around the Camera. These rooms house official documents which contain the deliberations of many experts and represent an accumulation of evidence, some of which has been used over the years to prevent disease and promote health.

He sighed heavily as the smell brought to mind the first report of the Royal Commission on Environmental Pollution, published in 1971. In it had been highlighted the problems of the illicit dumping of toxic waste – known as 'fly tipping' – on sites, such as waste ground, not registered to receive it. Although the problem had first been identified in 1963, the Government had not acted on this matter. Throughout 1971, the Royal Commission lobbied the Government to act, because of the potential danger to water supplies and the risk to public health. All to no avail, until one day a Midlands lorry driver called Lonnie Downes took the matter into his own hands. He had discovered that fellow drivers were being given a bonus of £20 a week to dump toxic waste (described as 'suds oil'). After complaining to the management, he was threatened with dismissal. Several weeks later, he was offered a promotion; Lonnie declined. He was offered £300 to leave the firm; again Lonnie declined. Instead, he went to the local branch of the Conservation Society, which sent a detailed report to the Secretary of State for the Environment. Despite this, the Government still did not want to act.

The Conservation Society then sent its findings to the press. The story was published in the Birmingham Sunday Mercury *on 10 January 1972. On 24 February that same year, 36 drums of sodium cyanide were found on a derelict piece of ground near Nuneaton where children were known to play. The Government finally acted: a bill was drafted and passed into law by 30 March 1972.*

Commentary

On this occasion, the evidence alone, even that contained within a scientifically respectable government report, was not enough to determine policy. Decisions taken by policy-makers and managers can be made either in response to public pressure or from an ideological position in which the scientific evidence may play a negligible part.

Making decisions about health services

When a proposal is made to introduce a new intervention, a healthcare decision-maker should:

- examine the evidence put forward by the proponent
- find other evidence, if it exists
- appraise the quality of the research evidence
- estimate the outcomes, both beneficial and adverse, of the innovation
- estimate the opportunity costs of introducing the innovation.

In general, there are two questions that must be asked when appraising the research evidence put forward to support the introduction of an innovation (Box 3.1).

Detailed advice on appraising the quality of research and the outcomes of research studies is given in Chapters 5 and 6, respectively.

3.1 Making decisions under pressure

The context of any decision a decision-maker may face can vary in complexity. Instances of the simplest type of decision-making are those in which an enthusiast wishes to introduce a new therapy, test or service and the decision-maker has to consider the effects of the innovation being proposed. There are, however, many other decisions that have to be made about more complex situations; for example, the need to find efficiency savings, or to re-organise a service because a lead consultant retires, or some equipment needs to be replaced.

3.1.1 Dealing with difficult decisions

In the competition for resources that exists in the modern world, services for which there is no evidence of effectiveness are in a weak position when competing with other services for which the evidence base is strong.

Margin Note 3.1

Absence of evidence of effectiveness is not *ipso facto* evidence of ineffectiveness

---

Box 3.1 General questions for the appraisal of research evidence

1. Is the design of this research study the most appropriate to answer my question?
2. How good is the quality of this particular research when compared with the best design of its type?

One example of difficult decision-making followed the publication of the conclusions from a systematic review of vision screening in children conducted by the Health Services Research Unit, University of Oxford, on behalf of the Health Technology Assessment Programme of the UK R&D Programme. Although no evidence of beneficial effects could be found, the proposal that the service be stopped was met with some concern, indeed, outrage.

How can the decision-maker deal with situations such as these?

3.1.2   Battalions of difficult decisions

When sorrows come, they come not as single spies,
But in battalions.

William Shakespeare, *Hamlet*, Act IV, Scene v

For the decision-maker who wishes to manage change, the fact that troubles come not as single spies but as whole battalions can be advantageous. If a single service must be cut, for example, a community hospital has to be closed or an A&E department has to be shut down, the general public and the media are able to focus on a single issue and present it negatively with potentially devastating consequences for the decision-maker. If, however, a decision to reduce investment in one particular service for which there is no evidence of effectiveness can be linked with five other options for increasing investment (three of which could be funded if the service currently provided could be scaled down) then this changes the context and enables the decision-maker to present the outcome in a positive way.

Thus, in making difficult decisions, the decision-maker should seek to avoid a situation in which a simple yes-or-no decision is required and instead identify various options, some of which could be funded by the limited resources available. One technique that is valuable in this situation is Programme Budgeting and Marginal Analysis (PBMA).

Programme budgeting allows decision-makers in a health service to identify the amount of money that has been invested in major health programmes, and to use that information to plan future investment.[1] It can be used together with marginal analysis – an economic appraisal technique that assesses incremental changes in costs and benefits when resources in programmes are increased, decreased or deployed differently – to identify the following:

- where resources are invested currently
- the effectiveness of current use of resources
- the most effective way of investing resources in future with respect to the needs of the population.[1]

Reference

1. Brambleby, P., Jackson, A. and Gray, J.A.M. (2008) *Better Allocation for Better Health and Healthcare: Annual Population Value Review* 2008. Second Iteration NHS National Knowledge Service, and Directorate of Commissioning and System Management, Department of Health, London.

3.2 Therapeutic and preventive interventions

3.2.1 Dimensions and definitions

A therapy is any intervention administered with the objective of improving the health status of patients or of populations. Drugs and surgical operations are obvious examples of a therapy, but preventive interventions, such as immunisation programmes or health promotion initiatives, are also therapies.

The criteria used to assess a therapy are:

- acceptability (Section 6.6.1.1)
- effectiveness (Section 6.4)
- safety (Section 6.5)
- patient satisfaction and patients' experience (Section 6.6)
- cost-effectiveness (Section 6.7)
- appropriateness (Section 6.9).

The term therapy usually refers to a single specific act that a professional undertakes or performs on either a single patient or all the individuals in a particular 'population'. However, it is also possible to apply the term to more

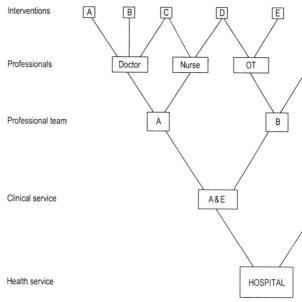

Fig. 3.1
The increasing complexity of therapeutic interventions, from the performance of a single therapeutic act to the introduction of a clinical service

complicated situations in which the effect of a series of therapeutic acts is tested, for example:

- a comparison of treatment by different professionals, e.g. doctor vs nurse, chiropractor vs orthopaedic surgeon
- a comparison of treatment by different teams within a clinical service
- a comparison of treatment by different types of clinical service.

This increasing complexity of therapeutic interventions, from the application of a single therapy to that of whole services, is shown in Fig. 3.1.

Screening, which is a combination of a diagnostic test and a therapy, is discussed in Section 3.4.

3.2.2   Searching

Any search for a therapy should have three or four main components (Table 3.1) based on the PICO (or PECO) formulation[1] (see Section 9.4.1). This search can be restricted to a relevant study design by using Publication Type or Clinical Queries in Medline (PubMed, OVID or Dialog interfaces).

Table 3.1 Components of a search for a therapy

Component	Example
The clinical problem (P)	Migraine
The therapy or intervention (I)	Behaviour therapy
The comparison (C) *optional*	Aspirin
The outcome (O)	Pain reduction

The clinical problem (P) is usually easy to specify.

The therapy (I) itself is more difficult to specify because it may be described in different ways. Try to include text words and index terms, and use synonyms.

The comparison (C) is optional, and can be used in the search if you are comparing two therapies.

The outcome(s) (O) should be considered because this is an additional way of focusing your search, but it will restrict your results.

The search results can be restricted to a certain study design – for therapy, the first step is to look for a systematic review or meta-analysis of studies by using the Publication Type Meta-Analysis [pt]. If this is unsuccessful, the next step is to look for trials by choosing the Publication Type Randomised Controlled Trial [pt].

Searching tips

➠ Use the therapy category or the systematic review search box on PubMed Clinical Queries to construct a quick, focused search for randomised controlled trials or systematic reviews:
http://www.ncbi.nlm.nih.gov/entrez/query/static/clinical.shtml.

➠ An overview of Clinical Queries can be obtained from the journal *Evidence-Based Medicine*.[2]

➠ Try your therapy search in the Cochrane Library (http://www.cochrane.org/), a high-quality electronic resource containing reliable systematic reviews and clinical trials.

3.2.3 Appraisal

3.2.3.1 The balance of good and harm

The randomised controlled trial (RCT) is the best method for assessing the effectiveness of a therapy (Section 5.4), but it should be incorporated in a systematic review of trials. However, even this powerful research method may not answer the question: 'Does this intervention do more good than harm?'

The harmful or adverse effects of therapy (often referred to as side-effects) are usually rarer than beneficial effects. Thus, a study that has been designed with sufficient power to detect a 5% improvement in the effectiveness of a new therapy when compared with an existing therapy may not be sufficiently powerful to detect any side-effects that may occur with a frequency of 1 in 1000. If the side-effect is mild, a skin rash, for example, this matters little, but if the side-effect is death this is serious. As such, RCTs designed to assess effectiveness often need to be complemented by cohort studies to assess safety (see Section 5.6). Therefore, more than one type of evidence is necessary to enable clinicians or those who pay for healthcare to assess the balance between good and harm conferred by a therapy.

It is also important for economic evaluations to be conducted alongside RCTs such that timely and reliable assessments of value for money are available to inform decisions on coverage and reimbursement [3–5] (see Section 6.7.3).

3.2.3.2 Assessing innovations in health service delivery

Although the RCT is considered to be the 'gold standard' for evaluating the effects of a therapy, such trials are more difficult to organise with increasing complexity of therapeutic intervention (Margin Fig. 3.1), either technically, because the number of services randomly allocated may be too few to ensure the trial has adequate power, or politically, because politicians may be reluctant to admit that a new policy should be subject to a trial – trials indicate equipoise and uncertainty (see Box 5.6). Consequently, studies of health service organisation and delivery are sometimes investigated using research methods other than the RCT, notably:

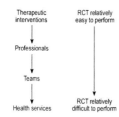

Margin Fig. 3.1

- the cohort study (see Section 5.6)
- the case-control study (see Section 5.5)
- controlled before and after study (see Section 5.7)
- interrupted time series (see Section 5.8).

Often, these methods require the analysis of large databases of health service utilisation. The use of these methods allows the following types of question to be addressed:

- What is the total mortality resulting from an operation, as distinct from the mortality observed in hospital?
- Is the outcome of care observed at one hospital or one type of hospital better than that which would be expected by chance?

If the mortality rate observed at one type of hospital is greater than that at another type, when controlled for case-mix and other potentially confounding variables, this may indicate the need to change policy or the management of the hospital system. If the mortality rate at one hospital is greater than that at other hospitals of the same type, this may indicate a problem with the quality of service delivery at that particular hospital (Section 6.8).

3.2.4 Getting research into practice

3.2.4.1 Therapy

Although there has been much discussion about the problems of implementing research evidence of the effectiveness of any new intervention within the health service, owing to the difficulty of influencing professional practice, this type of change is relatively simple because good-quality evidence is available and should dominate decision-making.

3.2.4.2 Innovations in health service delivery

As the subject of the decision changes from simple interventions, such as the administration of new drugs, to more complex interventions, such as changing the patterns of skill mix or of hospital provision (see Fig. 3.1), the availability of evidence decreases, not only in absolute but also in relative terms, that is, relative to the two other factors decision-makers have to take into account:

1. 'local' circumstances; for example, it may not be possible to change an emergency service so that care is delivered by consultants owing to the difficulties of recruiting and paying for the number of consultants required
2. the political context in which the service is delivered; for example, the introduction of nurse practitioners may be opposed by the public, or the closure of a low-volume local hospital service may be vigorously resisted by the community.

Resource constraints and political pressures do not, however, negate the need for evidence; on the contrary, the need for research-based knowledge is heightened even though these other factors may outweigh the scientific evidence when the final decision is taken.

The problems encountered when implementing complex interventions as a result of evidence-based management are illustrated by the adoption of stroke units, for which there is strong evidence of effectiveness. In a Cochrane Review, it was found that patients who receive organised stroke-unit care are more likely to survive their stroke, return home and make a good recovery.[6] However, for the adoption of any new service to be successful, it is vital not only to introduce the new service but also to dismantle the pre-existing service in order to fund the new service. Nonetheless, progress is possible. In the National Sentinel Stroke Audit in England, Wales and Northern Ireland, it was found that the number of hospitals with a stroke unit increased from 79% in 2004 to 91% in 2006,[7] demonstrating a continuing uptake of this complex intervention.

References

1. Richardson, W.S., Wilson, M.C., Nishikawa, J. et al. (1995) *The well-built clinical question: a key to evidence-based decisions.* ACP J. Club 123: A12–13.
2. Haynes, R.B. and Wilczynski, N. (2005) *Finding the gold in Medline: clinical queries.* Evid. Based Med. 10: 101–2.
3. Gold, M., Siegel, J., Russel, L. et al. (eds) (1996) *Cost-effectiveness in Health and Medicine.* Oxford University Press, New York.
4. Drummond, M. (2001) *Introducing economic and quality of life measurements into clinical studies.* Ann. Med. 33: 344–9.
5. Drummond, M.F., O'Brien, B., Stoddart, G.L. et al. (1997) *Methods for the Economic Evaluation of Health Care Programmes*, 2nd edn. Oxford University Press, Oxford.
6. Stroke Unit Triallists' Collaboration (2007) *Organised inpatient (stroke unit) care for stroke.* Cochrane Database of Systematic Reviews, 2007, Issue 1. Abstract available online at: http://www.cochrane.org/reviews/en/ab000197.html
7. Clinical Effectiveness and Evaluation Unit, Royal College of Physicians of London (2006) *National Sentinel Stroke Audit Phase I Organisational Audit 2006 Report for England, Wales and Northern Ireland.* Prepared on behalf of the Intercollegiate Stroke Working Party.

3.3 Tests

Gus and Wes had succeeded in elevating medicine to an exact science. All men reporting on sick call with temperatures above 102 were rushed to hospital. All those except Yossarian reporting on sick call with temperatures below 102 had their gums and toes painted with gentian violet solution and were given a laxative to throw away into the bushes. All those reporting on sick call with temperatures of exactly 102 were asked to return in an hour to have their temperatures taken again.

Joseph Heller, *Catch 22*, 1962

3.3.1 Dimensions and definitions

There are five common types of test:

- the presence or absence of a symptom – something a patient feels
- the presence or absence of a sign – something a clinician can detect
- laboratory results, expressed numerically (Margin Note 3.2, Margin Fig. 3.2)
- radiological images, interpreted perceptually
- pathological specimens, interpreted perceptually.

The term 'test' is often used as a synonym for diagnostic test, but tests may have a function other than that of diagnosis, for example:

- to monitor the effect of treatment, where the results are used to determine whether treatment should be continued, changed or stopped
- to provide information about prognosis (the future course of a disease)
- to indicate the presence or absence or degree of risk.

Screening is discussed separately in Section 3.4 because the process involves more than the performance of a test: the beneficial effects of screening tests must be balanced against the harmful or adverse effects of any intervention resulting from those screening tests.

Some of the criteria used to assess the efficacy of tests are the same as those used to assess that of therapies, namely, effectiveness, safety, acceptability and cost. The criteria specific to the assessment of tests are:

- sensitivity
- specificity
- the relationship between sensitivity and specificity
- predictive value
- likelihood ratio.

3.3.1.1 Sensitivity and specificity

Diagnostic tests are used for many purposes, but in their simplest form the results are either positive or negative: an individual is identified as either having the disease or not having the disease. However, few tests are perfect. Most people who do not have the disease will have a negative result (true-negatives), but some people with

Margin Note 3.2

A test is an assay which is given meaning by the application of knowledge to the result.

An assay is a measurement of a biochemical variable; the result is a number.

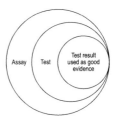

Margin Fig. 3.2

Margin Note 3.3

There is no test that is 100% sensitive and 100% specific

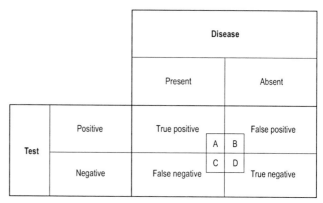

Fig. 3.2
The four types of test result

negative test results may actually have the disease
(false-negatives). Most people who do have the disease
will have a positive test result (true-positives), but some
people with positive test results will not have the disease
(false-positives). Thus, four types of test result may be
obtained as a combination of these two variables
(Fig. 3.2).

The balance between true-positives and false-positives
and between true-negatives and false-negatives is expressed
by two criteria which are used to judge all diagnostic tests,
namely:

- sensitivity
- specificity.

Sensitivity is the proportion of people with the disease
who are identified as having it by a positive test result.
Specificity is the proportion of people without the
disease who are correctly reassured by a negative test
result.

A method for calculating the sensitivity and specificity of
a diagnostic test is shown in Fig. 3.3.

3.3.1.2 Predictive values

Sensitivity and specificity are constant criteria that can
be applied to any diagnostic test irrespective of the
characteristics of the population on which the test is used.
However, the significance of a test result is determined
not only by the sensitivity and the specificity of the
test, but also by the prevalence of the condition in the
population upon which the test is used, which can alter
its predictive value.

		Disease	
		Present	Absent
Test	Positive	A	B
	Negative	C	D

Sensitivity $\frac{A}{A + C}$

Specificity $\frac{D}{B + D}$

Fig. 3.3
Calculation of the sensitivity and specificity of a diagnostic test

The predictive value of a test is an expression of the probability that the test result indicates the presence or absence of disease, therefore:

- the *positive predictive value* is the probability that a person with a positive test result actually has the disease
- the *negative predictive value* is the probability that a person with a negative test result does not actually have the disease.

Imagine conducting a diagnostic test that has a sensitivity of 90% and a specificity of 90% in two different populations of 1000 each, one in which there is a high prevalence of the disease and another in which there is a low prevalence. The results in Matrix 3.1 reflect the situation in hospital practice, in which 50% of the patients have the disease (high prevalence), and 90% of the people who have a positive test result will have the disease, therefore the test is said to have a positive predictive value of 90%. The results in Matrix 3.2 reflect the situation in general practice, in which only 10% of patients have the disease (low prevalence); even though the sensitivity of the test is the same, the positive predictive value is only 50%.

This difference in the predictive value of a test despite the constancy of sensitivity and specificity is the main reason that:

- hospital doctors believe that GPs miss 'easy' diagnoses
- GPs believe that hospital doctors over-investigate.

The criteria of sensitivity, specificity and predictive value are relevant for all tests whether numerical or perceptual.

Disease / Test	Present	Absent
Postive	450	50
Negative	50	450
Total	500	500

Matrix 3.1
Prevalence of disease - 50%, reflecting the situation in hospital practice

Disease / Test	Present	Absent
Postive	90	90
Negative	10	810
Total	100	900

Matrix 3.2
Prevalence of disease - 10%, reflecting the situation in general practice

3.3.1.3 Types of test result

Numbers

Some tests generate results in the form of numbers, for example, biochemical tests. When test results are expressed numerically, the meaning of those results will vary depending on whether the test has been used to identify:

- certain individuals within the range of a single population, for example, those who have raised blood pressure (Fig. 3.4)
- the presence of a condition in two populations, for example, those who do and those who do not have spina bifida, where the test results of each population will fall within a range of values and those two ranges will overlap (Fig. 3.5).

From Fig. 3.4, it can be seen how different test values can be chosen to distinguish between those identified as having 'normal' blood pressure and those identified as having 'high' blood pressure. From Fig. 3.5, it can be seen how the cut-off point between positive and negative can be

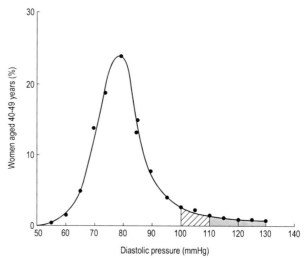

Fig. 3.4
Frequency distribution of diastolic pressure in females aged 40–49 years in a London population sample. The tinted area shows women known to be at risk and known to have a high probability of gaining benefit from treatment. The hatched area, representing pressures of 100–110 mmHg, shows women who are also at risk but have a lower probability of gaining from treatment. Women in the white area below the distribution curve have 'normal' blood pressures.
(Source: Pickering, 1974, *Hypertension: Courses, Consequences and Management*, 2nd edition. Churchill Livingstone, Edinburgh. with permission)

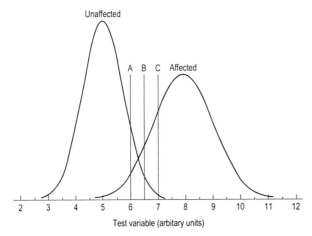

Fig. 3.5
Hypothetical example of the detection rate and false-positive rate of a screening test at three different cut-off levels: A, B and C. (Source: Cuckle and Wald, 1984, in Wald, N. J. (ed.) *Antenatal and Neonatal Screening*. Oxford University Press, Oxford)

varied. However, the choice of any numerical cut-off point within a data set, whether applied to a single population or to two populations, is arbitrary. The choice of a cut-off point is difficult because there is always a trade-off between sensitivity and specificity (see Section 3.3.1.4).

Words
Some tests, known as perceptual tests, are dependent upon the use of a human being as the instrument of measurement. Human perception is used to distinguish positive from negative, by:

- seeing – e.g. the analysis of X-rays or histopathological specimens
- hearing – e.g. the detection of heart murmurs
- touching or palpation – e.g. the detection of congenital dislocation of the hip.

Any test that involves human perception and judgement is bedevilled by variability of reporting on results. There are two forms of variability:

- intra-observer variability – the phenomenon in which the same observer classifies the same test result differently on two separate occasions
- inter-observer variability – the phenomenon in which different observers classify the same test results differently.

Within epidemiology, the phenomenon of inter-observer variability is widely accepted; it is also gaining acceptance by healthcare professionals. Indeed, this phenomenon should be recognised as an inevitable consequence of the use of perceptual tests. Unfortunately, within the legal system where 'expert' witnesses can be called by both the prosecution and the defence, inter-observer variability is interpreted categorically as one observer being 'right' and another being 'wrong'.

3.3.1.4 Between a rock and a hard place

As any threshold is an arbitrarily selected value, it is possible to change the threshold and therefore the balance between positive and negative results. At any particular threshold, the balance of false-positives and false-negatives will be different. This illustrates one of the central principles of testing, namely, that any increase in sensitivity is usually accompanied by a decrease in specificity (Margin Fig. 3.3) and vice versa. The greater the degree to which a service is designed never to miss a diagnosis, the greater will be the number of false-positive results generated. As sensitivity increases, a point is reached at which very small increases in sensitivity are accompanied by very large decreases in specificity, i.e. the number of false-positive results increases.

The consequences of this increase are:

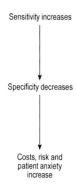

Sensitivity increases

Specificity decreases

Costs, risk and patient anxiety increase

Margin Fig. 3.3

- a greater number of patients made anxious
- the costs of treatment grow
- a greater number of patients will be harmed by the adverse effects of unnecessary treatments (see Margin Fig. 3.3).

The results of two studies demonstrate the disadvantage of increasing sensitivity; both examples illustrate the outcome of increasing the sensitivity of imaging tests, that is, an increase in the number of false-positive test results.

The sensitivity of magnetic resonance imaging (MRI) in the detection of pituitary adenoma (tumour) can be increased by the administration of certain chemicals to those undergoing imaging: in this study, the images from 100 healthy volunteers were mixed with those from 57 patients who had pituitary adenoma; the images were read by three experts independently. Ten per cent of the healthy volunteers were diagnosed as having adenoma, which is a very rare disease.[1]

In another study, the MR images of 98 asymptomatic people were mixed with those of 27 people who had back pain; the images were read by two experts independently. Sixty-four per cent of the asymptomatic individuals were classified as 'abnormal'.[2] In the accompanying editorial,[3] it was stated that: 'The recent increase in the rates of lumbar spine surgery may be related in part to the availability of new imaging techniques'.

3.3.1.5 Tests: the producer's perspective

The number of new tests developed, particularly biochemical tests, is increasing each year, and the rate of increase will accelerate as new genetic tests become available. Indeed, consumers in the USA can now order genetic tests, such as those for the BRCA1 and BRCA2 gene mutations, and other laboratory services direct through the World Wide Web without involving their doctor or health insurance plan. This is known as 'direct-to-consumer marketing', a strategy promoted by producers as increasing consumers' access to clinical testing and ensuring anonymity for those concerned about discrimination by employers or insurance companies on the basis of genetic predisposition to disease.[4]

To the manufacturer of a test, increased test accuracy is often sufficient to justify the introduction of a new product. Manufacturers rarely evaluate new tests or new versions of tests against such criteria as sensitivity or predictive value. The manufacturer is usually satisfied if:

- the chemical specification of the test has been improved: for example, if proteins can be separated with increased precision
- the performance of the test is easier and requires a lower level of skill from laboratory staff
- the cost of the test has been reduced.

Those clinicians responsible for developing tests focus primarily on increasing sensitivity, but this strategy carries a concomitant decrease in specificity (see Section 3.3.1.4).

3.3.1.6 Tests: the clinician's perspective

For the clinician, the test is never the first step in the process. The decision to request a test comes after two other processes, history-taking and examination, each of which has a likelihood ratio (Fig. 3.6).

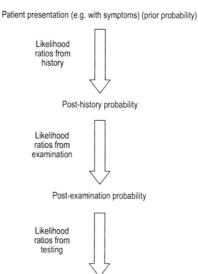

Fig. 3.6
Cascading likelihood ratios

In his important book on patient-centred diagnosis, Summerton[5] emphasises the importance of these steps and concludes by asking: 'Should commissioners of healthcare consider funding more primary clinical time as an alternative to yet more new diagnostic technologies?'[5]

3.3.1.7 Tests: the perspective of those who pay for healthcare

For the decision-maker in any health service, the perspective is different to that of the manufacturers and clinicians: although the manufacturers' and clinicians' criteria are relevant, other criteria are also important. Those who pay for healthcare need to know whether a marginal increase in sensitivity leads to better outcomes for the population as a whole or for individual patients only.

Any increase in the number of individuals having tests will result in an increase in the number of positive test results; some individuals with positive test results will have the disease, others will not (false-positives; Fig. 3.7). However, even if the false-positives are excluded and all the people who have a positive test actually have the disease, the effects of increasing the number of people tested may be simply to detect people with less severe disease (see Fig. 3.7).

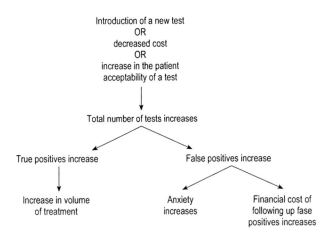

Fig. 3.7
The relationship between an increase in the volume of testing
(for various reasons) and the outcomes of that increase in testing

Research conducted in the USA has demonstrated that an increase in the number of tests performed increases the volume of treatment. In a cohort study of 12 coronary angiography service areas in New England in which the intensity of investigation by stress test of individuals with chest pain varied,[6] a positive relationship was found between total stress test rates and the rates of subsequent coronary angiography; a strong relationship was also shown between coronary angiography and revascularisation. Furthermore, in an analysis of the Medicare National Claims History files, which cover 30 million elderly Americans, it was found that investigation rates increased markedly over a 7-year period – from 50% to 300%.[7] These increases in the rates of diagnostic testing were associated with an increase in the rates of administration of relevant treatments (Table 3.2).

Table 3.2 Various investigations and the associated treatments: increased rates of testing lead to an increase in rates of intervention (Source: Verrilli and Welch[7])

Investigation	Treatment
Cardiac catheterisation	Cardiac revascularisation (CABG and PTCA)
Spinal imaging (CT and MRI)	Back surgery
Swallowing studies	Percutaneous gastrostomy
Mammography	Breast biopsy and excision
Prostate biopsy	Prostatectomy

One explanation could be that the increased rate of testing revealed exactly the same type of cases as had been diagnosed previously, but this explanation is not based on evidence. Another possibility is that an increase in testing, or an increase in test sensitivity, merely detects less severe cases, and the benefits obtained from increased expenditure on testing may decline as the volume of testing increases.

At the time of writing, in many biochemical laboratories, a greater number of tests are done to monitor chronic disease than those done to diagnose disease. Although many of these tests are relatively inexpensive, they may have significant consequences financially. For example, the calculation of the estimated glomerular filtration rate (EGFR) costs virtually nothing at a laboratory because an equation can be used that takes account of the patient's age, sex and, if necessary, the serum creatinine level. However, the consequence of performing this calculation is that more patients are now being diagnosed with chronic kidney disease (CKD). In some studies, as many as 10% of the population have been identified as having CKD, which has led to further investigation and referral.[8]

It is clear that increased testing is one of the major factors leading to an increase in the volume of treatment. Any attempt to control the volume of treatment that does not include controlling the development of diagnostic and disease monitoring services is doomed to failure.

However, it is also possible that biochemical laboratories have the capability to control the costs of health services in addition to improving value for money. For instance, it is more cost-effective for a laboratory to run a chronic disease management programme than to lat individual clinicians decide when repeat tests are required, achieved by ensuring that blood samples are accepted for analysis only if they have been requested by the laboratory.

3.3.2   Searching

Any search for a test should have three or four main components (Table 3.3) based on the PICO (or PECO) formulation[9] (see Section 9.4.1).

There may be a limited number of meta-analyses on tests; unfortunately, Medline does not provide a specific Publication Type to aid the retrieval of papers on tests.

Table 3.3 Components of a search for a test

Component	Example
The clinical problem (P)	Coeliac disease
The test (I)	Gliadin antibody test
The comparison (C) *optional*	Gold standard test
The outcome (O)	Sensitivity and specificity

The best single search term to use when retrieving papers on tests is "sensitivity" as a text word.[10]

In addition to this text word, Medical Subject Headings (MeSH) can be used when searching for papers on tests (MeSH fact sheet available online at http://www.nlm.nih.gov/pubs/factsheets/mesh.html). Relevant MeSH include the following:

- Sensitivity and Specificity/
- Predictive Value of Tests/
- False-Negative Reactions/
- False-Positive Reactions/
- Diagnosis, Differential/
- Diagnostic Test/
- Diagnostic Service/
- Routine Diagnostic Test/
- Diagnosis/.

Searching tips

➡ Use the diagnosis category on PubMed Clinical Queries to construct a quick focused search for papers on diagnostic tests, available online at: http://www.ncbi.nlm.nih.gov/entrez/query/static/clinical.shtml

➡ An overview of clinical queries can be obtained from the journal *Evidence-Based Medicine*.[11]

3.3.3   Appraisal

Appraisal is a two-stage procedure:

1. What is the best research method for appraising a test?
2. How good is any of the research found?

The best method for appraising a test is a large well-designed RCT that has patient outcomes, such as survival or quality of life, as end-points (Fig. 3.8A). Unfortunately, RCTs

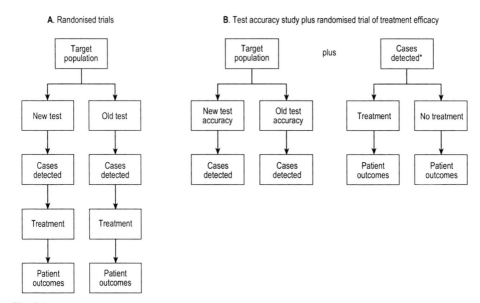

Fig. 3.8
Appraisal of new tests: (A) Evidence from a randomised controlled trial of a new test; (B) linked evidence of test accuracy and treatment efficacy. (Source: Lord et al.[13])

of tests are scarce because large trials are rarely feasible. As large trials are rarely feasible, there are several other types of evidence it may be useful to appraise:

- Systematic reviews of small studies in which meta-analysis of the data from the individual studies has been undertaken irrespective of whether the test results are presented as dichotomous (i.e. 'positive' or 'negative') or continuous. However, in a review of systematic reviews of diagnostic tests in cancer, Mallett et al.[12] concluded that the reliability and relevance of current systematic reviews of diagnostic tests are compromised by poor reporting and review methods.
- If there are no meta-analyses or systematic reviews available, as a compromise, results from individual research studies designed to investigate test performance as an end-point can be used.

Lord et al.[13] have developed a framework for deciding if evidence of test accuracy will suffice in the absence of evidence from an RCT of the test. They outline three categories of test attributes (Box 3.2), and propose a sequence of questions to help guide decision-making about whether evidence of test accuracy for each category will suffice.

Box 3.2 Categories of test attributes (Source: Lord et al.[13])

1. Safety and cost – i.e. the test is safer or costs less
2. Specificity – i.e. the test is more specific in that it excludes more cases of non-disease, and therefore avoids unnecessary treatment
3. Sensitivity – i.e. the test is more sensitive in that it detects more cases of disease and as such promotes more effective treatment

---

They suggest if there is already evidence from randomised trials showing that treatment of cases detected by the new diagnostic test improves patient outcomes, then evidence of increased accuracy *can* suffice (see Fig. 3.8B).

Lord et al. conclude that evidence from studies of accuracy *will* suffice if a new diagnostic test is safer or more specific but of a similar sensitivity to an old test. However, if a new test is more sensitive than an old test and extra cases of disease are detected (although the results from the treatment trials in which patients were enrolled who were detected using the old test may not apply to the extra cases detected) clinicians need to wait for results from randomised trials assessing treatment efficacy in patients detected by the new test. This is unless a new test detects the same spectrum and subtype of disease or the treatment response is similar across the disease subtype and spectrum.

Irwig et al.[14] have developed "Guidelines for Meta-analyses Evaluating Diagnostic Tests"; their checklist for evaluating meta-analyses of diagnostic tests is shown in Box 3.3, which can be used to supplement the general guidance on appraising systematic reviews (see Section 5.3.3).

For the appraisal of individual studies, the McMaster checklist[15] can be used (Box 3.4).

3.3.4   Getting research into practice

New tests, particularly biochemical tests, flood into clinical practice because there are no controls to restrict their introduction. It is rarely necessary to promote the use of any new test. To compound the situation, there is very little good-quality evidence of effectiveness for new tests that become available. The main challenge, therefore, is stopping starting (see Sections 2.5.1.2 and 7.6.3.2), i.e. controlling the introduction of new tests.

For a case-study of whether to introduce a new diagnostic test, see Section 9.6.1.

Box 3.3 Checklist for evaluating meta-analyses of diagnostic tests (Source: Irwig et al.[14])

- Is there a clear statement about:
  - the test of interest?
  - the disease of interest and the reference standard by which it is measured?
  - the clinical question and context?
- Is the objective to evaluate a single test or to compare the accuracy of different tests?
- Is the literature retrieval procedure described with search and link terms given?
- Are inclusion and exclusion criteria stated?
- Are studies assessed by two or more readers?
  - Do the authors explain how disagreements between readers were resolved?
- Is a full listing of diagnostic accuracy and study characteristics given for each primary study?
- Does the method of pooling sensitivity and specificity take account of their interdependence?
- When multiple test categories are available, are they used in the summary?
- Is the relation examined between estimates of diagnostic accuracy and study validity of the primary studies for each of the following design characteristics:
  - appropriate reference standard?
  - independent assessment of the test or tests and reference standard?
- In comparative studies, were all of the tests of interest applied to each patient or were patients randomly allocated to the tests?
- Are analytic methods used that estimated whether study design flaws affect diagnostic accuracy rather than just test threshold?
- Is the relation examined between estimates of diagnostic accuracy and characteristics of the patients and test?
- Are analytic methods used which differentiate whether characteristics affect diagnostic accuracy or test threshold?

Box 3.4 Methodological questions for appraising journal articles about diagnostic tests (Source: McMaster University[15])

The best articles evaluating diagnostic tests will meet most or all of the following eight criteria:

1. Was there an independent, 'blind' comparison with a 'gold standard' of diagnosis?
2. Was the setting for the study, as well as the filter through which study patients passed, adequately described?
3. Did the patient sample include an appropriate spectrum of mild and severe, treated and untreated disease, plus individuals with different but commonly confused disorders?
4. Were the tactics for carrying out the test described in sufficient detail to permit their exact replication?
5. Was the reproducibility of the test (precision) and its interpretation (observer variation) determined?
6. Was the term 'normal' defined sensibly? (Gaussian, percentile, risk factor, culturally desirable, diagnostic or therapeutic?)
7. If the test is advocated as part of a cluster or sequence of tests, was its contribution to the overall validity of the cluster or sequence determined?
8. Was the 'utility' of the test determined? (Were patients really better off for it?)

References

1. Hall, W.A., Luciano, M.G., Doppman, J.L. et al. (1994) *Pituitary magnetic resonance imaging in normal human volunteers: occult adenomas in the general population.* Ann. Intern. Med. 120: 817–20.
2. Jensen, M.C., Brant-Zawadki, M.N., Obuchowski, N. et al. (1994) *Magnetic resonance imaging of the lumbar spine in people without back pain.* N. Engl. J. Med. 331: 69–73.
3. Deyo, R.A. (1994) *Magnetic resonance imaging of the lumbar spine. Terrific test or tar baby? [Editorial]* N. Engl. J. Med. 331: 115–16.
4. Wolfberg, A.J. (2006) *Genes on the Web – direct-to-consumer marketing of genetic testing.* N. Engl. J. Med. 355: 6–8.
5. Summerton, N. (2007) *Patient-centred Diagnosis.* Radcliffe Publishing, Abingdon.
6. Wennberg, D.E., Kellett, M.A., Dickens, J.D. Jr et al. (1996) The association between local diagnostic testing intensity and invasive cardiac procedures. JAMA 275: 1161–4.
7. Verrilli, D. and Welch, H.G. (1996) The impact of diagnostic testing on therapeutic interventions. JAMA 275: 1189–91.
8. Levey, A.S., Coresh, J., Greene, T. et al. for the Chronic Kidney Disease Epidemiology Collaboration (2006) *Using standardised serum creatinine values in the modification of diet in renal disease; study equation for estimating glomerular filtration rate.* Ann. Intern. Med. 145: 247–54.
9. Richardson, W.S., Wilson, M.C., Nishikawa, J. et al. (1995) *The well-built clinical question: a key to evidence-based decisions.* ACP J. Club 123: A12–13.
10. Guyatt, G. and Rennie, D. (eds) (2002) *Users' Guides to the Medical Literature: Essentials of Evidence-Based Clinical Practice.* American Medical Association Press, Chicago, p. 43.

11. Haynes, R.B. and Wilczynski, N. (2005) *Finding the gold in Medline: clinical queries.* Evid. Based Med. 10: 101–2.

12. Mallett, S., Deeks, J.J., Halligan, S. et al. (2006) *Systematic reviews of diagnostic tests in cancer: review of methods and reporting.* Br. Med. J. 333; 413–19.

13. Lord, S.J., Irwig, L. and Simes, J.S. (2006) *When is measuring sensitivity and specificity sufficient to evaluate a diagnostic test, and when do we need randomized trials?* Ann. Intern. Med. 144: 850–5.

14. Irwig, L., Tosteson, A.N.A., Gatsonis, C. et al. (1994) *Guidelines for meta-analyses evaluating diagnostic tests.* Ann. Intern. Med. 120: 667–76.

15. McMaster University *Critical Appraisal Card* from Department of Clinical Epidemiology and Biostatistics. McMaster University, Hamilton, Ontario, Canada.

3.4 Screening

Screen: *an apparatus used in the sifting of grain, coal, etc. 1573.*

Shorter Oxford English Dictionary

Gentle Reader,

Empathise with Jock Armstrong and Will Taggart. They glared at one another across the row of straw which had been spewed forth from the Claas combine harvester, a massive mechanical monument, now still in the wheat of a Scottish harvest field.

'Look at the wheat on the ground, man,' roared Jock, 'You've set the holes in the screen too big so that you could hash on for the next job.'

'Ach, away man,' growled Will, his eyes shining forth in a face almost black with stour.

'I'm due at Balanin the night and she's blocked solid with chaff because the screen's set as small as they'll go.'

The peewit cried in the Galloway sky, its whooping call like a referee's whistle keeping the two opposing forces on either side of the line of straw: the farmer wanting the screen set so that not a single grain falls to earth; the contractor knowing that the smaller the holes, the more often will chaff, grain, stones and straw build up and cause first colic then complete obstruction in his combine harvester. And with him wanting to drive as fast as he can to the next farm to combine barley before the rain curtails harvesting (and income).

Commentary

Farmer or contractor; saving of grain or saving of time; sensitivity or specificity – the eternal tensions in any screening programme.

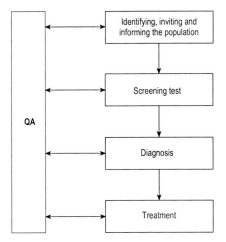

Fig. 3.9
The core components of all screening programmes

3.4.1 Dimensions and definitions

When screening is discussed, the term is usually understood to refer to a single test, for example, a cervical smear within a cervical screening programme. However, screening actually consists of all the steps in a programme from the identification of the population at risk to the diagnosis of the disease or its precursor in certain individuals to the treatment of those individuals (Fig. 3.9). In the case of cervical screening, the steps range from the identification of women in the age-group 24–64 years (the group known to benefit) to the accurate histopathological diagnosis and effective treatment of cervical cancer.

Thus, the effectiveness of any screening programme is determined by:

- the sensitivity of the series of tests applied to the population
- the effectiveness of the therapy offered to those individuals identified as having the condition.

Screening has two important characteristics that distinguish it from clinical practice:

- Someone other than the clinician is responsible for ensuring that the screening service covers the whole subset of the population identified as eligible for screening (in the UK, this is the Director of Public Health).

		Disease	
		Absent	**Present**
Harm from screening	**Does not occur**	Good outcome	True negative screening result
	Occurs	Acceptable provided the person was clear about the risk before accepting the invitation	Poor outcome

Matrix 3.3

- Some of the people who will be harmed in a screening programme do not have the disease for which they are being screened, whereas in clinical practice the patient seeking help for their symptoms or disease accepts the possibility of harmful or adverse effects of treatment because of the possibility of benefit (Matrix 3.3).

Margin Note 3.7

All screening programmes do harm

3.4.1.1 The changing balance of good and harm

Screening programmes, like any other intervention, have the potential to do both good and harm. However, the balance between good and harm will change with the frequency of testing and the quality of the programme. The beneficial effects of screening illustrate the law of diminishing returns[1] (Fig. 3.10A): in women aged 20–64 years, cervical screening at a frequency of once every 3 years reduces the incidence rate of cervical cancer by 91.2% compared with a reduction of 83.6% when the screening frequency is once every 5 years – an increase of only 7% in effectiveness.[2] The adverse effects of screening, or of any other intervention, usually follow a straight line (Fig. 3.10B): the greater the number of individuals involved in a screening programme, the greater the number experiencing side-effects (Fig. 3.10C). Thus, the ratio of good to harm changes as the number of screening tests performed increases. Indeed, a point is reached, referred to by Donabedian as the point of optimality, where the difference between benefit and harm starts to diminish (see Fig. 3.10C).

(a)

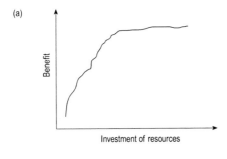

(b)

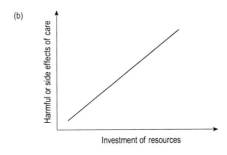

(c)

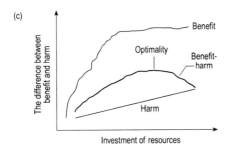

Fig. 3.10
(A) The law of diminishing returns – beneficial effects of screening
do not continue to increase in direct proportion to investment;
(B) the harmful or adverse effects of screening increase in direct
proportion to the resources invested; (C) the relationship between
the beneficial and adverse effects of screening – after a certain level
of investment, the health gain may start to decline.
(Source: Donabedian[1])

If the quality of the screening programme is low, the
benefits are reduced and adverse effects increase (Fig. 3.11);
if an adequate level of quality is not achieved, there may be
a point at which the harm done by screening is greater than
the good. Thus, the decision to introduce screening must be
taken with the greatest of care.

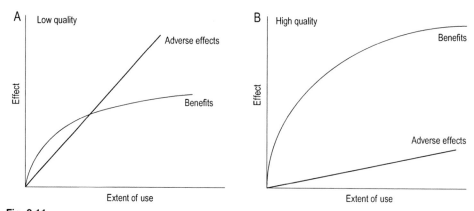

Fig. 3.11
The beneficial and harmful or adverse effects of a screening programme that is (a) of low quality, and (b) of high quality

3.4.2 Searching

Although it is difficult to use the standard PICO (or PECO) formulation[3] to identify the components of any search for a screening programme, the search can still be broken down into two main components to aid searching (Table 3.4).

To ensure identification of the most useful articles, include synonyms, and use generic text words and Medical Subject Headings (MeSH) for screening as well as the specific test such as:

- mammography
- mammogram
- screening
- detecting
- testing
- Mass Screening/
- Sensitivity and Specificity/
- Predictive Value of Tests/.

Some meta-analyses or systematic reviews on screening may be retrieved using the Publication Type Meta-Analysis [pt]; there is no specific Publication Type to retrieve studies on screening programmes.

Table 3.4 Components of a search for a screening programme

Component	Example
The health problem	Breast cancer
The principal test	Mammography

➠ Visit the National Library for Health (NLH) Screening Library, which undertakes to find, organise and provide access to the best available evidence on screening. Available online at: http://www.library.nhs.uk/screening/.

3.4.3 Appraisal

The first step is to identify the research design most likely to be helpful. In screening, the most helpful research design is the RCT or a systematic review of RCTs. Difficult as they may be to organise, RCTs of public health interventions such as screening should be subjected to the same rigorous appraisal as is applied to clinical interventions. Indeed, it could be argued that there is a need for stronger evidence to support the introduction of screening as a public health intervention because it is offered to healthy populations. As no intervention is without risk, some of the people who are subject to screening – a proportion of whom would not have developed the disease even if the intervention had not been introduced – will be put at risk.

Proponents of the introduction of any screening programme sometimes base their argument on cohort studies, which are designed to follow a series of people who have had a screening test and compare their survival with that of the general population. However, this is a poor method of evaluating screening, principally because of what is termed lead-time bias.

Imagine a disease that has a natural history of 10 years and causes symptoms after 5 years, which usually prompt the sufferer to visit a doctor; the survival time from the point of symptomatic diagnosis is 5 years (Fig. 3.12A).

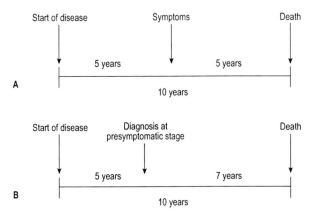

Fig. 3.12
The phenomenon of lead-time bias in screening

Box 3.5 Criteria for appraising screening developed in the 1960s (Source: Wilson and Jungner[4])

- The condition sought should be an important health problem.
- There should be an accepted treatment for patients with recognised disease.
- Facilities for diagnosis and treatment should be available.
- There should be a recognisable latent or early symptomatic stage.
- There should be a suitable test or examination.
- The test should be acceptable to the population.
- The natural history of the condition, including development from latent to declared disease, should be adequately understood.
- There should be an agreed policy on whom to treat as patients.
- The cost of case-finding (including diagnosis and treatment of patients diagnosed) should be economically balanced in relation to possible expenditure on medical care as a whole.
- Case-finding should be a continuing process and not a 'once and for all' project.

A test that enables a diagnosis to be made at an earlier, pre-symptomatic stage, for example, at 3 years, will apparently increase survival time by 2 years (Fig. 3.12B). This apparent increase in survival time does not necessarily mean that screening is effective; it may simply mean that the person with the pre-symptomatic disease identified by screening is aware of the condition for 7 years as opposed to 5 – this is referred to as lead-time bias. It is essential that any screening programme is evaluated within an RCT that has been designed with death as the outcome in order to control for lead-time bias.

The classic set of criteria for appraising screening tests was developed by Wilson and Jungner[4] in 1968 (Box 3.5). Although in the past these criteria were useful, they are now considered weak for several reasons:

1. First, there is insufficient emphasis on the adverse effects of screening and on the need to ensure that a programme does more good than harm. Although these considerations were important in the 1960s, in the context of a general public which is better informed, more assertive and more likely to sue if harm is done, it is essential to attend fully to the balance of good and harm. A 'Comment' in *The Lancet* by Szarewski and Sasieni[5] emphasises the importance of adhering to one of the basic tenets in medicine – at least do no harm. They feel this is especially important with respect to cervical screening in adolescents and

young women, given the evidence of considerable anxiety and psychosexual morbidity associated with cervical screening and colposcopy[6] and of the high rate of regression (>90%) within 36 months of low-grade abnormalities on the Pap smear.[7]

2. Second, Wilson and Jungner[4] state that an 'accepted treatment' should be available, but some 'accepted' treatments are either ineffective or of unproven efficacy.

3. Third, there is no discussion of the quality of the evidence upon which the decision to screen should be based.

A more suitable set of criteria for current use has been developed by the UK National Screening Committee (Box 3.6), based on those developed by Wilson and Jungner.[4]

3.4.4   Getting research into practice

Getting research into practice for a screening programme is a major undertaking, perhaps more so than for any other type of healthcare intervention. This is because the introduction of a new screening programme requires the concomitant introduction of a wide range of clinical interventions, together with the management and information support systems that will enable the quality of the programme to be assured. Any quality assurance programme must include:

• explicit agreed standards of good practice
• an information system that enables performance against those standards to be measured
• the authority to take action if standards are not achieved.

For a screening programme to do more good than harm requires not simply the demonstration that it is possible to achieve this outcome in a research setting, but also an emphasis on quality in practice that will allow the potential to be realised in any setting.

The decision to introduce screening is relatively easy; resolving the problems that may result from it can be much more difficult. For this reason, some aphorisms on screening are provided for the reader to ponder before succumbing to the temptations of screening (Box 3.7).

All these issues are discussed in greater detail in Raffle and Gray,[8] a practical handbook on screening.

> **Box 3.6** Criteria for appraising the viability, effectiveness and appropriateness of a screening programme (Source: UK National Screening Committee, available online at: http://www.screening.nhs.uk/)

Ideally, all the following criteria should be met before screening for a condition is initiated:

The condition

1. The condition should be an important health problem
2. The epidemiology and natural history of the condition, including development from latent to declared disease, should be adequately understood and there should be a detectable risk factor, disease marker, latent period or early symptomatic stage
3. All the cost-effective primary prevention interventions should have been implemented as far as practicable
4. If the carriers of a mutation are identified as a result of screening the natural history of people with this status should be understood, including the psychological implications

The test

5. There should be a simple, safe, precise and validated screening test
6. The distribution of test values in the target population should be known and a suitable cut-off level defined and agreed
7. The test should be acceptable to the population
8. There should be an agreed policy on the further diagnostic investigation of individuals with a positive test result and on the choices available to those individuals
9. If the test is for mutations the criteria used to select the subset of mutations to be covered by screening, if all possible mutations are not being tested, should be clearly set out

The treatment

10. There should be an effective treatment or intervention for patients identified through early detection, with evidence of early treatment leading to better outcomes than late treatment
11. There should be agreed evidence-based policies covering which individuals should be offered treatment and the appropriate treatment to be offered
12. Clinical management of the condition and patient outcomes should be optimised in all healthcare providers prior to participation in a screening programme

The screening programme

13. There should be evidence from high-quality randomised controlled trials that the screening programme is effective in reducing mortality or morbidity. Where screening is aimed solely at providing information to allow the person being screened to make an 'informed choice' (e.g. Down's syndrome, cystic fibrosis

Continued

Box 3.6—*Cont'd*

carrier screening), there must be evidence from high-quality trials that the test accurately measures risk. The information that is provided about the test and its outcome must be of value and readily understood by the individual being screened

14. There should be evidence that the complete screening programme (test, diagnostic procedures, treatment/intervention) is clinically, socially and ethically acceptable to health professionals and the public

15. The benefit from the screening programme should outweigh the physical and psychological harm (caused by the test, diagnostic procedures and treatment)

16. The opportunity cost of the screening programme (including testing, diagnosis and treatment, administration, training and quality assurance) should be economically balanced in relation to expenditure on medical care as a whole (i.e. value for money)

17. There should be a plan for managing and monitoring the screening programme and an agreed set of quality assurance standards

18. Adequate staffing and facilities for testing, diagnosis, treatment and programme management should be available prior to the commencement of the screening programme

19. All other options for managing the condition should have been considered (e.g. improving treatment, providing other services), to ensure that no more cost-effective intervention could be introduced or current interventions increased within the resources available

20. Evidence-based information, explaining the consequences of testing, investigation and treatment, should be made available to potential participants to assist them in making an informed choice

21. Public pressure for widening the eligibility criteria for reducing the screening interval, and for increasing the sensitivity of the testing process, should be anticipated. Decisions about these parameters should be scientifically justifiable to the public

22. If screening is for a mutation, the programme should be acceptable to people identified as carriers and to other family members

Bibliography

Department of Health (1998) *Screening of Pregnant Women for Hepatitis B and Immunisation of Babies at Risk.* Department of Health, London (Health Service Circular : HSC 1998/127).

Wilson, J.M.G., Jungner, G. (1968) *Principles and Practice of Screening for Disease.* Public Health Paper No. 34. World Health Organization, Geneva.

Cochrane, A.L. and Holland, W.W. (1971) *Validation of screening procedures.* Br. Med. Bull. 27: 3.

Sackett, D.L. and Holland, W.W. (1975) *Controversy in the detection of disease.* Lancet 2: 357–9.

Wald, N.J. (ed) (1984) *Antenatal and Neonatal Screening.* Oxford University Press, Oxford.

Holland, W.W., Stewart, S. (1990) *Screening in Healthcare.* Nuffield Provincial Hospitals Trust London.

Gray, J.A.M. (1996) *Dimensions and Definitions of Screening.* NHS Executive Anglia and Oxford, Research and Development Directorate, Milton Keynes.

Box 3.7   Aphorisms on screening

- A stitch in time does not necessarily save nine.
- The decision to introduce a new screening programme should be taken as carefully as the decision to build a new hospital.
- Never think about screening tests, only about screening programmes.
- Screening programmes shown to be efficacious in a research setting require an obsession with quality to be effective in a service setting.
- The public are over-optimistic about screening; professionals are over-pessimistic.
- Finding 'asymptomatic' disease by means of screening always increases the length of time a person knows s/he has the disease; this increased period of awareness should not be confused with increased survival.
- All screening programmes do harm; some can do good as well.
- The harm from a screening programme starts immediately; the good takes longer to appear. Therefore, the first observable effect of any programme, albeit an effective one, is to impair the health of the population.
- A screening programme without false-positives will miss too many cases to be effective.
- Like a tightrope walker above Niagara Falls, any screening programme must balance false-negatives and false-positives.
- A screening programme without false-negatives will cause unnecessary harm to a healthy population.
- For the distressed patient seeking help, the clinician does what s/he can; for the healthy person recruited to screening, only the best possible service will suffice.
- Screening programmes should be run with firm management. If quality falls, a screening programme that was doing more good than harm may then do more harm than good.
- Though insignificant to the population, a single false-positive can be of devastating significance to the individual.
- If a screening programme is *not* supported by a quality assurance system comprising standards, information and authority to act, it should be stopped.
- If a quality assurance programme is not generating at least one major public enquiry every 3 years, it is ineffective.
- At best, screening is a zero-gratitude business.

References

1. Donabedian, A. (2002) *An Introduction to Quality Assurance in Health Care*. Oxford University Press, Oxford.
2. Eddy, D.M. (1990) *Screening for cervical cancer*. Ann. Intern. Med. 113: 214–26.
3. Richardson, W. S., Wilson, M. C., Nishikawa, J. et al. (1995) *The well-built clinical question: a key to evidence-based decisions*. ACP J. Club 123: A12–13.
4. Wilson, J.M.G. and Jungner, G. (1968) *Principles and Practice of Screening for Disease*. World Health Organization, Geneva.

5. Szarewski, A. and Sasieni, P. (2004) *Cervical screening in adolescents – at least do no harm—[Comment]* Lancet 364: 1642–4.
6. Rogstad, K.E. (2002) *The psychological impact of abnormal cytology and colposcopy.* Br. J. Obstet. Gynaecol. 109: 364–8.
7. Moscicki, A.B., Hills, N., Shiboski, S. et al. (2001) *Risks for incident human papillomavirus infection and low-grade squamous intraepithelial lesion development in young females.* JAMA 285: 2995–3002.
8. Raffle, A.E. and Gray, J.A.M. (2007) *Screening: Evidence and Practice.* Oxford University Press, Oxford.

3.5   Health policy

3.5.1   Dimensions and definitions

> A policy is a course of action.

When classifying health policy, the usual approach is to use the determinants of health over which it is possible to exert an influence (Fig. 3.13):

- lifestyle
- the physical environment
- the biological environment
- the socio-economic environment
- health services.

There are two main reasons why health policy may be formulated and introduced:

1. to change the way in which health services are funded, organised or held accountable – healthcare policies
2. to improve health through changes in lifestyle or the physical, biological and/or social environments – public health policies.

Margin Note 3.8

Policy: a course of action adopted and pursued by a government, party, ruler, statesman, etc.; any course of action adopted as advantageous or expedient. (The chief living sense.)
Shorter Oxford English Dictionary

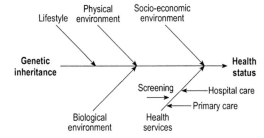

Fig. 3.13
The determinants of health

3.5.1.1 Healthcare policy

If health services are effective, it is possible to prevent
or reduce (by curing it) the prevalence of a disease or to
alleviate its burden by minimising the disability that disease
causes. Increasing the level of effectiveness within a health
service is governed by healthcare policy.

Changes to health services that might be introduced
through healthcare policy include:

- the delegation of responsibility for decision-making
  about the use of resources
- increasing the number of people involved in decisions
  about resources
- increasing incentives to achieve better value for money
- clarifying and strengthening accountability
- improving performance against targets
- improving patient care.

Although such changes are often political, that is,
decided upon by politicians, they will always have
managerial consequences; managers must ensure that policy
objectives are met using the resources available.

Managers can also introduce changes to health services to
improve:

- efficiency
- cost-effectiveness
- quality
- accountability
- safety
- acceptability.

For example, managers can:

- introduce schemes of quality improvement
- increase investment in training
- change managerial structures to increase professional
  involvement, to decrease the amount of time wasted by
  professionals in management, or both
- change the financial computing system
- introduce measures to involve patients in the process of care
- externalise certain services, such as cleaning or pathology.

However, such managerial changes have only indirect effects
on clinical decision-making, whereas politicians make policy
decisions that affect clinical practice directly. In the UK, one
such decision has been to influence GP prescribing habits by

excluding certain drugs from the list from which doctors can choose; another such decision has been the introduction of case management (a US term) or care management (a UK term) to improve the quality of care for severely mentally ill people.

3.5.1.2 Public health policy

The primary focus of public health policies is change in the physical, biological and/or socio-economic environments or in people's lifestyle.

Changes in the physical, biological and/or socio-economic environments or in people's lifestyle are the main factors influencing:

- the incidence of disease, i.e. the number of new cases of a disease in the population
- the prevalence of the disease, i.e. the number of cases of a disease in the population at any one point in time.

3.5.2   Searching

Although it is difficult to use the standard PICO (or PECO) formulation[1] to identify the components of any search for health policies, the search can still be broken down into two main components, and combined with terms for health policy (Table 3.5).

Combine these terms with the MeSH terms Health Policy/, Public Policy/ or Policy Making/, and/or use the text words "policy", "policies" and "recommendations".

Searching tips

➡ It may be productive to search the specialist databases HMIC or PAIS, or to visit the National Library for Health (NLH) Health Management Library, available online at: http://www.library.nhs.uk/healthmanagement/

3.5.3   Appraisal

3.5.3.1 Appropriate study designs for evidence about healthcare policies

For healthcare policy, it may be possible to find evidence from RCTs, such as the one that failed to demonstrate a

Table 3.5   Components of a search for a health policy

Component	Example
The health problem	Obesity
The intervention	Physical activity

beneficial effect of case management in people who had severe mental illness.[2,3] However, for healthcare policies that influence the financing and organisation of a health service, the evidence most easily available is that derived from descriptive studies or non-randomised studies, such as interrupted time series (Section 5.8) or controlled before and after studies (Section 5.7) of health service interventions (accepted for inclusion by the Cochrane Review Group Effective Practice and Organisation of Care).

For public health policies, the evidence may be available from more conventional scientific study designs, such as:

- the case-control study (Section 5.5)
- the cohort study (Section 5.6).

3.5.3.2 Natural experiments as sources of evidence about healthcare policy

There is a common belief that research on health policy or approaches to health service management is difficult to translate from one country to another because of the myriad socio-economic, cultural, and political differences. Although it is true that it is often not possible to transfer a policy or managerial option directly from one country to another, research on health policy and management conducted in different countries can be illuminating.

If the healthcare systems are similar, any initiatives or innovations are of interest; if the healthcare systems are different, it is useful to regard the difference as a 'natural' experiment. In a 'natural' experiment, differing approaches to the same problem can be compared despite the fact that those approaches were not planned in a research setting but arose by reason of different circumstances.

Even when the socio-economic, cultural, and political circumstances of a country are very different to those of one's own, there is much to be learned. Anthropological studies, such as that by Frankel described in *The Huli Response to Illness*,[4] can provide many insights into the human response to disease, illness and treatment, which may be helpful to policy-makers and managers. Indeed, managers and policy-makers may have underestimated the potential for learning from research conducted in other countries and within different cultures.

3.5.3.3 Appraising research on public health policies

When appraising research evidence on a policy, there are two key questions to ask:

- How valid is the evaluation?
- How relevant is the policy to the local service?

If the evaluation of a policy was carried out in a different country, the issue of relevance is important.

There are two aspects to relevance in this situation:

1. the feasibility of introducing a particular policy into one's own country
2. the practicability of introducing the intervention associated with the implementation of that policy into one's own country.

For example, legislation passed in the USA is of limited relevance elsewhere in the world, and vice versa, but the potential effects of legislation on professional behaviour or managerial decision-making are relevant and it may be possible to reproduce those in other countries, albeit through different legislation or by other means.

A checklist of useful questions for the appraisal of research designed to evaluate public health or healthcare policy is shown in Box 3.8.

Box 3.8 Checklist for the appraisal of research designed to evaluate public health or healthcare policy

- Were the explicit policy objectives clearly stated?
- Did the research workers identify and articulate any implicit objectives of the policy under investigation?
- Were valid outcome measures identified for each of the explicit and implicit objectives?
- Was data collection complete?
- Were data collected before and after the introduction of the new policy?
- Was the follow-up of sufficient length to allow the effects of policy change to become evident?
- Were any other factors that could have produced the changes (other than the policy) identified in the key criteria and discussed?
- Were possible sources of bias in the research workers acknowledged in the paper or in any accompanying editorial?

3.5.4   Getting research into practice

As individuals usually have strong views about what is
right in terms of policy or management, there may be greater
exception to implementing knowledge derived from research
into policy-making and management than that encountered
when promoting the adoption of research findings in clinical
practice. If a policy has been based primarily on an ideology,
or if a management change stems from the conviction of
an individual manager, then evidence that such a policy
or management change is ineffective or counterproductive
is likely to meet with resistance. A policy-maker may be
defensive about challenges to his/her ideology, and the
manager may regard any challenges as a personal affront.
It is important, however, that a double standard is not
introduced, namely, that policy-makers and managers exhort
clinicians to implement research findings in clinical practice
when they themselves are either not actively searching for
evidence or failing to implement knowledge derived from
research when it is presented to them.

References

1. Richardson, W.S., Wilson, M.C., Nishikawa, J. et al. (1995) *The well-built
   clinical question: a key to evidence-based decisions.* ACP J. Club 123: A12–13.
2. Marshall, M. (1996) *Case management: a dubious practice. [Editorial]* Br. Med.
   J. 312: 523–4.
3. Marshall, M., Gray, A., Lockwood, A. et al. (2007) *Case management
   for people with severe mental disorders.* Cochrane Database of Systematic
   Reviews, 2007 Issue 1. John Wiley and Sons, Ltd. Abstract available online
   at: http://www.cochrane.org/reviews/en/ab000050.html
4. Frankel, S. (1986) *The Huli Response to Illness.* Cambridge University Press,
   Cambridge.

Gentle Reader,

Empathise with Jair de Jesus Mari, professor of psychiatry in São Paulo. September is hot in São Paulo, sometimes oppressively so. However, it was not the heat that bothered Jair in 1994. He was frustrated with the process of publishing scientific papers. For more than a year, he had laboured to summarise all the trials of psychosocial family interventions in schizophrenia that could be found by hand-searching psychiatric journals. His review, based on six trials, was submitted to a prestigious journal in August 1993 and published in August 1994,[1] after a delay that was torment to him. He had received praise from colleagues, and felt satisfied when he finally saw his review in print.

One month later it was out of date; two further trials, both from China, had been published in another journal. He swore (the equivalent of 'bloody hell' in Portuguese). What should he do now? Write a letter to the first journal? Perhaps, but what he really wanted was to revise the meta-analysis and base the revision on all eight trials, and anyway, readers who saw the letter would not necessarily have the original article to hand. What is more, letters are not peer-reviewed so they are not necessarily taken seriously by readers. Jair de Jesus Mari faced an insoluble dilemma.

Commentary

Jair's dilemma cannot be solved on paper, but it is possible to resolve it electronically.

All decision-makers should have computer access to the best information about the effectiveness of any intervention, that is, a systematic review of trials based on a complete search of the literature, which also:

- *can be updated quickly when new evidence appears*
- *has summaries of the original trials available*
- *includes practical implications, as well as scientific conclusions*
- *has a responsive 'letters' column in which all comments/criticisms and the author's replies are available instantaneously.*

The Cochrane Library provides such a facility; the review by Pharoah et al.[2] meets all of the above criteria.

References

1. Mari, J.J. and Streiner, D. (1994) *An overview of family interventions and relapse in schizophrenia.* Psychol. Med. 23: 565–78.
2. Pharoah, F., Mari, J., Rathbone, J. et al. (2007) *Family intervention for schizophrenia.* Cochrane Database of Systematic Reviews 2007, Issue 1. John Wiley and Sons. Abstract available online at: http://www.cochrane.org/reviews/en/ab000088.html

Finding good-quality evidence

The decision-maker wishing to find evidence on which to base a decision is confronted by many obstacles, shown in Fig. 4.1 and discussed below. The steps that can be taken collectively to overcome these obstacles are also shown in Fig. 4.1; however, the individual searcher can also take action to negotiate these obstacles.

4.1.1   The relevance gap: absence of high-quality evidence

Despite years of research, the available evidence is not best suited to the needs of healthcare decision-makers. The research agenda tends to be dictated by those who invest in research and development.

Patsopoulos et al.[1] identified those clinical medicine articles from 1994 to 2003 that had been cited most often by the end of 2004, and assessed changes in not only authors' affiliations but also sources of funding. They found that for 60% of the most frequently cited articles funding was from government or other public sources, and for 36% funding was from industry. However, they also found that the proportion of most frequently cited articles funded by industry had increased over time, and by 2001 was equal to the proportion funded by government or public sources. Indeed, 65 of 77 most frequently cited randomised controlled trials received funding from industry, and this proportion increased significantly with time ($P = 0.003$). Patsopoulos et al. suggest that academics may be losing control of the clinical research agenda to industry.

In a thoughtful article in *The Lancet*, David Melzer argued that owing to the possibility of a return on capital investment, pharmaceutical companies are willing to invest in the research and development of new drugs.[2] One of the outcomes of this strategy is that in evidence-based decision-making priority is increasingly being given to

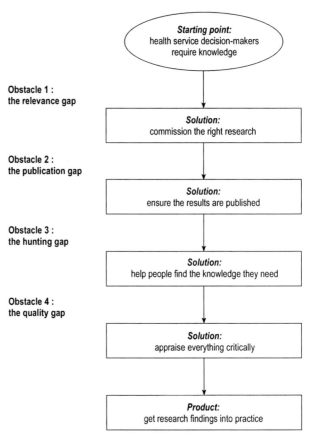

Fig. 4.1
The evidence gaps

drugs rather than, for example, psychological treatments or group therapy because there is better evidence available about drugs. As Melzer points out, 'methods of treatment of the human or animal body by surgery or therapy or of diagnosis practised in the human or animal body' are excluded from patent protection, therefore there is no incentive for companies to invest in research to develop and evaluate them.

Knowledge management solutions
In the UK, one of the main functions of the NHS research and development programmes is the identification of NHS requirements for research-based knowledge. The intention is to narrow the 'relevance gap' and address the imbalances resulting from pharmaceutical company funding strategies by commissioning specific research that will provide answers to the questions healthcare decision-makers, and

patients, want answered. Liberati and Magrini[3] have called
for pharmaceutical companies to agree to collaborate on an
explicitly prioritised research agenda in which questions
about care are more relevant than drug-specific issues. In
addition, Garattini et al.[4] have identified a role for research
ethics committees in assessing carefully clinical protocols with
respect to issues such as the use of placebos, comparators
and doses, and therapeutic end-points in order for these
committees to act in the best interests of the patient.

The creation of systematic reviews, and the organisation
of these reviews into health technology assessment reports,
improves the quality of the evidence. The number of
systematic reviews is increasing, stimulated by the work of
the Cochrane Collaboration.

The searcher's solution
Many healthcare decisions must be made for which there
is no high-quality evidence. However, the absence of high-
quality evidence does not make evidence-based decision-
making impossible; in this situation, what is required is the
best evidence available, not the best evidence possible.

4.1.2   The publication gap: failure to publish research results

Any searcher must find the sources of evidence. Although
much is made of the 'grey literature', that is, the results of
studies not published in scientific journals, the main source
of evidence is the published literature. However, this is
incomplete for several reasons:

- the 'sloppy' researcher – too many researchers fail to
  write up and submit their findings for publication,
  known as submission bias
- the 'disheartened' researcher, less motivated to complete
  and submit for publication negative results – an example
  of submission bias
- the 'coy' pharmaceutical company, nervous of revealing
  results that may not show the company's products in the
  most advantageous light and as a consequence reporting
  results selectively (i.e. publishing the more favourable
  results only and ignoring intention-to-treat analyses[5]) –
  another example of submission bias
- the 'biased' editor, keener to publish positive than
  negative results – known as publication bias[6]
- the under-representation of journal content about the
  health needs of resource-poor populations – known as

'ethnic' or country-of-origin bias, 'where the scientific, medical and public health priorities of the rich world are presented as the norm'.[7]

The factors determining the non-publication of research results tend to produce a positive bias in the published literature as a whole, and country-of-origin bias tends to produce a positive bias in the English language literature.

Knowledge management solutions

The compulsory registration of all randomised controlled trials at their commencement will counteract the incompleteness of the published literature because it will then be possible to trace unpublished studies.

Horton[7] has suggested the following to combat the effects of ethnic or country-of-origin bias in journals:

- reviewing the composition of journal editorial boards
- calling for research from resource-poor settings
- commissioning editorials and reviews about developing world health issues.

Although these suggestions are helpful, it is also important to address a fundamental inequity in research funding, namely that 90% is channelled into diseases that affect only 10% of the world's population. This is known as the 10/90 gap.[8] Thus, it is vital not only to increase the quantity but also to improve the quality of research originating in developing countries.[7]

The searcher's solutions

It is difficult for the searcher to compensate for publication bias. For research workers, it is appropriate to search for unpublished data, but for busy decision-makers it is not an effective use of time. The best solution is to search for a systematic review (one that involves a search of both published and unpublished literature), and to be aware of the phenomenon of positive bias in its various guises when appraising research articles (see Table 6.2). To compensate for country-of-origin bias, any search should not be restricted to the English language only, and a Medline search should be complemented by searches of other databases to include articles from journals published in other languages and in other countries, e.g. EMBASE.

4.1.3   The hunting gap: difficulties in finding published research

There are many electronic databases, but the two principal sources for medical and health research are Medline and

EMBASE. However, these databases do not cover all medical research areas.

Knowledge management solutions

In the UK, one of the aims in the establishment of the National Library for Health (NLH) was to provide easy access to the best current knowledge for clinicians, managers, and patients (http://www.library.nhs.uk).

One of the objectives of the Cochrane Collaboration is to make the results of more trials available to searchers. This objective is fulfilled in two main ways:

- by incorporating any trials found from hand-searching journals and from searches of Medline and EMBASE into Cochrane Reviews
- by compiling the Cochrane Database of Systematic Reviews.

Although systematic reviews are worthy documents, they can be daunting. Therefore, novel types of publication are needed to systematise knowledge for clinicians. Haynes[9] originally classified knowledge into four categories (the '4S' model), representing different levels of detail, as follows:

1. systems
2. synopses, i.e. structured abstracts
3. syntheses and systematic reviews
4. studies.

Prompted by the Haynes model, a '6S' model was developed in the UK, in which the four 'S' categories of knowledge were refined into six. However, we found the constraint of an 'S' too Procrustean, and have further developed the model to become the 'Types of Evidence' model, which includes 7 categories of knowledge (Fig. 4.2). Whichever system of categorisation is used, the need to provide summaries of all the knowledge about a particular topic has now been recognised.

In addition to the preparation of easy-to-read summaries of evidence, it is possible to harness the power of the Internet not only to allow knowledge to be pulled by the clinician or patient when needed but also for clinicians to be prompted when a decision has to be made or when vital knowledge should be pushed at them. This approach has been adopted in England to create a National Knowledge Service (NKS) (Fig. 4.3).

The searcher's solution

The use of specialist databases (Margin Note 4.1) can minimise but not resolve the problems posed by the limitations of electronic databases. Access to the Cochrane

Margin Note 4.1
Specialist databases

Nursing and allied health

- CINAHL, available online at http://www.ovid.com/site/catalog/DataBase/40.jsp?top=2&mid=3&bottom=7&subsection=10

Health management policy

- Health Management Information Consortium, HMIC (Source: UK Department of Health, Nuffield Institute for Health and King's Fund Library), available online at: http://www.ovid.com/site/catalog/DataBase/99.jsp?top=2&mid=3&bottom=7&subsection=10
- Health Management Specialist Library, available online at: http://www.library.nhs.uk/healthmanagement

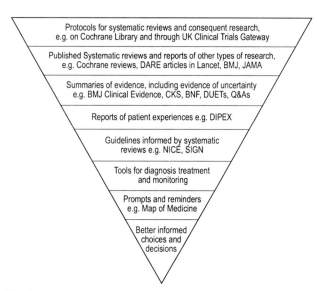

Fig. 4.2
'Types of Evidence' model for the classification of knowledge

Library diminishes the problems of searching for RCTs; users should consult the Cochrane Database of Systematic Reviews and PubMed, which now indexes systematic reviews clearly.

4.1.4   The quality gap: the need for critical appraisal

During the last decade, as the deficiencies in the design, analysis and reporting of trials have been documented, the need to develop standards for the practice and documentation of trials has been recognised.

4.1.4.1 *Flaws in the methodology and reporting of research*

There are several potential sources of bias in published papers:

- flaws in the methodology of the research, such as in randomisation, introduce a positive bias known as methodological bias[10]

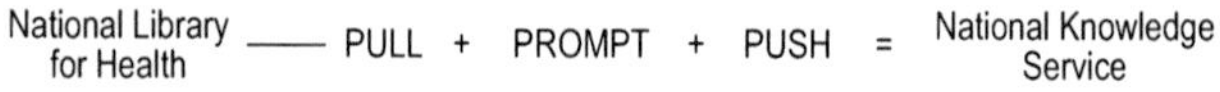

National Library —— PULL + PROMPT + PUSH = National Knowledge
for Health   Service

Fig. 4.3
Elements comprising the National Knowledge Service (NKS) in England

- incomplete reporting of outcomes – statistically significant outcomes have a higher odds of being reported than non-significant outcomes for both efficacy and harm, which may over-estimate the benefits of an intervention[11]
- inconsistencies between primary outcomes as stated in the trial protocol and the primary outcomes as published, which may also over-estimate the benefits of an intervention[11]
- multiple or duplicate publication – reporting the results of the same study in at least two publications.[12]

Knowledge management solutions

The CONSORT Statement was first published in 1996[13] to improve the quality of randomised controlled trials, and the QUOROM Statement was published in 1999[14] to improve the quality of reporting of meta-analyses of randomised controlled trials. The CONSORT Statement has been revised and extended as the field has evolved.[15–17]

If the advice in these statements is widely implemented, they should help to improve the quality of research findings and the way in which they are reported, and to minimise the positive bias that currently hinders decision-makers and others who must interpret research results. The editorial policy of leading journals such as *The Lancet* and the *British Medical Journal* is to follow both the QUOROM and CONSORT guidelines, and other journal editors will be bound to follow the example of these role models as those who pay for journals become increasingly aware of these sources of bias and the deficiencies in the published literature.

However, in 2001, Moher et al.[15] reported that the CONSORT Statement had not yet resulted in a standardised approach to reporting trials and concluded that:

> *there are substantial risks of exaggerated claims of treatment effects arising from post-hoc emphases across multiple analyses. Sub-group analyses are particularly prone to over-interpretation and one is tempted to suggest 'don't do it' (or at least 'don't believe it') for many trials.*[15]

Moreover, in three studies undertaken over eight years, Clarke et al.[18] have shown that the results of new randomised trials have not been presented in the context of updated systematic reviews of other relevant studies, and thus there is a failure to comply with the CONSORT Statement requirement that data from a new trial should be interpreted in the light of the totality of the available evidence.

Chan et al.[11] recommend that, to ensure transparency, all planned RCTs are registered and their protocols be made publicly available prior to trial completion.

A list of initiatives promoting standards to improve the quality of reporting research results are shown in Margin Note 4.2.[13–17,19–23]

In March 2006, the EQUATOR Network was set up to improve the quality of healthcare by promoting the transparent and accurate reporting of health research – for further information, see Margin Note 4.3.

The searcher's solutions

It is important for the searcher to be aware of sources of bias within published research articles, and to appraise critically both the study design and the reporting of results. It is also important to be aware that the peer-review process has flaws (see Section 4.1.4.3) and is not a guarantee that these sources of bias will have been identified before publication.

The searcher should consult the Cochrane Database of Systematic Reviews and the Database of Reviews of Effectiveness.

4.1.4.2 Misleading abstracts

A review of abstracts in the world's best medical journals showed that between 18% and 68% of the abstracts were inaccurate, that is, either they were inconsistent with the data in the main text or they contained data not given in the main text.[24]

Knowledge management solutions

In the QUOROM Statement,[14] standards for the reporting of meta-analyses are set out, including the way to structure abstracts. These guidelines should facilitate an improvement in the quality of abstracts of trials and meta-analyses.

The searcher's solution

Every research article found requires critical appraisal. Advice to bear in mind when reading abstracts is as follows:

• if the abstract is unstructured, be suspicious[25]

• if the abstract highlights negative findings, it may not be biased; if it highlights positive findings, appraise the methods section carefully before accepting the results as good-quality evidence.

4.1.4.3 Peer review: the death of another sacred cow

> Mantra: *Indian 1808. [Sanskrit mantra lit. 'instrument of thought', f. man to think.] A sacred text or passage, esp. one from the Vedas used as a prayer or incantation.*
>
> Shorter Oxford English Dictionary

> *The only thing that will stop you publishing an article is a shortage of postage stamps.*
>
> Traditional research proverb

It is naïve to assume that, because a paper reaches a particular conclusion, it must be certainly true. Yet many people seem to consider that publication of any piece of research in a peer-reviewed journal provides sufficient credibility for decision-making. It doesn't.

Moore and McQuay 2006[26]

For a research article to be published in one of the hallmark journals, it must undergo the process of peer review, in which the paper is sent to one or more experts in the field for comment before it is accepted for publication. Goodman et al.[27] showed that peer review can improve the quality of medical research reporting, and during the late 1990s 'peer review' reached the status of a mantra such that publication of an article in a peer-reviewed journal was taken as an automatic guarantee of the quality of research. However, it is now clear that there are flaws in the process, and it is necessary to be much more critical of peer review as a hallmark due to the various sources of bias that continue to appear in the research reports published in peer-reviewed journals.

There are four main flaws with the peer-review process:

1. the failure to spot poor literature retrieval, where research studies are based on an inaccurate assessment of the current state of knowledge[28,29]
2. the failure to detect statistical problems[30] (Margin Note 4.4)
3. the failure to identify unsystematic systematic reviews[31,32] (Margin Note 4.5)
4. the failure to recognise duplicate publication.[33]

Knowledge management solution
One attempt to resolve some of these problems is to make the peer-review process open, for example, by identifying the peer reviewers and any conflicts of interest they might have. However, it would appear from the study by van Rooyen et al.[34] that open peer review has no effect, either beneficial or adverse, on:

- the quality of peer reviews
- the peer reviewers' recommendations.

Despite this finding, the editor of the *British Medical Journal* introduced a system of open peer review in 1999 'for largely ethical reasons',[35] emphasising that, although evidence-based decision-making means making a decision based on evidence, values and resources must also be taken into account. Although peer review as a process will continue to be used, in future it must be more rigorous, evidence-based and open.[36]

Margin Note 4.4
Statistical problems identified in 50 clinical trials
(Source: Assmann et al.[30])

Statistical problems identified in 50 clinical trials published in a three-month period in the four major journals – the *British Medical Journal*, the *Journal of the American Medical Association*, *The Lancet* and the *New England Journal of Medicine*:[30]

- About half the trials used significance tests for baseline comparison inappropriately
- Methods of randomisation were often poorly described
- Two-thirds of reports presented sub-group findings but most without appropriate statistical tests for interaction
- Many reports placed too much emphasis on sub-group analysis that commonly lacked statistical power

Margin Note 4.5
Unsystematic 'systematic reviews'
(Source: McAlister et al.[32])

- Failure to satisfy criteria of good quality
- Failure to describe how evidence was identified, evaluated or integrated
- Failure to support the recommendations for treatment on the basis of randomised controlled trials

Margin Note 4.6

Caveat lector

The only approach that is workable, honest and open may be to provide the reader with:

- as much information as possible about the methods used to arrive at the conclusion in the written document
- the skills to appraise research information so that it is possible for each individual to ascertain if the information is fit for their purpose, and relevant to the decision being made

The searcher's solution

The searcher can find research reports that are less likely to contain bias by searching for systematic reviews.

References

1. Patsopoulos, N.A., Ioannidis, J.P.A. and Analatos, A.A. (2006) *Origin and funding of the most frequently cited papers in medicine: database analysis.* Br. Med. J. 332: 1061–4.

2. Melzer, D. (1998) *Patent protection for medical technologies: why some and not others?* Lancet 351: 518–9.

3. Liberati, A. and Magrini, N. (2003) *Information from drug companies and opinion leaders. [Editorial]* Br. Med. J. 326: 1156–7.

4. Garattini, S., Bertele, V. and Bassi, L.L. (2003) *How can research ethics committees protect patients better? [Education and debate]* Br. Med. J. 326: 1199–202.

5. Melander, H., Ahlqvist-Rastad, J., Meijer, G. et al. (2003) *Evidence-b(i)ased medicine – selective reporting from studies sponsored by pharmaceutical industry: review of studies in new drug applications.* Br. Med. J. 326: 1171–3.

6. Easterbrook, P.J., Berlin, J.A., Gopalan, R. et al. (1991) *Publication bias in clinical research.* Lancet 337: 867–72.

7. Horton, R. (2003) *Medical journals: evidence of bias against the diseases of poverty.* Lancet 361: 712–13.

8. Global Forum for Health Research (2002) *The 10/90 Report on Health Research.* Global Forum for Health Research, Geneva.

9. Haynes, R.B. (2005) *The 4S evolution of services for finding current best evidence.* Evid. Based Nurs. 8: 4–6.

10. Schulz, K.F., Chalmers, I., Grimes, D.A. et al. (1994) *Assessing the quality of randomization from reports of controlled trials published in obstetrics and gynecology journals.* JAMA 272: 125–8.

11. Chan, A.-W., Hrobjartsson, A., Haahr, M.T. et al. (2004) *Empirical evidence for selective reporting of outcomes in randomized trials. Comparison of protocols to published articles.* JAMA 291: 2457–65.

12. Gøtzsche, P.C. (1989) *Multiple publication of reports of drug trials.* Eur. J. Clin. Pharmacol. 36: 429–32.

13. Begg, A., Cho, M., Eastwood, S. et al. (1996) *Improving the quality of randomised controlled trials. The CONSORT Statement.* JAMA 276: 637–9.

14. Moher, D., Cook, D.J., Eastwood, S. et al. for the QUOROM Group (1999) *Improving the quality of reports of meta-analyses of randomised controlled trials: the QUOROM Statement.* Lancet 354: 1896–1900.

15. Moher, D., Schultz, K.F., Altman, D. et al. for the CONSORT Group (2001) *The CONSORT Statement: revised recommendations for increasing the quality of parallel group randomized trials.* Lancet 285: 1987–91.

16. Altman, D.G., Schultz, K.F., Moher, D. et al. for the CONSORT Group (2001) *The revised CONSORT Statement for reporting randomized trials: exploration and elaboration.* Ann. Intern. Med. 134: 663–94.

17. Ioannidis, J.P.A., Evans, S.J.W., Gøtzsche, P.C. et al. for the CONSORT Group (2004) *Better reporting of harms in randomized trials: an extension of the CONSORT Statement.* Ann. Intern. Med. 141: 781–8.

18. Clarke, M., Hopewell, S. and Chalmers, I. (2007) *Reporting of clinical trials should begin and end with up-to-date systematic reviews of other relevant evidence: case study.* J. R. Soc. Med. 100: 187–90.

19. Bossuyt, P.M., Retisma, J.B., Bruns, D.E. et al. (2004) *Towards complete and accurate reporting of studies of diagnostic accuracy: the STARD initiative.* Fam. Pract. 21: 4–10.

20. Pocock, S.J., Collier, T.J., Dandreo, K.J. et al. (2004) *Issues in the reporting of epidemiological studies: a survey of recent practice.* Br. Med. J. 329: 883.

21. Stroup, D.F., Berlin, J.A., Morton, S.C. et al. for the Meta-analysis of Observational Studies in Epidemiology (MOOSE) Group (2000) *Meta-analysis of observational studies in epidemiology: a proposal for reporting.* JAMA 283: 2008–12.

22. Des Jarlais, D.D., Lyles, C., Crepaz, N. and the TREND Group (2004) *Improving the reporting quality of nonrandomized evaluations of behavioural and public health interventions. The TREND Statement. [Commentary].* Am. J. Public Health 94: 361–6.

23. Elwyn, G., O'Connor, A., Stacey, D. et al. (2006) *Developing a quality criteria framework for patient decision aids: online international Delphi consensus process.* Br. Med. J. 333: 417.

24. Pitkin, R.M., Branagan, M.A. and Burmeister, L.F. (1999) *Accuracy of data in abstracts of published research articles.* JAMA 281: 1110–11.

25. Ad Hoc Working Group for Critical Appraisal of the Medical Literature (1987) *A proposal for more informative abstracts of clinical articles.* Ann. Intern. Med. 106: 598–604.

26. Moore, A. and McQuay, H. (2006) *Bandolier's Little Book of Making Sense of the Medical Evidence.* Oxford University Press, Oxford.

27. Goodman, S.N., Berlin, J., Fletcher, S.W. et al. (1994) *Manuscript quality before and after peer review and editing at Annals of Internal Medicine.* Ann. Intern. Med. 121: 11–21.

28. Chalmers, I. and Clarke, M. (1998) *Discussion sections in reports of controlled trials published in general medical journals: islands in search of continents.* JAMA 280: 280–2.

29. Clarke, M., Alderson, P. and Chalmers, I. (2002) *Discussion sections in reports of controlled trials published in general medical journals.* JAMA 287: 2799–801.

30. Assmann, S.F., Pocock, S.J., Enos, L.E. et al. (2000) *Subgroup analysis and other (mis)uses of baseline data in clinical trials.* Lancet 355: 1064–9.

31. Jadad, A.R., Moher, M., Browman, G.P. et al. (2000) *Systematic reviews and meta-analyses of treatment of asthma: critical evaluation.* Br. Med. J. 320: 537–40.

32. McAlister, F.A., Clark, H.D., van Walraven, C. et al. (1999) *The medical review article revisited: has the science improved?* Ann. Intern. Med. 131: 947–51.

33. Tramer, M.R., Reynolds, D.J.M., Moore, R.A. et al. (1997) *Impact of covert duplicate publication on meta-analysis: a case study.* Br. Med. J. 315: 635–40.

34. Van Rooyen, S., Godlee, F., Evans, S. et al. (1998) *Effect of open peer review on quality of reviews and on reviewers' recommendations: a randomised trial.* Br. Med. J. 318: 23–7.

35. Smith, R. (1998) *Opening up BMJ peer review.* Br. Med. J. 318: 4–5.

36. Godlee, F. and Jefferson, R. (eds) (1999) *Peer Review in Health Sciences.* BMJ Publishing Group, London.

4.2   Coping alone

In managing the acquisition of knowledge there are two principal modes:

- pro-active
- reactive.

A pro-active style of knowledge management is to scan the literature regularly and thereby search for potentially relevant knowledge (predominantly a scanning activity). A reactive style of knowledge management is based on the principle that no decision-maker will ever be able

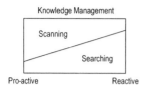

Knowledge Management

Scanning

Searching

Pro-active   Reactive

Margin Fig. 4.1

to anticipate all the questions that are likely to arise and therefore it is more effective to develop good searching skills and use them as and when required (predominantly a searching activity). Each decision-maker must strike a balance between the two types of activities and define a mode of knowledge management most appropriate to needs and circumstances (Margin Fig. 4.1).

4.2.1 Becoming a better scanner

When preparing a scanning strategy, use the checklist of questions shown in Box 4.1.

4.2.2 Becoming a better searcher

There are two steps that can be taken to improve searching skills (see also Section 9.4.2):

1. Undertake formal training; ask the librarian if there are any searching training courses available.
2. Elicit the support of a librarian; first enrol for an induction session, then search with the librarian, and finally ask the librarian to review some searches completed without support to obtain feedback on sensitivity and precision.

4.2.3 Becoming better at critical appraisal

Training in critical appraisal is now widely available (see, for example, Section 9.7.3 and Margin Box 9.3). If there is no access to formal training, take the following steps:
- Consult the book *Users' Guides to the Medical Literature: A Manual for Evidence-Based Clinical Practice* (2002), edited

---

Box 4.1 Useful prompts in the preparation of a scanning strategy

- How many hours each week do I want to spend scanning for new knowledge?
- What sources of knowledge do I want to scan regularly?
- What sources of information will I exclude?
- How can I ensure that I do not miss important new knowledge using this strategy?
- What checklists can I use to ensure that I stick to my scanning objectives? (A weekly checklist is useful.)
- Is there anyone else who could develop, or has developed already, a scanning strategy with whom I could share the load?
- How can I review the benefits and weaknesses of this strategy at the end of the year?

by Guyatt and Rennie and published by the American Medical Association (AMA) Press.

- Set up a problem-based journal club in order to work with colleagues to find and appraise articles relating to decisions that have to be made.

4.2.4   Use it or lose it

Any decision-makers within a health service who find, appraise and use evidence will contribute to changing the culture of the organisation in which they work (see Section 7.2). This course of action provides an example to other people who will discuss the evidence found and begin to search for evidence themselves. As such, the skills of searching for, appraising and retrieving evidence will be strengthened, not only within individuals but also throughout the organisation.

4.3   A knowledge service for the 21st century

Gentle Reader,

Visualise the Radcliffe Camera (the building our young public health physician walked past in Chapter 3), which rises like a giant pannetone at the heart of one of Oxford's most beautiful squares. It is part of the Bodleian Library, to which it is connected by an underground railway (large enough only for small goblins). Deep underground are the stacks which house not only many treasures but also, as the Bodleian is a copyright library and receives every book published in Britain, an odd miscellany. For instance, on emerging from the underground passage through which one can walk from the New Bodleian to the Radcliffe Camera, one is greeted by the sight of the entire output of Mills & Boon, a publisher of romantic novels known in the trade as 'bodice-rippers'.

Commentary

The Bodleian Library epitomises the library of the 20th century; however, with the advent of the World Wide Web, a completely different type of service is developing to serve the needs of those seeking for knowledge in the 21st century.

*What information consumes is rather obvious:
it consumes the attention of its recipients. Hence a wealth
of information creates a poverty of attention and a need to
allocate that attention efficiently among the overabundance
of information sources that might consume it.*

Herbert Simon in *Computers, Communications
and the Public Interest* (1971)

Margin Note 4.7

Eight ubiquitous problems in health systems

(Adapted from Pang et al.[1])

- Errors and mistakes
- Poor-quality healthcare
- Waste of resources
- Variations in policy and practice
- Patients' poor experience of healthcare
- Over-enthusiastic adoption of interventions of low value
- Failure to get new evidence and interventions of high value into practice
- Failure to manage ignorance and uncertainty

Knowledge is the enemy of disease, and just as clean water has played, and continues to play, a vital part in controlling communicable diseases such as cholera across the world, access to 'clean', clear knowledge is essential to the control of disease in the 21st century.[1] Access to clean, clear knowledge will also help to minimise or prevent the major healthcare problems experienced in all healthcare systems[1] (Margin Note 4.7, and Prologue).

There are two aspects to clean, clear knowledge:

1. the need for new knowledge
2. applying existing knowledge in ways to improve healthcare, especially for underprivileged groups, communities or populations.

Although the immediate response may be to identify gaps in the knowledge base, applying what we already know is likely to have a greater impact on health and disease than any new drug or technology introduced within the next 10 years.[1] There are large gaps in knowledge application, and resources are needed to link reliable knowledge with effective decision-making and health policy development. Common problems associated with applying existing knowledge are shown in Box 4.2. Furthermore, even if existing knowledge is applied, it may not be used to maximum benefit.

The challenge is to ensure that everyone has access to clean, clear knowledge, a public health need as important as access to clean clear water. To achieve this, every country needs a national library for health containing knowledge relevant to the health problems of that country. The knowledge about health problems needs to be 'purified' (using systems of quality assurance), organised and actively disseminated, the aim being to deliver best current

---

Box 4.2 Problems with applying existing knowledge (Source: Pang et al.[1])

Existing knowledge might not be:

- relevant to the local context
- of adequate quality
- accessible
- easily usable

---

knowledge to those who need it in the health system, including patients.

Further functions of a national library for health are:

- identifying gaps in knowledge
- supporting research designed to address the knowledge gaps
- highlighting ways to use various types of knowledge and inform decisions about health policy.

Reference

1. Pang, T., Gray, M. and Evans, T. (2006) *A 15th grand challenge for global public health. [Comment]* Lancet 367: 284–6.

Further reading

Haynes, R.B. and Wilczynski, N. (2005) *Finding the gold in Medline: clinical queries.* Evid. Based Med. 10: 101–2.

Sanders, S., and Del Mar, C. (2005) *Clever searching for evidence.* Br. Med. J. 330: 1162–3.

Gentle Reader,

Empathise with the epidemiologist. He stood in the dock, cool, calm and collected. The judge entered, adjusted her robes, peered over her half-moon spectacles, and imposed, by all the non-verbal signals commonly used in that particular form of theatre, her presence on the court.

'How do you plead?' she said, 'Guilty or not guilty?'

The epidemiologist replied, 'How should I know until I have heard the evidence?'

Commentary

This story, the only prologue intended to be humorous which can be found by the editorial team despite exhaustive searching, highlights the appropriate question that should always be asked when any proposition is made: 'How do I know until I have heard the evidence?'. However, hearing the evidence alone is insufficient. It is always important to make judgements about quality. A witness may be able to recount an impressive version of what happened but if he or she is not reliable then the evidence will be of little use.

Appraising the quality of research

Research is a process of enquiry that produces knowledge. It is related to other activities, such as audit, but has several distinguishing features (Box 5.1).

Research can be classified into one of two categories:

1. that which increases the understanding of health, ill health, and the process of healthcare
2. that which enables an assessment of interventions that could be used to try to promote health, prevent ill health, or improve the process of healthcare.

These two categories of research are linked. The former provides a base of knowledge from which ideas can be generated for preventing ill health or managing disease more effectively and efficiently – sometimes called hypothesis-generating research; the latter is used to evaluate the effects of putting such ideas into practice – sometimes called hypothesis-testing research. In this book, the focus is primarily on hypothesis-testing research because it is of greatest use to decision-makers.

5.1.1   Hypothesis-testing research

There are two methods for testing a hypothesis:

1. observational
2. experimental.

1. Observational research
In observational research, the researcher observes a population or group of patients or manipulates data about those subjects. The subject data used by the researcher can be:

- data which are already available
- data which are collected additionally, from interviews either with patients or with healthcare professionals, or from datasets such as cancer registries and death certificates.

> **Box 5.1** The distinguishing features of research as defined in the NHS R&D programme in the UK
>
> - To provide **new knowledge** necessary for the improvement of the performance of the NHS in enhancing the health of the nation.
> - To generate results that are **generalisable**, i.e. that will be of value to those in the NHS who face similar problems but who are outwith the particular locality or context of the research project.
> - To have been designed to follow a clear, well-defined study **protocol**.
> - To have had the study protocol **peer reviewed**.
> - To have obtained the approval, where necessary, of the relevant **ethics committee**.
> - To have defined arrangements for **project management**.
> - To report findings such that they are open to critical examination and accessible to all who could benefit from them – this will normally involve **publication**.

Qualitative research (Section 5.10), surveys (Section 5.9) and case-control studies (Section 5.5) are all forms of observational research. An observational study can be conducted:

- on variations already known to exist among different types of healthcare professional or service – sometimes called a 'natural experiment'
- as part of an evaluation of a change in health service delivery that has been introduced as a result of policy or a managerial innovation or by a commercial company.

2. Experimental research
In experimental research, the intervention under investigation is performed at the instigation of the researcher. The most powerful type of experimental study is the RCT (Section 5.4).

It should be noted that:

- cohort studies (Section 5.6) can be either observational or experimental
- although systematic reviews can be performed on any type of research, the term is most often used to describe reviews of RCTs.

An economic appraisal can be built into both methods of testing an hypothesis (see Section 6.7).

Frequently, there are disputes between the proponents of experimental research ('trialists') and the proponents of observational or qualitative research; however, the focus on areas of disagreement has hidden the fact that there are many areas of agreement. A letter published in the *British Medical Journal*, written in response to an editorial,[1] contains a useful summary of the contribution of observational research (Box 5.2),[2] which should be seen as complementary to experimental research trials and not presented falsely as being in opposition.

Indeed, for the Christmas 1997 edition of the *British Medical Journal*, the editor asked two leading researchers, in a spirit of peace and goodwill, to write a joint leader which was entitled 'Choosing the best research design for each question. It's time to stop squabbling over the "best" methods'.[3] Sackett and Wennberg wrote:

Each method should flourish, because each has features that overcome the limitations of the others when confronted with questions they cannot reliably answer …

But focusing on the shortcomings of somebody else's research approach misses the point. The argument is not about the inherent value of the different approaches and the worthiness of the investigators who use them. The issue is, which way of answering the specific question before us provides the most valid, useful answer? Health and healthcare would both be better served if investigators

---

Box 5.2 Important roles for observational methods (Source: Black[2])

1. Some interventions, such as defibrillation for ventricular fibrillation, have an impact so large that observational data are sufficient to show it.
2. Infrequent adverse outcomes would be detected only by RCTs so large that they are rarely conducted. Observational methods such as post-marketing surveillance of medicines are the only alternative.
3. Observational data provide a realistic means of assessing the long-term outcome of interventions beyond the time-scale of many trials. An example is long-term experience with different hip joint prostheses.
4. Whatever those who question the value of healthcare interventions might think, many clinicians often will not share their concern and will be opposed to an RCT; observational approaches can then be used to show clinical uncertainty and pave the way for such a trial.
5. Despite the claims of some enthusiasts for RCTs, some important aspects of healthcare cannot be subjected to a randomised trial for practical and ethical reasons. Examples include the effect of volume on outcome, the regionalisation of services, a control of infection policy in a hospital, and admission to an intensive care unit. To argue that these topics could theoretically be evaluated by an RCT is of little practical help in advancing knowledge.

redirected the energy they currently spend bashing the research approaches they do not use into increasing the validity, power, and productivity of the ones they do.

Since 1997, there have been further developments in the way that observational research is viewed and valued in relation to experimental research:

> Observational studies and randomized trials (or meta-analyses of them) will tend to agree when they fulfil criteria of quality, validity, and size. This is important because it begins to set the rules of how we investigate difficult areas of care, where randomized trials may be difficult or impossible, or where ethical considerations overrule doing them. If we are careful observational studies can give the same result as a randomized trial.[4]

5.1.2   Fraud in medical research

The underlying assumption in this chapter is that any research published is genuine. However, it is now recognised that fraud in medical research is more common than was previously imagined. Lock and Wells cover this topic comprehensively.[5] Fraud has been defined by the US Food and Drugs Administration (FDA) as follows:

> … the deliberate reporting of false or misleading data or the withholding of reportable data. There are three general types of fraud:
>
> Altered Data – generating biased data or changing data that are otherwise legitimately obtained. Examples are changing laboratory clinical data, altering animal weights, breaking the study blind and/or study randomization.
>
> Omitted Data – not reporting data that have an impact on study outcomes. Examples include removing subjects from the study for bogus reasons, not reporting or disguising adverse effects (events/experiences), and replacing animals on trial.
>
> Manufactured Data – fabricating information or creating results without performing the work. Examples are filling in values in the case report form (e.g. blood pressure, lab values, X-ray reports) for which no data were obtained, photocopying data from one patient for another, and creating fictitious patients (as cited in Schwarz, 1997[6]).

References

1. Sheldon, T.A. (1994) *Please bypass the PORT*. Br. Med. J. 309: 142–3.
2. Black, N. (1994) *Experimental and observational methods of evaluation*. Br. Med. J. 309: 540.

3. Sackett, D.L. and Wennberg, J.E. (1997) *Choosing the best research design for each question. It's time to stop squabbling over the 'best' methods. [Editorial]* Br. Med. J. 315: 1636.

4. Moore, A. and McQuay, H. (2006) *Bandolier's Little Book of Making Sense of the Medical Evidence.* Oxford University Press, Oxford, page 214.

5. Lock, S. and Wells, F. (eds) (1997) *Fraud and Misconduct in Medical Research,* 2nd edn. BMJ Books, London.

6. Schwarz, J.A. (1997) *Detection, handling and prevention of fraud in clinical studies in Europe.* Drugs Made Ger. 40: 8–15.

5.2   Choosing the right research method

This chapter has been designed to help decision-makers in any health service appraise information arising from research. In this context, there are two fundamental categories of research:

- primary research, in which the focus is on patients or populations
- secondary research, in which the focus is on *reviewing* primary research.

The suitability of various research methodologies for evaluating different types of intervention is summarised in Matrix 5.1, and that for evaluating different outcomes in Matrix 5.2. Often, for a complete evaluation, the results from more than one type of research method need to be used.

5.3   Systematic reviews (Margin Fig 5.1)

Secondary research has long been viewed as 'second class'. The consequence was that a research worker who might devote hours to polishing an article describing primary research to be read by other researchers would, when preparing a review,

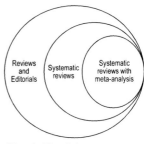

Margin Fig. 5.1

Matrix 5.1

Intervention	Type of research						
	Qualitative research	Case control	Cohort	Controlled before and after studies	Interrupted time series	RCT	Systematic review
Diagnosis			✓			✓✓	✓✓✓
Treatment		✓ For surgical interventions	✓	✓	✓	✓✓	✓✓✓
Screening						✓✓	✓✓✓
Managerial innovation	✓	✓	✓	✓	✓	✓✓	✓✓✓

Matrix 5.2

Outcome	Qualitative research	Surveys	Case control	Controlled before and after study	Interrupted time series	Cohort	RCT	Systematic review
				Type of research				
Effectiveness of an intervention			✓				✓✓	✓✓✓
Effectiveness of health service delivery	✓	✓		✓	✓	✓	✓✓	✓✓✓
Safety	✓	✓	✓			✓	✓✓	✓✓✓
Acceptability	✓	✓					✓✓	✓✓✓
Cost-effectiveness							✓✓	✓✓✓
Appropriateness	✓	✓		✓				✓✓✓
Quality	✓	✓	✓	✓	✓	✓		✓✓✓
Aetiology: causation of disease		✓	✓					

take a handful of articles from a filing cabinet and throw them into a weekend bag. Sadly, this attitude has been detrimental, not only to science but also to the public health.

However, there is now a growing body of evidence that highlights numerous flaws in the design and reporting of primary research, most of which result in an exaggeration of the beneficial effects of an intervention (see Table 6.2). To improve the quality of reporting of controlled trials, the CONSORT Statement recommended that the results of any single trial should be discussed and appraised in the context of all available research evidence on that particular topic. To investigate whether this recommendation was being acted upon, Clarke, Chalmers and co-workers have analysed the discussion section of randomised trials published at three time-points – May 1997,[1] May 2001[2] and May 2005[3] – in the following five general medical journals:

1. *The Lancet*
2. *British Medical Journal*
3. *Annals of Internal Medicine*
4. *Journal of the American Medical Association*
5. *New England Journal of Medicine.*

The results of this analysis are presented in Table 5.1, showing the number of reports:

- found in each of the three months
- that were the first trial to address a particular question
- that contained an updated systematic review integrating the new results

Table 5.1 Analysis of the discussion sections in reports of RCTs published in five general medical journals at three time-points (Source: Clarke et al.[3])

	May 1997 (1)	May 2001 (2)	May 2005 (3)
No. reports found and assessed	26	33	18
No. first trials addressing the question	1 (4%)	3 (9%)	3 (17%)
No. containing an updated systematic review integrating the new results	2 (8%)	0 (0%)	0 (0%)
No. in which previous review was discussed but the results were not integrated	4 (15%)	3 (9%)	5 (28%)
No. in which no apparent systematic attempt was made to set the results in the context of other trials	19 (73%)	27 (82%)	10 (56%)

- in which a previous review was discussed but the results were not integrated
- for which no apparent systematic attempt had been made to set the results in the context of other trials.

Clarke et al.[3] concluded that there is no evidence of progress between 1997 and 2005 in the proportion of trial reports published in general medical journals which discussed new results within the context of up-to-date systematic reviews of relevant evidence from other controlled trials. They also observed that although the proportion of trials in which reference is made to systematic reviews in the discussion section has increased, for the majority of reports there is a failure to do this.

There have also been developments in the methods used for preparing systematic reviews, including those needed to identify the unexpected effects of treatments[4] and those for incorporating into a review the results of research describing and analysing the experiences of people giving and receiving treatments.[5]

5.3.1 Dimensions and definitions

A review of primary research, sometimes referred to as secondary research, can cover:

- only one type of research method – for example, a review of surveys or of RCTs
- a combination of different research methods – for example, a review of the literature on the relationship between abuse (sexual and physical) and gastrointestinal illness that included surveys, and case-control and cohort

studies, revealed an association between these two problems.[6]

There are four kinds of review:

- traditional or unsystematic reviews, a category that includes editorials
- systematic reviews
- systematic reviews that include meta-analysis
- Cochrane Collaboration Reviews.

The main differences between traditional and systematic reviews are highlighted in Matrix 5.3, and those between systematic reviews and Cochrane Collaboration Reviews are shown in Matrix 5.4. Although traditional or unsystematic reviews may be readable and convenient to obtain, they can often be misleading, principally because they are unscientific.[7]

Economic evaluation can be a component of any of the types of review described above (see Section 6.7), but it is not necessarily included in a traditional or unsystematic review.

5.3.1.1 Meta-analysis

In a systematic review, the data from individual studies may be pooled and re-analysed using established statistical

Matrix 5.3 The main differences between traditional or unsystematic reviews and systematic reviews

Characteristics	Traditional or unsystematic review	Systematic review
Strategy used to search for primary sources	Limited, usually to one electronic database, e.g. Medline	Well-defined search of published and unpublished literature
Explicit description of search strategy	Not included	Included
Abstraction of data from primary sources	Subjective and haphazard choice	Systematic appraisal of quality of all papers identified using explicit quality criteria
Analysis of results from primary sources	Variety of techniques used	Systematic analysis using validated methods, e.g. correcting for heterogeneity

Matrix 5.4 The main differences between systematic reviews and Cochrane Collaboration reviews

Characteristics	Systematic review	Cochrane Collaboration review
Strategy used to search for primary sources	Search of published literature, which might include hand-searching	Search of published and unpublished literature by hand
Dynamics of review process	Singular – limited to within a certain time frame, i.e. no updating	Iterative – regular updating as further studies published
Degree of consumer involvement	None	Consumers participate in all stages of the process

methods. This technique is called meta-analysis, but a systematic review in which this technique is employed is sometimes also called a 'meta-analysis'. Ioannidis and Lau have characterised the potential of meta-analysis as an:

… objective methodological engine, which enables information to be prospectively incorporated into a continuum of a large body of evidence.[8]

There are two types of meta-analysis, categorised according to the source of the data analysed:

- MAL meta-analysis, in which the data analysed are abstracted from published papers in the literature, i.e. it is data concerning groups of patients
- MAP meta-analysis, in which the data analysed are individual patient data obtained directly from the authors of published papers; a MAP meta-analysis may also include unpublished data obtained from drug companies or other sources.

Stewart and Clarke found MAP meta-analyses to be more accurate than MAL meta-analyses;[9] however, in this comparison, the patients included in the individual patient data analysis were followed for a longer period of time. As MAP meta-analysis is a laborious and time-consuming process, it is probably more cost-effective to undertake MAL meta-analysis, and then, in exceptional cases, decide whether it is necessary or appropriate to undertake MAP meta-analysis.

5.3.2   Searching

When searching for a systematic review, there is a sequence of five simple steps to follow, as shown below.

Step 1: Is there a review in the Cochrane Database of Systematic Reviews (CDSR)? If not, proceed to Step 2.

Step 2: Is there a review in the Database of Abstracts of Reviews of Effectiveness (DARE)? If not, proceed to Steps 3, 4 and 5.

Step 3: Search Medline using the Publication Type Meta-Analysis [pt]. To search more comprehensively for systematic reviews in Medline, Hunt and McKibbon[10] advocate the use of either a simple or comprehensive search strategy (sometimes called a search filter or 'hedge'). These strategies have been incorporated into a single search filter to retrieve citations identified as systematic reviews or meta-analyses in PubMed – use the systematic review search box in PubMed Clinical Queries to type in your clinical topic and then click 'Go'. Available online at: http://www.ncbi.nlm.nih.gov/entrez/query/static/clinical.shtml

Step 4: Search EMBASE. The Scottish Intercollegiate Guidelines Network (SIGN) has produced a search filter for retrieving systematic reviews in EMBASE, available online at:

http://www.sign.ac.uk/methodology/filters.html#systematic. Combine this filter with your search topic.

Step 5: Search other specialist databases if required.

5.3.3 Appraisal

As healthcare decision-makers and other stakeholders increasingly make use of the findings from systematic reviews as a source of evidence, it is vital to appraise their methodological quality. The examples below demonstrate the need for critical appraisal before accepting the findings from a systematic review or meta-analysis as reliable evidence.

Jadad et al.[11] used the Oxman and Guyatt index to evaluate the quality of reporting and of the review for 50 systematic reviews and meta-analyses on the treatment of asthma, 12 of which were published in the Cochrane Library and 38 in peer-review journals. Using this index, they found that:

- 40 of the reviews had 'serious or extensive flaws'
- all 6 reviews associated with industry had 'serious or extensive flaws'
- of the 10 most rigorous reviews, seven were published in the Cochrane Library.

McAlister et al.[12] followed up Cindy Mulrow's work of almost a decade earlier, in which she had highlighted the lack of scientific soundness in summarising evidence for review articles,[7] and they assessed the methodological quality of all reviews of clinical topics published in six general medical journals during 1996. Of 158 review articles, they found that:

- only two satisfied all 10 methodological criteria of good quality
- less than one-quarter described how evidence was identified, evaluated or integrated.

In addition, of the 111 reviews in which treatment recommendations were made, only 45% cited randomised controlled clinical trials to support their recommendations.

Moher et al.[13] investigated the characteristics of systematic reviews, including emerging aspects not previously examined, that were written in English and indexed in Medline during November 2004. They identified 300 systematic reviews, which involved more than 33 700 separate studies including one-third of a million participants. Descriptive analysis of the systematic reviews against 51 items revealed:

- 71% ($n = 213$) were categorised as 'therapeutic'
- 53% ($n = 161$) reported combining results statistically and of these 91.3% (147/161) assessed consistency across the studies
- only 17.7% ($n = 53$) reported being updates of previously completed reviews
- none ($n = 0$) had a registration number
- 40.7% ($n = 122$) did not state funding sources
- only 23.1% reported assessing for publication bias
- far superior reporting standards for Cochrane reviews when compared with non-Cochrane therapeutic reviews.

5.3.3.1 Systematic reviews

A systematic review of all the evidence available is always more reliable than any single piece of evidence; a review of the relationship between abuse and gastrointestinal illness demonstrates this.[6] However, as systematic reviews can vary in quality, each one must be carefully appraised. A checklist of questions that can be used for the appraisal of systematic reviews is given in Box 5.3.[10]

A source of bias in systematic reviews has been found by Misakian and Bero,[14] which arises from delays in the publication of, and failure to publish, non-significant results. These authors assert that this time-lag in publication

---

Box 5.3 Checklist for the appraisal of systematic reviews (Source: Hunt and McKibbon[10])

1. Did the review article address a focused question?
2. Is it likely that important, relevant studies were missed?
3. Were the inclusion criteria to select articles appropriate?
4. Was the validity of the included studies assessed?
5. Were the assessments of studies reproducible?
6. Were the results similar from study to study?
7. What are the overall results and how precise are they?
8. Will the results help in caring for patients?

provides an argument for the regular updating of reviews as practised by the Cochrane Collaboration.

Once the quality of a review has been appraised, it is then possible to consider its relevance to the local population and the decision that has to be made.

5.3.3.2 Systematic reviews including meta-analysis

If meta-analysis comprises part of any review, the process of appraisal must be more stringent. Meta-analysis is a powerful tool; performed correctly, it produces helpful evidence consistent with, but having narrower confidence intervals than, that from single trials (see Section 6.1.3). However, it is important to be aware that meta-analysis can produce a different conclusion to that generated by the performance of a large RCT. LeLorier et al. found that the outcomes of 12 large RCTs were not predicted accurately 35% of the time by the meta-analyses that had been published previously on the same topic.[15] Moreover, in a review including meta-analysis of magnesium treatment for myocardial infarction, Teo et al. concluded that this therapy was 'effective, safe and simple',[16] whereas in a large RCT known as ISIS-4 (the fourth International Study of Infarct Survival) it was found that magnesium was ineffective.[17] These examples illustrate two main points:

- that the findings from single large RCTs are a superior source of evidence to those from systematic reviews of small trials *if* the large RCT was conducted in the context of a systematic review of previous trials[1]
- the limitations of meta-analysis.[18]

In an editorial accompanying the paper of LeLorier et al., Bailar concluded that meta-analysis may still be improved.[19] One of the ways in which it is possible to improve the quality of both systematic reviews and meta-analyses was investigated by Moher et al., who found that the quality of the individual trials subjected to meta-analysis had an influence on the interpretation of benefit of the intervention under investigation.[20]

There are two further reasons why the results of meta-analyses should be treated with caution.

1. Meta-analyses can be based solely on data from trials found by electronic searches of Medline, which:
   – does not cover all of the world's biomedical journals
   – finds only those trials that are published, which are usually biased towards the positive.[21]

2. The data from the trials included in a meta-analysis are often heterogeneous, that is, there are important differences among them. Although there are statistical techniques that can be used to minimise the effects of heterogeneity, it still presents a problem.[22]

In the light of these potential sources of bias and error in meta-analyses, as for all other research methodologies, the quality of any meta-analysis should be appraised critically. A checklist of questions for the appraisal of reviews that include a meta-analysis is shown in Box 5.4;[23] these questions should be used in conjunction with those shown in Box 5.3.

In 1999, Moher et al.[24] published guidelines to improve the quality of reporting of systematic reviews of randomised controlled trials, known as the QUOROM Statement. The Statement includes 18 items, eight of which are evidence-based. Biondi-Zoccai et al.[25] investigated compliance of systematic reviews on the same clinical topic (the use of acetylcysteine in the prevention of contrast-associated nephropathy) with the QUOROM checklist and the scores on the Oxman and Guyatt quality index. They found compliance with the QUOROM checklist to be relatively high although shorter manuscripts had significantly lower scores. There was no association between QUOROM and Oxman and Guyatt scores, mainly due to the greater emphasis in the latter on selection bias and validity assessment.

5.3.4   Uses and abuses

The systematic review is the best source of evidence for decision-makers. An editorial by Mulrow et al.[26] in the *Annals of Internal Medicine* introduced a series of articles on systematic reviews, which together provide a useful overview of this research methodology and its application. One article of particular interest to those who make

---

Box 5.4 Checklist for the appraisal of review articles that include meta-analysis

- Was the searching technique limited to an electronic search of Medline?
- Are the results of the individual trials widely divergent?
  It is not appropriate to pool trials in a meta-analysis if the level of heterogeneity is too great.
- Are all the individual trials in the meta-analysis small?
  If so, be very cautious.[23]

Box 5.5 Stages in the use of systematic reviews by consumers and policy-makers (Source: Bero and Jadad[27])

- Awareness of the existence of systematic reviews.
- Perception of the advantages and disadvantages of using them.
- Identification of individual reviews.
- Critical evaluation.
- Incorporation into decisions.
- Participation in the design, evaluation, and dissemination of findings.

---

decisions about groups of patients and populations is by Bero and Jadad,[27] in which the authors describe how policy-makers and consumers can use the evidence from systematic reviews in decision-making (Box 5.5). They conclude that as systematic reviews provide an objective summary of large amounts of information they can be a useful decision-making tool for policy-makers to help them decide what healthcare to provide, and for consumers to help them make decisions about healthcare. Bero and Jadad highlighted the scarcity of evidence about the impact of the use of systematic reviews on decision-making by policy-makers and consumers, and recommended that strategies to increase the use of systematic reviews should be evaluated for their usefulness.

Major advances have now been made in what is known as 'knowledge translation':

- In Canada, the Canadian Institute for Advanced Research has supported and guided a change in government decision-making to enable evidence-based policy-making.[28]
- In England, the Cabinet Office has been promoting evidence-based policy-making across all government departments.
- The World Health Organization promotes knowledge translation throughout its work protecting and improving global health.

One of the first examples of the extensive use of the findings from systematic reviews in a textbook was that written by McQuay and Moore on pain relief.[29] Since then, other such texts have been published. Two that are notable cover the subjects of surgery[30] and stroke[31] in an evidence-based way.

References

1. Clarke, M. and Chalmers, I. (1998) *Discussion sections in reports of controlled trials published in general medical journals. Islands in search of continents?* JAMA 280: 280–2.

2. Clarke, M., Alderson, P. and Chalmers, I. (2002) *Discussion sections in reports of controlled trials published in general medical journals.* JAMA 287: 2799–801.

3. Clarke, M., Hopewell, S. and Chalmers, I. (2007) *Reports of clinical trials should begin and end with up-to-date systematic reviews of other relevant evidence: a status report.* J. R. Soc. Med. 100: 187–90.

4. Glasziou, P., Vandenbrouke, J. and Chalmers, I. (2004) *Assessing the quality of research.* Br. Med. J. 328: 39–41.

5. Thomas, J., Harden, A., Oakley, A. et al. (2004) *Integrating qualitative research with trials in systematic reviews.* Br. Med. J. 328: 1010–12.

6. Drassman, D.A., Talley, N.J., Alden, K.W. et al. (1995) *Sexual and physical abuse and gastrointestinal illness.* Ann. Intern. Med. 123: 782–94.

7. Mulrow, C.W. (1987) *The medical review article: state of the science.* Ann. Intern. Med. 106: 485–8.

8. Ioannidis, J.P.A. and Lau, J. (1998) *Can quality of clinical trials and meta-analyses be quantified?* Lancet 352: 590.

9. Stewart, L.A. and Clarke, M.J. (1995) *Practical methodology of meta-analyses (overviews) using updated individual patient data.* Stat. Med. 14: 2057–79.

10. Hunt, D.L. and McKibbon, K.A. (1997) *Locating and appraising systematic reviews.* Ann. Intern. Med. 126: 532–8.

11. Jadad, A.R., Moher, M., Browman, G.P. et al. (2000) *Systematic reviews and meta-analysis on treatment of asthma: critical evaluation.* Br. Med. J. 320: 537–40.

12. McAlister, F.A., Clark, H.D., van Walraven, C. et al. (1999) *The medical review article revisited: has the science improved?* Ann. Intern. Med. 131: 947–51.

13. Moher, D., Tetzlaff, J., Tricco, A.C. et al. (2007) *Epidemiology and reporting characteristics of systematic reviews.* PLoS MEDICINE 4(3): e78:0447–0455.

14. Misakian, A.L. and Bero, L.A. (1998) *Publication bias and research on passive smoking. Comparison of published and unpublished studies.* JAMA 280: 250–3.

15. LeLorier, J., Gregoire, G., Benhaddad, A. et al. (1997) *Discrepancies between meta-analyses and subsequent large randomised controlled trials.* N. Engl. J. Med. 337: 536–42.

16. Teo, K.K., Yusuf, S., Collins, R. et al. (1991) *Effects of intravenous magnesium in suspected acute myocardial infarction: overview of randomised trials.* Br. Med. J. 303: 1499–503.

17. ISIS-4 Collaborative Group (1995) *ISIS-4: a randomised factorial trial assessing early oral captopril, oral mononitrate, and intravenous magnesium sulphate in 58,050 patients with suspected acute myocardial infarction.* Lancet 345: 669–85.

18. Yusuf, S. and Flather, M. (1995) *Magnesium in acute myocardial infarction. ISIS4 provides no grounds for its routine use. [Editorial]* Br. Med. J. 310: 751–2.

19. Bailar, J.C. III (1997) *The promise and problems of meta-analysis.* N. Engl. J. Med. 337: 559–60.

20. Moher, D., Pham, B., Jones, A. et al. (1998) *Does quality of reports of randomised trials affect estimates of intervention efficacy reported in meta-analyses?* Lancet 352: 609–13.

21. Easterbrook, P.J., Berlin, J.A., Gopalan, R. et al. (1991) *Publication bias in clinical research.* Lancet 337: 867–72.

22. Thompson, S.G. and Pocock, S.J. (1991) *Can meta-analyses be trusted?* Lancet 338: 1127–30.

23. Egger, M. and Smith, G.D. (1995) *Misleading meta-analysis: lessons from an 'effective, safe, simple' intervention that wasn't. [Editorial]* Br. Med. J. 310: 752–4.

24. Moher, D., Cook, D.J., Eastwood, S. et al. for the QUOROM Group (1999) *Improving the quality of reports of meta-analyses of randomised controlled trials: the QUOROM Statement.* Lancet 354: 1896–1900.

25. Biondi-Zoccai, G.G.L., Lotrionte, M., Abbate, A. et al. (2006) *Compliance with QUOROM and quality of reporting of overlapping meta-analyses on the role of acetylcysteine in the prevention of contrast associated nephropathy: case study.* Br. Med. J. 332: 202–9.

26. Mulrow, C.D., Cook, D.J. and Davidoff, F. (1997) *Systematic reviews: critical links in the great chain of evidence.* Ann. Intern. Med. 126: 389–91

27. Bero, L.A. and Jadad, A.R. (1997) *How consumers and policymakers can use systematic reviews for decision making.* Ann. Intern. Med. 127: 37–42.

28. Kindig, D., Day, P., Fox, D. M. et al. (2003) *What new knowledge would help policymakers better balance investments for optimal health outcomes?* Health Serv. Res. 38: 1923–38.

29. McQuay, H.J. and Moore, A. (1998) *An Evidence-Based Resource for Pain.* Oxford University Press, Oxford.

30. Meakins, J.L. and Gray, J.A.M. (guest eds) (2006) *Evidence-based surgery. An issue of surgical clinics.* Surg. Clin. North Am., vol. 86, no. 1. Sanders.

31. Warlow, C.P, Dennis, M.S., van Gijn, J. et al. (1996) *Stroke: A Practical Guide to Management.* Blackwell Science, Oxford.

The interested reader should also consult the Cochrane Database of Systematic Reviews (CDSR), the Cochrane Review Methodology Database, and the *Reviewers' Handbook,* which are all part of the Cochrane Library.

5.4   Randomised controlled trials

The RCT is a very beautiful technique, of wide applicability, but as with everything else there are snags.
Archie Cochrane, *Effectiveness and Efficiency, 1989*

5.4.1   Dimensions and definitions

The primary use for an RCT is to evaluate the effectiveness of an intervention, usually a treatment regimen, but it is also possible to apply it to diagnostic interventions, screening programmes or managerial innovations. The defining features of an RCT are shown in Box 5.6.

Errors in an RCT may arise as a result of bias or by chance. Bias is manifest as a systematic error that favours either the treatment or the control group. The error is referred to as systematic because if it occurs once it will occur repeatedly due to a flaw in the design or management of the trial. The features of an RCT are designed to minimise bias. Error due to chance is random. Therefore, trials must be carefully designed to ensure that they have sufficient

Box 5.6 The defining features of an RCT

- There must be equipoise, that is, genuine doubt prior to the trial about whether one option is better than another.
- The individuals who might benefit from the intervention are randomly allocated to receive that intervention or not; the latter form the control group, and receive a placebo or the 'standard' treatment.
- All entrants to the trial are followed up in treatment and control groups.
- Individuals in the treatment group remain in that group irrespective of whether they actually receive the intervention; for example, in a trial of breast cancer screening those randomly allocated to receive screening remain in that group even if they do not attend for treatment – this is called randomisation on an 'intention-to-treat' basis.
- The assessment of outcome is made by an assessor who is unaware of the patient's status; this is know as 'blind' assessment.
- All patients are included in the analysis.
- In some types of RCT, such as drug trials, both doctor and patient may be 'blind', i.e. unaware of whether the patient is a member of a treatment group or of the control group – such a trial is known as 'double blind'.

power to detect a difference between treatment and control groups, if one exists, or to demonstrate that there is no effect if the treatment is ineffective (Box 5.7).

The feature that distinguishes an RCT from a controlled trial is the random allocation of subjects to receive the intervention under investigation.

For a book about RCTs that is clear, concise and easy to read, consult Jadad (see Further Reading at the end of this section).

5.4.1.1 Mega trials

To detect a small improvement in health outcome, for example, 5%, a very large trial is needed. Although at first sight it might appear that a 5% improvement is clinically insignificant, for common diseases, such as myocardial infarction, a 5% improvement is of great importance. Large trials, sometimes called 'mega trials', can be designed to demonstrate these small differences in outcome; such trials have made a significant contribution to the management

Margin Note 5.1
History of the RCT

For an excellent history of the RCT, refer to the James Lind Library (an electronic resource) where all the key documents in the evolution of the RCT are presented under the descriptor of 'a fair test', available online at: http://www.jameslindlibrary.org/

Box 5.7 Power rules

- The smaller the effect expected in the treatment being tested, the larger the trial necessary to have sufficient power to detect it.
- The larger the trial, the greater its power.

Matrix 5.5 The distinguishing features between trials and mega trials

Characteristics	RCT	Mega trial
Number of subjects	Tens or hundreds	As many as 20,000 each in the treatment and control groups
Number of professionals	Less than ten	Many investigators, sometimes hundreds
Location	Single centre	Multiple centres in several countries
Entry criteria	Restrictive	Simple – wide variety of different types of patient included
Treatment regimen	Only that under investigation	Other treatments in addition to that under investigation may be administered

of cardiovascular disease.[1] The main differences between a trial and a mega trial are shown in Matrix 5.5.

Some of the characteristics of a mega trial can be seen as limitations, for example, the administration of additional treatments may lead to any effect of the experimental therapy being obscured.[2] Any such effects must be borne in mind during the appraisal of mega-trial findings. In contrast, some workers feel that certain characteristics that could be regarded as weaknesses, such as simple entry criteria, actually reflect the situation in clinical practice.

5.4.1.2 Patient preference in trials

A methodological development of particular importance is the incorporation of patient preference into trials in which the patient's participation in the process of treatment, and therefore his/her motivation, is essential for the intervention to be effective. In drug trials, patient preference is not a significant factor (all the patient has to do is swallow the pills), but in other types of treatment, for example, a study of subcutaneous continuous infusion pumps in the management of diabetes, patient preference needs to be built into the design of the trial.[3]

5.4.1.3 'N of 1' trials

The 'N of 1' trial is a single-patient controlled trial used in the specific circumstances of the care of a patient whose condition, depression for instance, fluctuates widely and is affected by a multiplicity of factors such that the effect of treatment is difficult to assess.[4] In such a situation, after consultation with the doctor, the patient might agree to an 'N of 1' trial. During the trial, personnel in the pharmacy will switch the patient's therapy between active and placebo treatments several times. To be conclusive, the therapy may need to be switched as many as 10 times. Neither doctor nor patient is aware of the switches, i.e. they are 'blind'. The doctor and patient will meet at review consultations, but the assessment of treatment outcome is made by a third party, who is also 'blind', i.e. not aware of when the patient was receiving the active drug or the placebo.

5.4.2 Searching

It is possible to search Medline specifically for RCTs. Combine your clinical problem, intervention and outcome search terms with the Publication Type Randomized Controlled Trial [pt], or if using PubMed, use the Therapy category on Clinical Queries (see Section 3.2.2).

Problems can be experienced when searching for trials, because of the limited coverage of Medline and some imprecise indexing. However, these are diminishing as the work of the Cochrane Collaboration progresses. Hand-searching of journals, including those covered by Medline and EMBASE, has revealed many more trials, which are now easily available in the Cochrane Controlled Trials Register, via the Cochrane Library – in October 2006, there were 477 942 RCTs available.

5.4.3 Appraisal

During the 1970s, although the RCT was regarded as the 'gold standard' for demonstrating the effectiveness of a therapy, there was a growing awareness that this research method also had limitations:

- A survey of 71 negative RCTs showed that the majority of these trials were too small, that is, had insufficient power, to detect important clinical differences, a fact of which the authors seemed unaware.[5]
- A study of 206 RCTs showed that randomisation, one of the main design features of an RCT necessary to prevent bias, was poorly reported. Moreover, in those trials for which randomisation was not described, the effect of treatment was exaggerated by an amount greater than the true effect of the treatment (Table 5.2).[6]

Table 5.2 Methodological quality and estimates of treatment effects in controlled trials (trials with poor evidence of randomisation were compared with trials with adequate randomisation) (Source: Schulz et al.[6])

Methodological issue	Exaggeration of odds ratio (%)
Inadequate method of treatment allocation	Larger by 41%
Unclear method of treatment allocation	Larger by 30%
Trials not double blind	Larger by 17%

- In one review of 196 double-blind trials, it was stated that: 'Doubtful or invalid statements were found in 76% of the conclusions or abstracts'.[7] Bias consistently favoured the new drug in 81 trials and the control in only one trial.[7]
- In a critical appraisal of the relationship between the methodological quality, and other characteristics, of 51 reviews of spinal manipulation as a treatment for low back pain and the conclusions about the effectiveness of this intervention,[8] it was found that one of the factors associated with a positive conclusion (the outcome in 34 reviews) was the presence of a spinal manipulator on the review team.

From these examples, it can be seen that the results of RCTs, like any other research findings, need careful appraisal using explicit criteria.

There are many factors that have been shown to bias a trial, and various checklists of quality criteria have been produced, but these are usually of most use to research workers. Chalmers[9] has identified the three most important factors as follows:

1. inadequate randomisation
2. failure to blind the assessor of outcome
3. failure to follow up all the patients in the trial.

These criteria are epidemiological and can be used to assess the quality of a trial. Jadad et al.[10] have developed the Oxford five-point scoring system using these factors in order to assess the quality of clinical trials (Box 5.8). This is a simple scale to use, and trials that receive a score of three or more are relatively free of bias and can be trusted.

Other more extensive sets of criteria can be used to assess these and other factors such as the size of the effect found in a trial (Box 5.9). However, depending on the way in which they are presented, numerical scoring systems can conceal the main threats to validity, and it is often simpler to list them. Furthermore, the level of agreement between different scoring systems can be poor.[11]

Box 5.8 The Oxford Scoring System for assessing the quality of clinical trials
(Source: Jadad et al.[10])

This is not the same as being asked to review a paper. It should not take more than 10 minutes to score a report and there are no right or wrong answers. Please read the article and try to answer the following questions:

1. Was the study described as randomized (this includes the use of words such as randomly, random, and randomization)?
2. Was the study described as double-blind?
3. Was there a description of withdrawals and drop-outs?

Scoring the items

Give a score of 1 point for each 'yes' and 0 points for each 'no'. There are no in-between marks. Give an additional point if:

- On question 1, the method of randomization was described and it was appropriate (table of random numbers, computer generated, coin tossing, etc.)
- On question 2, the method of double-blinding was described and it was appropriate (identical placebo, active placebo, dummy, etc.)

Deduct 1 point if:

- On question 1, the method of randomization was described and it was inappropriate (patients were allocated alternately or according to date of birth, hospital number, etc.)
- On question 2, the study was described as double-blind but the method of blinding was inappropriate (e.g. comparison of tablet vs injection with no double dummy).

Advice on using the scale

1. Randomization

If the word randomized or any other related words such as random, randomly, or randomisation are used in the report, but the method of randomization is not described, give a positive score to this item. A randomization method will be regarded as appropriate if it allows each patient to have the same chances of receiving each treatment and the investigators can not predict which treatment is next. Therefore methods of allocation using date of birth, date of admission, hospital numbers, or alternation should not be regarded as appropriate.

2. Double-blinding

A study must be regarded as double-blind if the word double-blind is used (even without description of the method) or if it is implied that neither the care-giver nor the patient can identify the treatment being assessed.

3. Withdrawals and drop-outs

Patients who were included in the study but did not complete the observation period or who were not included in the analysis must be described. The number and the reasons for withdrawal must be stated. If there are no withdrawals, it should be stated in the article. If there is no statement on withdrawals, this item must be given a negative score (0 points).

Box 5.9 Checklist for appraising randomised controlled trials (©CASP)

The 10 questions are adapted from: Guyatt, G.H., Sackett, D.L. and Cook, D.J. *Users' guides to the medical literature. II. How to use an article about therapy or prevention.* JAMA (1993) 270: 2598–601, and JAMA (1994) 271: 59–63. The checklist is available online at: http://www.phru.nhs.uk/learning/casp_rct_tool.pdf

Screening questions

1. Did the study ask a clearly focused question?

Consider if the question is 'focused' in terms of:
  – the population studied
  – the intervention given
  – the outcomes considered.

2. Was this a randomised controlled trial (RCT) and was it appropriately so?

Consider:
  – why this study was carried out as an RCT
  – if this was the right research approach for the question being asked.
Is it worth continuing?

Detailed questions

3. Were participants appropriately allocated to intervention and control groups?

Consider:
  – how participants were allocated to intervention and control groups. Was the process truly random?
  – whether the method of allocation was described. Was a method used to balance the randomisation, e.g. stratification?
  – how the randomisation schedule was generated and how a participant was allocated to a study group
  – if the groups were well balanced. Are any differences between the groups at entry to the trial reported?
  – if there were differences reported that might have explained any outcome(s) (confounding).

4. Were participants, staff and study personnel 'blind' to participants' study group?

Consider:
  – the fact that blinding is not always possible
  – if every effort was made to achieve blinding
  – if you think it matters in this study
  – the fact that we are looking for 'observer bias'.

5. Were all of the participants who entered the trial accounted for at its conclusion?

Consider:
  – if any intervention-group participants got a control-group option or vice versa
  – if all participants were followed up in each study group (was there loss to follow-up?)
  – if all the participants' outcomes were analysed by the groups to which they were originally allocated (intention-to-treat analysis)

- what additional information would you like to have seen to make you feel better about this?

6. Were the participants in all groups followed up and data collected in the same way?

Consider:
- if, for example, they were reviewed at the same time intervals and if they received the same amount of attention from researchers and health workers; any differences may introduce performance bias.

7. Did the study have enough participants to minimise the play of chance?

Consider:
- if there is a power calculation. This will estimate how many participants are needed to be reasonably sure of finding something important (if it really exists and for a given level of uncertainty about the final result).

8. How are the results presented and what is the main result?

Consider:
- if, for example, the results are presented as a proportion of people experiencing an outcome, such as risks, or as a measurement, such as mean or median differences, or as survival curves and hazards
- how large this size of result is and how meaningful it is
- how you would sum up the bottom-line result of the trial in one sentence.

9. How precise are these results?

Consider:
- if the result is precise enough to make a decision
- if a confidence interval is reported; would your decision about whether or not to use this intervention be the same at the upper confidence limit as at the lower confidence limit?
- if a P value is reported where confidence intervals are unavailable.

10. Were all important outcomes considered so the results can be applied?

Consider whether:
- the people included in the trial could be different from your population in ways that would produce different results
- your local setting differs much from that of the trial
- you can provide the same treatment in your setting.

Consider outcomes from the point of view of:
- the individual
- the policy maker and professionals
- the family/carers
- the wider community.

Consider whether:
- any benefit reported outweighs any harm and/or cost. If this information is not reported can it be filled in from elsewhere?
- policy or practice should change as a result of the evidence contained in this trial.

Since 1966, a set of guidelines has been developed on an iterative basis to improve the quality of reporting of randomised controlled trials,[12-15] known as the CONSORT Statement. To find the most up-to-date information on CONSORT, visit the website: http://www.consort-statement.org/.

5.4.3.1 Subgroup analysis

It is tempting for the investigators involved in any trial or meta-analysis to analyse data from subgroups of patients to look for treatment effects, particularly if the overall result of the trial is negative. This technique is known as subgroup analysis or data 'dredging'.

Subgroup analysis can be an important part of the analysis of a comparative clinical trial, but it is common for the results to be over-interpreted, which can lead to further 'mis-guided' research and/or sub-optimal patient care.[16] Lagakos' recommendations[16] about the proper conduct of subgroup analysis are shown in Table 5.3.

Any effects of treatment demonstrated by subgroup analysis should be viewed with caution and the analysis appraised carefully using the checklist developed by Oxman and Guyatt[17] (Box 5.10).

5.4.4 Uses and abuses

An RCT is the best way of evaluating the effectiveness of an intervention, but it is open to misuse.

Table 5.3 Dos and don'ts of reporting subgroup analyses (Source: Lagakos[16])

Dos	Don'ts
• Report the number of subgroup analyses, which were pre-specified and which were post-hoc, and whether any were suggested by the data	
For within-subgroup comparisons	*For within-subgroup comparisons*
• Give an estimate of the magnitude of the treatment difference and a corresponding confidence interval	• Best not to present P values
• Confidence intervals should be interpreted as providing a plausible range of treatment differences consistent with the trial results	• Confidence intervals should not be used to infer whether a treatment difference in a subgroup is statistically significant (on the basis of whether the interval excludes the hypothesis of equality between treatment groups)

> **Box 5.10 Guidelines for deciding whether apparent differences in subgroup response are real (Source: Oxman and Guyatt[17])**
>
> - Is the magnitude of the difference clinically important?
> - Was the difference statistically significant?
> - Did the hypothesis precede rather than follow the analysis?
> - Was the subgroup analysis one of a small number of hypotheses tested?
> - Was the difference suggested by comparisons within rather than between studies?
> - Was the difference consistent across studies?
> - Is there indirect evidence that supports the hypothesized difference?

5.4.4.1 Interpretation and presentation

A research-based fact is like an uncut diamond, valuable but of little use. The decision-maker has to be able to apply that fact. A checklist of questions that can be used to determine the applicability of research findings is shown in Box 5.11.

However, the application of any research information is beset with difficulties because the results of an RCT done on a sample of the whole population must be extrapolated to the local population for which the decision-maker is responsible. This involves judgement, and there are two pervasive but subtle influences that bear upon a decision-maker's judgement and the way in which s/he might apply research findings to the local population.

1. Cultural effects: interpretation
Cultural factors influence the interpretation of research information. In general, physicians in the USA have been quicker to adopt innovations in high technology than their counterparts in the UK. This difference can be illustrated by the differing attitudes towards clot-busting agents.[18] In the USA, tissue plasminogen activator (tPA) is the drug of choice; in the UK, it is streptokinase. However, it can be seen from Fig. 5.1 that tPA is no more effective than streptokinase, but it is 10 times more expensive; moreover, streptokinase has fewer adverse effects (Fig. 5.2).[18] American culture fosters the attitude that a novel intervention should

> **Box 5.11 Checklist for assessing the applicability of research findings**
>
> - How wide are the confidence intervals?
> - What were the exclusion and inclusion criteria?
> - How similar were the patients in the trial to the 'local' patient group?
> - Could the quality of service provided in the trial be reproduced locally?

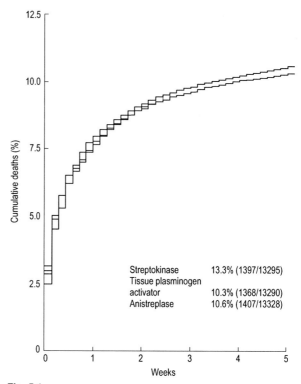

Fig. 5.1
Mortality as an outcome following treatment with one of three thrombolytic agents as compared in the ISIS-3 trial
(Source: O'Donnell,[18] with permission, BMJ Publishing Group)

be tried if there is no evidence against its use, whereas the attitude in the UK is that a new intervention should not be introduced until there is strong evidence in favour of its use: New World vs Old; Gung-ho vs Stick-in-the-Mud.

The way in which health services are financed, and individual clinicians are paid, influences decision-making. For this reason, those who pay for healthcare are beginning to introduce 'pay for performance'. One such scheme in general practices in the UK increased the provision of support for smoking cessation and was associated with a reduction in smoking prevalence among diabetes patients in a primary care setting.[19]

2. The framing effect: presentation
If a picture is set off by a good frame, it will sell more easily – an experience-based aphorism from the antiques trade. The same applies to research findings: decision-makers are influenced not only by the data but also by the way in which those data are presented. This phenomenon, known as the framing effect, has been recognised by psychologists

Margin Note 5.2
Aphorisms about the presentation of research results

• For those who want to influence others, use relative risk reduction as the means of presenting data.
• For those who are likely to be influenced by data presentation, never, ever, accept information on the basis of relative risk reduction alone.

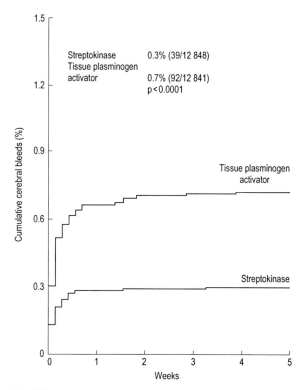

Streptokinase 0.3% (39/12 848)
Tissue plasminogen
activator 0.7% (92/12 841)
p<0.0001

Tissue plasminogen
activator

Streptokinase

Fig. 5.2
Rates of cerebral bleeds with streptokinase and tissue plasminogen activator in ISIS-3 (Source: O'Donnell,[18] with permission, BMJ Publishing Group)

for years. Indeed, the way in which the pharmaceutical industry presents data to clinicians increases the probability of positive interpretation and therefore of prescribing.

Evidence of the existence of the framing effect is growing. The results of studies in Canada[20] and Italy[21] have shown the degree to which clinicians are influenced by data presented in terms of relative risk reduction. The framing effect has also been shown to influence purchasers. Fahey et al.[22] provided 182 executive and non-executive members of 13 health authorities, family health services authorities, or health commissions with the results from a randomised trial on breast cancer screening and those from a systematic review on cardiac rehabilitation. However, both sets of results were presented in four different ways, as shown in Table 5.4.[22]

From the 140 questionnaires returned, it was found that the willingness to fund either programme was influenced significantly by the way in which the data were presented. Relative risk reduction stimulated a significantly higher inclination to purchase, followed by the number needed

Table 5.4 The framing effect: presentation of the same information in four different ways for two programmes (Source: adapted from Fahey et al.[22])

Method of data presentation	Mammography	Cardiac rehabilitation
Relative risk reduction	34%	20%
Absolute risk reduction	0.06%	3%
Percentage of event-free patients	99.82% vs 99.8%	84% vs 87%
Number needed to treat (NNT)	1592	31

to treat (NNT). It is intriguing to note that only three respondents, 'all non-executive members claiming no training in epidemiology', recognised that the four different modes of presentation of the two sets of data summarised the same results in both cases.

5.4.4.2 Reporting trial end points

All trials have a primary objective, for example, the prevention of stroke by the treatment of high blood pressure, in which the occurrence of stroke is measured as the primary end point. However, because it may take years before it is possible to measure the treatment effect on the primary end point, it is tempting for workers to report the effect on secondary end points, which in this example would be the level of blood pressure. The practice of basing treatment recommendations on an analysis of secondary end points should be treated with great caution (Casebook 5.1).[23]

Further reading

Jadad, A.R. (1998) *Randomised Controlled Trials. A User's Guide.* BMJ Books, London.

Casebook 5.1 Primary or secondary end points? (Source: Messerli[23])

In the Antihypertensive and Lipid-Lowering Treatment to Prevent Heart Attack Trial (ALLHAT), the primary end point was coronary heart disease. It was found that chlorthalidone (chlortalidone), lisinopril and amlodipine had identical effects on the primary end points, and yet the major conclusion of the trial was that thiazide diuretics are superior in preventing one or more major forms of cardiovascular disease and should be preferred for first-line antihypertensive therapy. This conclusion was based on an analysis of secondary end points and cost.

As the ALLHAT investigators pointed out themselves, secondary end points are 'soft' data and should not be used as a basis for main conclusions or lead to a drug class being recommended as preferred.

References

1. Yusuf, S., Collins, R. and Peto, T.R. (1984) *Why do we need some large sample randomised trials?* Stat. Med. 3: 409–20.

2. Woods, K.L. (1995) *Mega-trials and the management of myocardial infarction.* Lancet 346: 611–14.

3. Brewin, C.R. and Bradley, C. (1989) *Patient preferences and randomised controlled trials.* Br. Med. J. 299: 313–15.

4. Guyatt, G., Sackett, D., Tayler, W. et al. (1986) *Determining optimal therapy – randomised trials in individual patients.* N. Engl. J. Med. 314: 889–92.

5. Freiman, J.A., Chalmers, T.C., Smith, H. et al. (1978) *The importance of Beta, the type II error, and sample size in the design and interpretation of the randomised controlled trial.* N. Engl. J. Med. 299: 690–4.

6. Schulz, K.F., Chalmers, I., Hayes, R.J. et al. (1995) *Empirical evidence of bias: dimensions of methodological quality associated with estimates of treatment effects in controlled trials.* JAMA 273: 408–12.

7. Gøtzsche, P.C. (1989) *Methodology and overt and hidden bias in reports of 196 double blind trials of non-steroidal anti-inflammatory drugs in rheumatoid arthritis.* Control. Clin. Trials 10: 31–56. *Erratum* Control. Clin. Trials 10: 356.

8. Assenfeldt, W.J.J., Koes, B.W., Knipschild, P.G. et al. (1995) *The relationship between methodological quality and conclusions in reviews of spinal manipulation.* JAMA 264: 1942–8.

9. Chalmers, I. (1995) *'Applying overviews and meta-analyses at the bedside': discussion.* J. Clin. Epidemiol. 48: 67–70.

10. Jadad, A.R., Moore, R.A., Carroll, D. et al. (1996) *Assessing the quality of reports of randomized clinical trials: is blinding necessary?* Control. Clin. Trials 17: 1–12.

11. Juni, P., Altman, D.G. and Egger, M. (2001) *Systematic reviews in health care: assessing the quality of controlled clinical trials.* Br. Med. J. 323: 42–6.

12. Begg, A., Cho, M., Eastwood, S. et al. (1996) *Improving the quality of randomized controlled trials. The CONSORT Statement.* JAMA 276: 637–9.

13. Moher, D., Schultz, K.F., Altman, D. et al. for the CONSORT Group (2001) *The CONSORT Statement: revised recommendations for increasing the quality of parallel group randomised trials.* Lancet 285: 1987–91.

14. Altman, D.G., Schultz, K.F., Moher, D. et al. for the CONSORT Group (2001) *The revised CONSORT Statement for reporting randomized trials: exploration and elaboration.* Ann. Intern. Med. 134: 663–94.

15. Ioannidis, J.P.A., Evans, S.J.W., Gøtzsche, P.C. et al. for the CONSORT Group (2004) *Better reporting of harms in randomized trials: an extension of the CONSORT Statement.* Ann. Intern. Med. 141: 781–8.

16. Lagakos, S.W. (2006) *The challenge of subgroup analyses – reporting without distorting.* N. Engl. J. Med. 354: 1667–9.

17. Oxman, A.D. and Guyatt, G.H. (1992) *A consumer's guide to subgroup analyses.* Ann. Intern. Med. 116: 78–84.

18. O'Donnell, M. (1991) *The battle of the clotbusters.* Br. Med. J. 302: 1259–61.

19. Millett, C., Gray, J., Saxena, S. et al. (2007) *Impact of a pay-for-performance incentive on support for smoking cessation and on smoking prevalence among people with diabetes.* Can. Med. Assoc. J. 176: 1705–10.

20. Naylor, C.D., Chen, E. and Strauss, B. (1992) *Measured enthusiasm: does the method of reporting trial results alter perceptions of therapeutic effectiveness?* Ann. Intern. Med. 117: 916–21.

21. Bobbio, M., Demichelis, B. and Giustetto, G. (1994) *Completeness of reporting trial results: effect on physicians' willingness to prescribe.* Lancet 343: 1209–11.

22. Fahey, T., Griffiths, S. and Peters, T.J. (1995) *Evidence-based purchasing: understanding results of clinical trials and systematic reviews.* Br. Med. J. 311: 1056–60.

23. Messerli, F.H. (2003) *ALLHAT, or the Soft Science of the Secondary End Point.* Ann. Intern. Med. 139: 777–80.

5.5   Case-control studies

For two decades from the 1970s, the case-control study, a major type of observational study, was eclipsed by the RCT as the 'gold standard' in the evaluation of effectiveness, but during the 1990s its distinct and essential contribution regained recognition. Well-conducted observational studies have an important contribution to make, particularly in the evaluation of surgical treatments,[1] and to aetiology or the study of the causation of disease.

5.5.1   Dimensions and definitions

The starting point of a case-control study is outcome. Individuals selected for the control group have the same characteristics or exposures as the individuals in the study group except for the characteristic or exposure that is the subject of the hypothesis. In a case-control study of a cancer, for example, the study group comprises those who have the cancer; the characteristics of these individuals, e.g. age and gender, are matched with those of the controls, with the exception that the individuals in the control group do not have the cancer.

However, a study in which the outcomes for men who received an intervention, such as prostate cancer screening, simply by virtue of being eligible for a private service, are compared with those of men of the same age who have not had the intervention simply because they were not eligible is *not* a case-control study; it is a badly designed and invalid trial.

Case-control studies have several advantageous features:

- they can be less expensive than RCTs (although some case-control studies are expensive because they involve a large number of subjects)
- they can sometimes be completed relatively quickly.

A case-control study can be used to investigate the following problems:

- the causation of disease
- the adverse effects of treatment.

5.5.1.1 Study of the causation of disease

In a case-control study of people who had lung cancer, it was found that smoking was the main cause of lung cancer: a large proportion of those who had lung cancer smoked, while only a very small proportion of the control group, none of whom smoked, developed lung cancer.[2]

5.5.1.2 Study of the adverse effects of treatment

As the beneficial effects of treatment are usually more
common than the adverse effects, an RCT with sufficient
power to detect the beneficial effects will probably not be
powerful enough to detect adverse effects. Adverse effects
can be detected either by following patients over many
years in a cohort study (Section 5.6) or within a case-control
study (current section).

In a study of the adverse effects of treatment for high
blood pressure,[3] 623 hypertensive patients who were
members of a group health cooperative and who had had
a first fatal or first non-fatal myocardial infarction were
compared with 2032 hypertensive patients, matched for
age, sex and calendar year, who had not had a myocardial
infarction. The following patients were excluded: those who
had been members of the cooperative for less than
1 year; those who did not have a diagnosis of hypertension;
those who had had a prior myocardial infarction; those
whose infarction had been a complication of a procedure or
surgery. Patients entered into the study had to have
been taking antihypertensive medicines for at least
30 days – preliminary analysis had shown that the recent
starting of beta-blockers and calcium-channel blockers
was strongly associated with a risk of myocardial
infarction. Initial analysis included only those patients
who were free of clinical cardiovascular disease. A strong
association between acute myocardial infarction and dose
of calcium-channel blocker, administered either alone or
in combination with a diuretic, was found. The risk at the
highest doses of calcium-channel blockers was three times
that at the lowest doses. It is interesting that the authors of
this case-control study then performed a systematic review
of RCTs,[4] which underlines the usefulness of evaluating a
therapy using several different research methods.

5.5.2   Searching

Usually, the first step in any search strategy is to search for
RCTs (see Sections 5.4.2 and 3.2.2). However, as the results
of RCTs alone will not necessarily give all the outcomes
of an intervention, it is always useful to search for case-
control studies. Medline does not have a specific Publication
Type for case-control studies; the best way to retrieve case-
control studies is to 'explode' (i.e. include this term together
with all subordinate terms) the Medical Subject Heading
(MeSH) Case Control Studies/. It is important to be aware

that, as with all study design MeSH, its use will generate methodological articles on how to conduct or evaluate a case-control study as well as examples of case-control studies. As most optimal strategies contain both MeSH and text terms, it is also advisable to use the term "case control" as a text word (i.e. in title or abstract). Do not conduct a text word search for the phrase "case control studies" because terms such as "case control design" will be missed.

5.5.3   Appraisal

Case-control studies are prone to bias: in a major review of case-control studies, 35 different sources of bias were identified.[5] For the user of research information or a decision-maker, these 35 sources of bias can be distilled into three questions, as follows.

1. Was the selection of control subjects based on a set of criteria that matched the controls with the case subjects on every criterion except the presence of the disease or risk factor being studied?
2. Were measurements on the control subjects free from bias, e.g. was the observer performing the assessment aware of the patient's status as a case or as a control subject?
3. Was there recall bias, i.e. did people with the disease have a better recall of past events associated with the disease?

5.5.4   Uses and abuses

The main uses of case-control studies are:

- the identification of the causes of disease
- the identification of rare effects of treatment, usually side-effects.

The main abuse of a case-control study is using it as the sole method of evaluation for the effectiveness of an intervention. The most appropriate methodology to use for this research question is an RCT, which should always be applied first.

References

1. Meakins, J.L. (2006) *Evidence-Based Surgery*. In: Meakins, J. L. and Gray, J. A. M. (guest eds) *Evidence-Based Surgery, An Issue of Surgical Clinics of North America*. Surg. Clin. North Am., vol. 86, no. 1, pages 1–16. Sanders.

2. Doll, R. and Hill, A.B. (1952) *The study of the aetiology of carcinoma of the lung.* Br. Med. J. ii: 1271–86.
3. Psaty, B.M., Heckbert, S.R., Koepsell, T.D. et al. (1995) *The risk of myocardial infarction associated with antihypertensive drug therapies.* JAMA 274: 620–5.
4. Furberg, C.D., Psaty, B.M. and Meyer, J.V. (1995) *Nifedipine. Dose-related increase in mortality in patients with coronary heart disease.* Circulation 92: 1326–31.
5. Sackett, D.L. (1979) *Bias in analytic research.* J. Chron. Dis. 32: 51–63.

5.6   Cohort studies

Cohort 1489 [a. F. cohorte, ad. L. cohortem (cohors), f. co- + hort-, …] 1. Rom. Antiq. A body of from 300 to 600 infantry; the tenth part of a legion. 2. transf. A band of warriors 1500. 3. fig. A company, band 1719.

Shorter Oxford English Dictionary

5.6.1   Dimensions and definitions

In a cohort study, a group of people is investigated over a particular period of time; any changes that occur during that period are recorded. A cohort study can be either retrospective, for example, a review of all cases of breast, colorectal or prostate cancer treated in seven Californian hospitals between 1980 and 1982,[1] or prospective, that is, the identification of a group of healthy people or patients in order to follow them from one point in time to another.

In a cohort study, subject data can be those collected routinely or those collected specifically for the purpose of the study, or a combination of both.

A cohort study can be used to investigate the following situations:

- the outcome of treatment when it is not possible to perform an RCT for ethical reasons; for example, a study to determine the outcome of prostatectomy.[2] The findings from a cohort study enable quality standards such as the re-admission rate[3] to be based on evidence
- different approaches to health service delivery and management that cannot be evaluated in an RCT, either because the number of units is too small to confer adequate power upon the trial or because health service policy-makers or managers will not allow their service to be included in such a trial

- 'natural experiments', that is, either when changes are made in the organisation or delivery of healthcare for political or managerial reasons, or where different patterns of care exist in similar settings by reason of history and tradition.

Cohort studies have been used to investigate:

- staffing changes: for example, in a study of the effect of introducing on-site physician staffing to intensive care units in hospitals other than teaching centres, it was found that survival improved among patients who had an intermediate likelihood of death[4]
- the relationship between volume and quality – for some types of intervention an association has been found, particularly for those that are more complex[5,6]
- the relationship between status and organisation of a hospital, such as teaching vs non-teaching or public vs private, and clinical outcome; although these relationships are complicated, important results can be obtained: for example, in one study, a 'positive correlation between higher mortality rates and hospitals located in States with strict prospective reimbursement programs' was found[7]
- the relationship between the organisation of a clinical service and clinical outcome: for example, better coordination was shown to be associated with lower mortality in intensive care,[8] and the admission of severely injured patients directly to an operating theatre was shown to reduce 'mortality, morbidity and suffering' in a cohort of patients followed for 9 years after a change in hospital organisation[9]
- the relationship between professional qualification and clinical outcome – in one study, higher levels of qualification were associated with better outcome,[5] but this finding may reflect a failure to train less highly qualified staff adequately.

It is possible to organise RCTs to assess the benefits of different types of service, such as a geriatric assessment service,[10] or of different methods of healthcare financing (for example, in one RCT the clinical outcomes of a health maintenance organisation and of a fee-for-service organisation were compared[11]). However, for many questions about the relationship between the funding and organisation of healthcare and patient outcomes, a well-conducted cohort study is one of the most appropriate types of research design. It is also possible to use interrupted time series (see Section 5.8) or a controlled before and after study (see Section 5.7) to investigate such questions.

In the funding or commissioning of research, the balance between promoting direct experimentation, through RCTs, and supporting observational studies, such as a survey of 'high cost patients in 17 acute-care hospitals',[12] must be reviewed continually.

5.6.1.1 The role of clinical databases

In a leader in the *British Medical Journal*, Black[13] called for the development of 'high quality clinical databases' which could provide a basis for either observational studies, such as cohort studies, or for RCTs. Databases in which all the cases of a particular type are collected – for example, patients who have leukaemia or all those who have been through intensive care – allow the entire population that has had a particular disorder, or experienced a particular level of care, to be identified and followed up. In Norway and Sweden, registers have now been developed to allow the follow-up of patients who have had a hip replacement. In fact, the Swedish register enables over 80 000 operations to be reviewed.[14] With the computerisation of patient records, such as the National Programme for IT (NPfIT) in England, the ease with which it is possible to undertake such follow-up will be greatly increased.

Some workers would also argue that such databases provide a better framework for research than RCTs, in which the focus is often on selected subsets of the population.

5.6.2   Searching

The best single Medline term for retrieving cohort studies is to explode the Medical Subject Heading (MeSH) Cohort Studies/ and combine it with your subject of interest. In many cases, it may not be necessary to search specifically for cohort studies because a search undertaken in the subject of interest will uncover them.

5.6.3   Appraisal

There are three study design features that are pivotal in the appraisal of any cohort study.

1. The recruitment of individuals
The most important aspect of recruitment is completeness: all of the subjects in a defined time-period should be recruited. If any sampling procedure has been applied to recruitment, such

as the recruitment of patients admitted either on weekdays or between 09.00 and 17.00 hours, it should create suspicion that the study results are biased. It can also be useful to ask: 'What happened to the patients who were not recruited?' It might be that the more severe cases were referred elsewhere, or those undertaking referral may have referred only mild cases to the hospitals in the study.

2. Study criteria

The criteria used to assess the outcomes of care must be valid. For example, in-patient mortality is not a valid criterion of the quality of hospital care because of variations in duration of patient stay; it is better to use a criterion such as 30- or 60-day mortality. If criteria other than mortality are used, the instruments used to measure variables, such as pain or quality of life, should be validated.

3. Analysis of results

In the analysis of results, the severity of illness should always be taken into account and receive explicit mention in the paper. For example, in studies of intensive care, there is a validated system for assessing the severity of a patient's condition, known as APACHE (acute physiology and chronic health evaluation).[8]

It is also important to control for the effects of co-morbidity, that is, the presence of other diseases that might have influenced outcome.[1] Robust techniques have been developed to do this and must have been applied to the clinical outcome if the results are to be accepted as valid.[15–17]

A checklist of questions that can be used in the appraisal of the findings of any cohort study is shown in Box 5.12.

Box 5.12 Checklist for appraising cohort studies

- Is clear information given about the way in which the cohort was recruited?
- Were any steps or decisions taken that could have included or excluded more severe cases?
- If mortality is a criterion, what steps were taken to ensure that all deaths were identified?
- If other criteria were used, have the instruments used for measurement been validated?
- Was the severity of disease taken into account in the analysis?
- Was the presence of other diseases (co-morbidity) taken into account in the analysis?

5.6.4   Uses and abuses

It is appropriate to use cohort studies:

- to assess changes in health service management or organisation
- to identify uncommon or adverse effects of treatment.

The main abuse of a cohort study is to assess the effectiveness of a particular intervention when a more appropriate method would be an RCT.

References

1. Greenfield, S., Aronow, H.U., Elashoff, R.M. et al. (1988) *Flaws in mortality data. The hazards of ignoring comorbid disease.* JAMA 260: 2253–5.
2. Fowler, F.J., Wennberg, J.E., Timothy, R.P., et al. (1988) *Symptom status and quality of life following prostatectomy.* JAMA 259: 3018–22.
3. Henderson, J., Goldacre, M.J., Graveney, M.J. et al. (1989) *Use of medical record linkage to study re-admission rate.* Br. Med. J. 299: 709–13.
4. Theodore, C.M., Phillips, M.C., Shaw, L. et al. (1984) *On-site physician staffing in a community hospital intensive care unit.* JAMA 252: 2023–7.
5. Kelly, J.V. and Hellinger, F.J. (1986) *Physician and hospital factors associated with mortality of surgical patients.* Med. Care 24: 785–800.
6. Kelly, J.V. and Hellinger, F.J. (1987) *Heart disease and hospital deaths: an empirical study.* Health Serv. Res. J. 22: 369–95.
7. Shortell, S.M. and Hughes, E.F.X. (1988) *The effects of regulation, competition and ownership on mortality rates among hospital inpatients.* N. Engl. J. Med. 318: 1100–7.
8. Knaus, W.A., Draper, E.A., Douglas, M.S. et al. (1986) *An evaluation of outcome from intensive care in major medical centers.* Ann. Intern. Med. 104: 410–18.
9. Fischer, R.P., Jelense, S. and Perry, J.F. Jr (1978) *Direct transfer to operating room improves care of trauma patients.* JAMA 240: 1731–2.
10. Stuck, A.E., Siu, A.L., Wieland, G.D. et al. (1993) *Comprehensive geriatric assessment: a meta-analysis of controlled trials.* Lancet 342: 1032–6.
11. Ware, J.E., Rodgers, W.H., Davies, A.R. et al. (1986) *Comparison of health outcomes at a health maintenance organisation with those of fee-for-service care.* Lancet i: 1017–22.
12. Schroeder, S.A., Showstack, J.A. and Roberts, H.E. (1979) *Frequency and clinical description of high-cost patients in 17 acute-care hospitals.* N. Engl. J. Med. 300: 1306–9.
13. Black, N. (1997) *Developing high quality clinical databases.* Br. Med. J. 315: 381–2.
14. Malchau, H., Herberts, P., Eisler, T. et al. (2002) *The Swedish Total Hip Replacement Register.* J. Bone Joint Surg. Am. 84(Suppl. 2): 2–20.
15. Knaus, W.A. and Nash, D.B. (1988) *Predicting and evaluating patient outcomes.* Ann. Intern. Med. 109: 521–2.
16. Seagroatt, V. and Goldacre, M.J. (1994) *Measures of early postoperative mortality beyond hospital fatality rates.* Br. Med. J. 309: 361–5.
17. Jencks, S.F. and Dobson, A. (1987) *Refining case-mix adjustment. The research evidence. [Special article]* N. Engl. J. Med. 317: 679–86.

5.7.1   Dimensions and definitions

A controlled before and after study is a quasi-experimental study design that can be used to investigate complex interventions.

In a controlled before and after study, there are at least two study groups:

- an intervention group
- a control group comparable to the intervention group.

Data are collected in both groups both before and after an intervention is administered to the intervention group. Apart from the intervention, the control group should experience the same secular, and any other sudden, changes as the intervention group. The scores on the outcome measure of interest between the intervention group and the control group before an intervention takes place are then compared with the scores in both groups after the intervention has occurred. This is referred to as the change score, and any observed differences between the groups are assumed to be due to the intervention (Fig. 5.3).

It is important that:

- data collection in the intervention and control groups is contemporaneous both before and after the intervention is applied to the intervention group

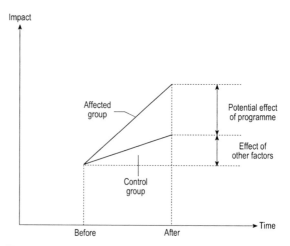

Fig. 5.3
Key attributes of a controlled before and after study design

- methods of data collection are the same for the intervention and control groups
- the control group is comparable to the intervention group in terms of population characteristics, performance and setting, which may include factors such as the reimbursement system, the level of care, and academic status. The inclusion of more than one comparable control group can help limit any confounding by site.

The reliability of the estimate of any effect is influenced by the existence of any unidentified differences between the intervention and control groups.

5.7.2   Searching

In many cases, it may not be advisable to search specifically for controlled before and after studies because a search undertaken in the subject of interest will uncover them. There are no search filters available to assist you in searching for before-after study designs, and including search terms to try and identify these types of studies may be restrictive. However, certain terms can be used to enable retrieval of appropriate studies:

- the Publication Type Comparative Study [pt]
- the MeSH Cross-Over Studies/ or Prospective Studies/
- the free text terms "before-after" or "crossover".

Using a combination of the above in your search will retrieve the highest number of appropriate study designs.

5.7.3   Appraisal

The main potential source of bias in a controlled before and after study is the degree to which the control group or groups is comparable to the intervention group. The level of comparability between the groups can be assessed by examining the baseline data. The greater the degree of imbalance between baselines, the greater will be the potential for bias.

Other potential sources of bias include:

- data collection in terms of contemporaneity and method(s)
- assessment of outcomes
- selection of outcome measures.

> **Box 5.13 Checklist of factors to consider when appraising the results of a controlled before and after study (Source: adapted from Cochrane Effective Practice and Organisation of Care Review Group)**
>
> 1. Was the control group (or groups) comparable to the intervention group in terms of:
>   – population characteristics?
>   – performance?
>   – setting?
> 2. Was data collection contemporaneous in the intervention and control groups?
> 3. Was the same method of data collection used in the intervention and control groups?
> 4. Were follow-up data collected for 80–100% of participants?
> 5. Was the assessment of outcomes blinded?
> 6. Are the outcome measures reliable?
> 7. Is it unlikely that the control group received the intervention?

A checklist for the appraisal of the results of a controlled before and after study is given in Box 5.13.

5.7.4   Uses and abuses

The main use of a controlled before and after study is to assess the impact of changes in health service organisation or policy. For instance, the effect on hospitalisation utilisation rates of capitation plus incentive payments was assessed in a controlled before and after study.[1] In this study, 39 physicians converted from fee-for-service to capitation payments during 1985–89 and 7 physicians remained with fee-for-service. Annual hospitalisation rates for all physicians were measured:

- 3 years before capitation
- 1 year before capitation
- 3 years after capitation.

The pattern of hospitalisation utilisation rates was found to be similar for both methods of payment.

The main methodological weakness of a controlled before and after study design is the difficulty in identifying a comparable control group. For example, it is possible that the intervention and control groups could experience different policy changes and/or other secular trends, which can be identified by differences in baseline measures between the two groups.

Reference

1. Hutchison, B., Birch, S., Hurley, J. et al. (1996) *Do physician payment mechanisms affect hospital utilization? A study of Health Service Organizations in Ontario.* Can. Med. Assoc. J. 154: 653–61.

5.8   Interrupted time series

5.8.1   Dimensions and definitions

An interrupted time series is a quasi-experimental study design that can be used to investigate complex interventions immediately and over time when randomisation is not possible or practical, such as a change in policy.

In an interrupted time series, the impact and/or effectiveness of an intervention on a population can be assessed against the pre-intervention trend (Fig. 5.4).[1] It is important that:

- the time at which the intervention occurs is clearly specified
- data are collected at a number of time-points to capture the point at which the intervention is expected to have an effect
- data collected before the intervention should enable any underlying trend to be observed

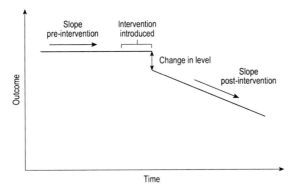

Fig. 5.4
Key attributes of an interrupted time series study design
(Source: England[1])

Margin Note 5.3
Types of interrupted time series (ITS) study design
(Source: England[1])

- Simple ITS – one experimental group with multiple observations before and after the intervention.
- ITS with a non-equivalent, no-intervention control group.
- ITS with non-equivalent dependent variables – data collection involves variables that should be affected by the intervention and those that should not.
- ITS with removed intervention – subjecting an experimental group to an intervention and taking measurements, and then removing the intervention and taking measurements.
- ITS with switching replications – involves two non-equivalent experimental groups: when one acts as a control the other receives the intervention and then when the previous control group receives the intervention the previous intervention group acts as the control.
- Short ITS – involves a total of <40 measurements pre-test and post-test.

- data collected after the intervention should allow any underlying secular trend to be observed in addition to the effect of the intervention.

Analysis using an interrupted time series design can be prospective or retrospective.

5.8.2 Searching

In many cases, it may not be advisable to search specifically for interrupted time series study designs because a search undertaken in the subject of interest will uncover them. There are no search filters available to assist you in searching for time series studies, and including search terms to try and identify these types of studies may be restrictive. However, certain terms can be used to enable retrieval of appropriate studies:

- the MeSH Time Factors/ or Time/
- the free text terms "interrupted time series" or simply "time series" (less restrictive).

Using a combination of the above in your search will retrieve the highest number of appropriate study designs.

5.8.3 Appraisal

The first step in appraising an interrupted time series is to be able to identify the point at which the intervention occurred. In addition, there should be at least three pre-intervention and three post-intervention data points, depending on the type of intervention.
Interrupted time series can be affected by:

- residual selection bias
- external influences on outcome
- secular changes
- maturation effects, for example, if the intervention being evaluated is a technique requiring training and a set of skills.

A checklist for reviewing an interrupted time series study is shown in Box 5.14.

5.8.4 Uses and abuses

The main use of an interrupted time series is to assess the effect of an area-wide intervention, for example, guideline

---

Box 5.14 Checklist of factors to consider when appraising the results of a interrupted time series study (Source: adapted from Cochrane Effective Practice and Organisation of Care Review Group)

1. Was the intervention independent of other changes? Consider the following sources of bias:
   - seasonal (were any potential seasonal factors identified and removed during analysis?)
   - historical (were there appropriate controls to assess the effect of factors other than the intervention on the results? Did any other events occur that might impact on the outcomes?)
   - selection (was the intervention group representative of the study population? Did the composition of the intervention group change at the time of the intervention?)
   - instrumentation (was there a change in the way data were recorded or observed?)
   - construct (were the outcome measures appropriate? This is particularly important if archive data were used for the baseline.)
   - external (can the outcome be generalised and applied to other conditions or populations?)
   - maturational (was the effect of experience measured and accounted for in evaluating the effect of the intervention?)
   - Statistical (how many data points were collected before and after the intervention?)
2. Were the data analysed appropriately?
3. Was the reason for the number and spacing of pre- and post-intervention points given?
4. Was the shape of the intervention effect specified?
5. Was the intervention unlikely to have affected data collection?
6. Was the assessment of the outcome blinded?
7. How complete is the data set?
8. Is the outcome measure reliable?

---

implementation strategies in primary care or a mass media campaign. It is not possible to assess the impact of any concurrent events on the outcomes of interest.

Reference

1. England, E. (2005) *How interrupted time series can evaluate guideline implementation*. Pharm. J. 275: 344–7.

5.9   Surveys

5.9.1   Dimensions and definitions

A survey is an investigation of what is happening at a
point in, or during a period of, time. For example, in a
survey of 61 US hospitals in which the approaches to
quality improvement were investigated in relation to an
objective measure of clinical efficiency (length of stay),
it was found that the most important determinant of
quality was the management culture within a hospital
rather than the specific quality improvement techniques
utilised.[1]

To increase the power of a survey, it can be combined
with statistical analysis. For example, in a study of the
factors that promoted or hindered physician satisfaction
with the hospital in which they worked, regression analysis
was conducted on the survey results.[2]

However, the best way to increase the validity of a
survey is to repeat it either after a period of time has elapsed
or after some intervention has been undertaken: this type
of study, in which a group of people, patients or service
providers is followed over a period of time, is called a
cohort study (see Section 5.6). Surveys, however, give the
fastest return on investment.

5.9.2   Searching

The appropriate technique for searching for surveys
will depend on the subject of the survey that you
require. It is common practice to use the Medical Subject
Heading (MeSH) Health Surveys/ but it may need to be
supplemented by an additional MeSH (e.g. Mortality/,
Birth Rate/, Vital Statistics/, Demography/, Morbidity/,
Incidence/, Prevalence/). It is also possible to use the
subject of the survey, such as a disease with a subheading
such as epidemiology or mortality (e.g. Coronary Disease/
epidemiology), or an intervention with a subheading such
as statistics and numerical data, trends or utilisation (e.g.
Coronary Angiography/statistics and numerical data).
The MeSH Health Care Surveys/ can be used to search for
statistical measures of utilisation and other aspects of the
provision of healthcare services including hospitalisation
and ambulatory care.

5.9.3 Appraisal

Gentle Reader,

Visualise Great Tew, a village that lies on the side of an Oxfordshire hill, where the cottages are thatched and the pub serves real ale. In 1066, it was owned by the Bishop of Bayeux, who was landlord to 42 souls. Fascinating detail about the mills, meadows and pasturage of Great Tew can be found in the Domesday Book, the first great survey of England, when King William I 'sent men all over England to find out … what or how much each landowner held … in land and livestock and what it was worth'.

The survey commissioners were required to take evidence on oath, and four Frenchmen and four Englishmen from each hundred were sworn to verify the detail. In addition, a second set of commissioners was sent out 'to shires they did not know, or they were themselves unknown, to check their predecessors' survey and report culprits to the King'.

Commentary

Not only was the survey of 1085 thorough, but King William also recognised that the quality of a survey, even the most comprehensive conducted by the highest authority, needed to be appraised.

A checklist for the appraisal of surveys is shown in Box 5.15.

5.9.4 Uses and abuses

The appropriate uses of a survey are:
- to obtain a snapshot of a service at a specific point in time
- to study complicated situations
- to determine the acceptability of an intervention to patients.

Box 5.15 Checklist for the appraisal of a survey

- How was the population to be surveyed chosen? Was it the whole population or a sample?
- If a sample, how was the sample chosen? Was it a random sample or was it stratified to ensure that all sectors of the population were represented?
- Was a validated questionnaire used? Did the authors of the survey mention the possibility of different results being obtained by different interviewers, if interviewers were used?
- What procedures were used to verify the data?
- Were the conclusions drawn from the survey all based on the data or did those carrying out the survey infer conclusions? *Inference is acceptable, but it must be clearly distinguished from results derived solely from the data.*

Although it is possible to identify the existence of problems during a survey, it is difficult to determine the cause(s) of those problems; additional research is often required in such a situation.

It is not possible to use a survey to measure any changes over time.

References

1. Shortell, S.M., O'Brien, J.L., Carman, J.M. et al. (1995) *Assessing the impact of continuous quality improvement/total quality management: concept versus implementation.* Health Serv. Res. J. 30: 377–401.
2. Burns, L.R., Andersen, R.M. and Shortell, S.M. (1990) *The effect of hospital control strategies on physician satisfaction and physician hospital conflict.* Health Serv. Res. J. 25: 527–60.

5.10 Qualitative research

5.10.1 Dimensions and definitions

Qualitative research can be used to gain an understanding of health and health services, and as such has a role to play in a science-based health service. The basic disciplines of qualitative research are social anthropology and sociology.

The other types of research methodologies described in this chapter (Sections 5.4–5.9) are examples of quantitative research, the basic disciplines of which are epidemiology, biostatistics, psychology and economics. Although each of these two types of research is fiercely defended by its proponents, there is much common ground for agreement and increasingly health service professionals are beginning to understand that both qualitative and quantitative research are necessary.

Qualitative research has two main functions:

1. To comprise part of a research programme that has qualitative and quantitative components. Sometimes quantitative research is preceded by qualitative work; for example, in the design of a study to identify the reasons why different services have different rates of intervention – in this case, it is appropriate to conduct structured or semi-structured interviews with lead consultants and managers to help design the quantitative research protocol. Similarly, in the preparation of patient questionnaires, it is often useful to discuss with focus groups of patients what they perceive to be

the useful outcomes of treatment, otherwise outcomes chosen by clinicians and research workers might bear little relation to what is important to patients.

2. To complement quantitative research; for example, to capture information that complements data obtained from patient questionnaires, and which can increase the validity of the information obtained using quantitative methods.

However, qualitative research should not be regarded as merely a complement and supplement to quantitative research. It can often be used to generate hypotheses for the solution of a problem, which can then be tested using either quantitative methods, by building on the findings of the qualitative research, or a combination of qualitative and quantitative methods. The relationship between qualitative and quantitative research methods is shown in Fig. 5.5.

The defining features of a qualitative research study are shown in Box 5.16. The types of question best answered by qualitative research are shown in Box 5.17, most of which are related to people's behaviour, beliefs and attitudes.

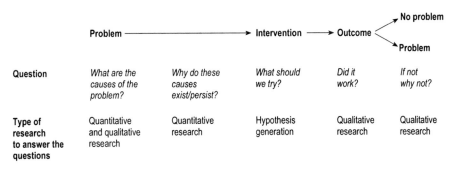

Fig. 5.5
The relationship between quantitative and qualitative research

---

Box 5.16 The defining features of a qualitative research study

- An explicit peer-reviewed protocol.
- Ethics committee approval.
- A theoretical framework.
- A clear project-management protocol.
- A means of identifying whether there are biases in the collection of information or drawing of conclusions.

> **Box 5.17 Examples of questions it is appropriate to address using qualitative research methods**
>
> • Why is it that people continue to smoke when the evidence about the harmful effects of smoking is incontrovertible and known to a proportion of those who smoke?
> • Why do people not take the medicine prescribed for them?
> • Why do clinicians adopt innovations of unproven effectiveness and of unknown effect while failing to adopt innovations of proven effectiveness?
> • Why are nurses and doctors not able to work with one another with ease?
> • What difference has the involvement of doctors in management made to the management of health services?

5.10.2   Searching

Medline has no Medical Subject Headings (MeSH) that adequately encompass the concept of qualitative research. It is probable that a higher yield of qualitative research articles will be obtained when searching nursing and allied health databases, such as CINAHL or the British Nursing Index. CINAHL uses a number of methodological index terms to describe qualitative research articles.

There have been few formal evaluations of the effectiveness of different search strategies (i.e. search 'filters') for retrieving qualitative research. In one study, three different search filters were compared for their capacity to retrieve qualitative research from CINAHL,[1] and it was found that a combination of strategies including thesaurus (e.g. Interviews/) and free text (e.g. "qualitative", "findings", "grounded theory") terms is necessary to maximise recall; the outcome of using a high-recall search strategy is poor precision.

5.10.3   Appraisal

The first step in appraisal is to determine whether the use of qualitative research in a study was appropriate.[2] The second step is to judge the quality of the qualitative research. As there are now good sources of information about qualitative research methods, it is possible to draw up criteria that can be used to judge quality. A checklist for the appraisal of qualitative research is shown in Box 5.18.

Box 5.18 Checklist for the appraisal of qualitative research

- Was the research question clearly identified?
- Was the setting in which the research took place clearly described?
- If sampling was undertaken, were the sampling methods described?
- Did the research workers address the issues of subjectivity and data collection?
- Were methods to test the validity of the results of the research used?
- Were any steps taken to increase the reliability of the information collected, for example, by repeating the information collection with another research worker?
- Were the results of the research kept separate from the conclusions drawn by the research workers?
- If quantitative methods were appropriate as a supplement to the qualitative methods, were they used?

5.10.4 Uses and abuses

The main use of qualitative research is to gain an understanding of the working of any health service, which is particularly important to those who must make decisions about groups of patients or populations.

The main abuse of qualitative research methods is to evaluate the effectiveness or safety of an intervention; in this situation, it is necessary to use quantitative methods.

References

1. Shaw, R.L., Booth, A., Sutton, A.J. et al. (2004) *Finding qualitative research: an evaluation of search strategies*. BMC Med. Res. Methodol. 4: 5.
2. Mays, N. and Pope, C. (1996) *Qualitative Research in Health Care*. BMJ Publishing Group, London.

5.11   Decision analysis

In evidence-based healthcare, although decisions are based on a careful appraisal of the best evidence available, how is that evidence incorporated into the decision-making process? One approach is to discuss any evidence in the context of information on the resources available and the needs or values of the population under consideration. A more systematic approach is to describe the evidence that must be taken into account in addition to estimating the impact of any of the various options available – this approach is known as decision analysis.

5.11.1   Dimensions and definitions

Lilford and Royston[1] have described decision analysis as:

> … the bridge from knowledge to action. To inform action, empirical or theory-based knowledge about the effects of actions must be set into a 'real-world' context where some facts are uncertain, where information must be brought together from disparate sources and where decisions must be based not only on professional expertise but also on patient preferences. Decision Analysis provides a framework for doing this and can thus help bridge the gap between knowledge and action. The Decision Analysis bridge can be traversed in both directions: one way to help translate existing knowledge into action; the other to indicate what new knowledge is needed to inform action.

Decision analysis is a technique that enables a quantification to be made of the effects or impacts of the different options involved in any decision. However, most decisions are not a simple choice between option A or option B because option A and option B may have different consequences. Decision analysis usually involves:

- establishing a set of objectives and settling upon the relative importance of each, that is, their utility or value
- identifying alternative courses of action
- establishing the likely outcomes of these actions, together with the probability of each of them occurring.

The analysis of a decision can be expressed as a 'decision tree' in which the consequences of various decisions are displayed together with the probability of each event occurring. To construct a decision tree, it is necessary to use the appropriate computer software. It is also important to base any decision tree on robust information about the natural history of the condition under discussion, and on good evidence about the effects of different interventions.

Once a decision tree has been constructed, it is possible to incorporate values. Patients or members of the public can be asked to assign values to the good and bad outcomes of a decision, otherwise known as utilities and disutilities, respectively. A decision tree for screening for Down's syndrome for a population of 100000 pregnancies is shown

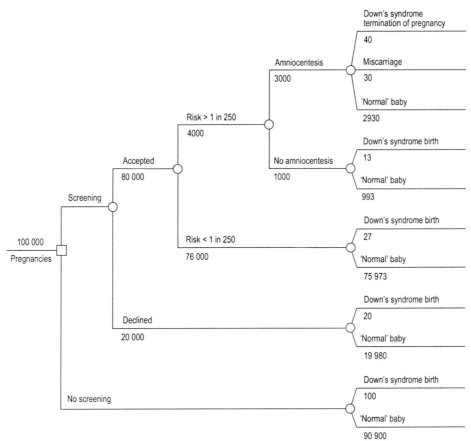

Fig. 5.6
Decision tree for Down's syndrome screening for a population of 100 000 pregnancies (Source: Thornton and Lilford,[2] with permission, BMJ Publishing Group)

in Fig. 5.6.[2] Values were assigned to the outcomes by women who participated in the study. A value of 0 was given to a healthy live-birth and a value of 1 to a Down's syndrome live-birth; miscarriage as a result of amniocentesis and a termination because of Down's syndrome were each given a weighting of 0.3.

To calculate the course of minimum expected disutility for any branch of a decision tree, the probabilities are multiplied by the disutilities. To use the example shown in Fig. 5.7: without screening, 100 Down's syndrome babies would be born. On the basis of various assumptions (shown in Fig. 5.7), screening would detect 40 Down's syndrome babies (terminations) and 30 women would miscarry

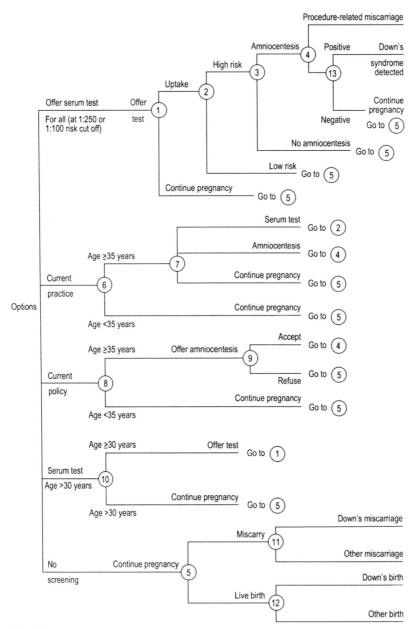

Fig. 5.7
Decision tree for five screening policies for detecting Down's syndrome before birth
(Source: Fletcher et al.,[3] with permission, BMJ Publishing Group)

healthy babies as a result of amniocentesis. Therefore the
expected disutility of a screening programme is:

40 terminations because of Down's syndrome + 30 miscarriages
because of amniocentesis × 0.3 = 21

The expected disutility of not screening for Down's
syndrome is:

40 Down's syndrome births × 1.0 = 40

Thus, screening results in a net gain of 19 'utility units'.
The same technique can also be used to compare different
screening policies. The decision tree in Fig. 5.7 shows the
impacts of five different screening policies for detecting
Down's syndrome before birth,[3] the decision analysis of which
included financial cost but not disutilities. It also included
sensitivity analysis, which enables the effect of variations in
one or more of the variables, such as the cost of ultrasound or
the specificity of the serum test, to be examined.

A case-study of a decision analysis used to investigate the
management options for large dental restoration is given in
Section 9.6.2.

5.11.2   Searching

Search for decision analysis articles using the Medical
Subject Heading (MeSH) Decision Support Techniques/.

5.11.3   Appraisal

A checklist of questions useful in the appraisal of the quality
of a decision analysis is shown in Box 5.19.

Critical appraisal of a decision analysis will necessitate
an assessment of the original parameters used to perform
the analysis. For example, the decision analysis in which the
impacts of various screening policies for detecting Down's
syndrome were compared[3] was subject to the following
criticisms:

- the assumption of an uptake of 75% for amniocentesis
  was overoptimistic[4]
- age-specific values for sensitivity and specificity were not
  used[5]
- the costs were overestimated[6]
- the detection rates and the false-positive rates were too low.[7]

> **Box 5.19** Checklist for the appraisal of a decision analysis
>
> - What proportion of the branches in the decision tree represent good data based on good-quality research?
> - If utilities have been used, were they based on surveys of people with the health problem, surveys of a sample of the general population, or estimates of the author's personal values?
> - Has sensitivity analysis been performed to determine whether the estimate of effectiveness used in the decision analysis is higher or lower than the true level of effectiveness?
> - Has sensitivity analysis been performed to determine whether the estimate of the incidence of side-effects is higher or lower than the true incidence of side-effects?
> - Has sensitivity analysis been performed to test the analysis at estimates of financial cost higher or lower than the cost estimates used in the decision analysis?
> - Has sensitivity analysis been used to test the effect of higher or lower utilities being assigned to different options?
> - Have all the costs that should be taken into account been included?

Although Fletcher et al. dealt with these criticisms,[8] they pointed out that:

> One of the advantages of using decision analysis as a tool for considering the consequences of different screening policies is that the assumptions and numerical values on which the model's predictions are based are explicit. If there is debate about the assumptions or the numbers that should be used in the calculations it is easy to recalculate the model with the new numbers.

A critical approach to decision analysis therefore does not necessarily reveal flaws in the technique, but instead helps to clarify any assumptions that may have been implicit or 'fudged' (Fig. 5.8), and can be used to improve the decision analysis through an iterative process.

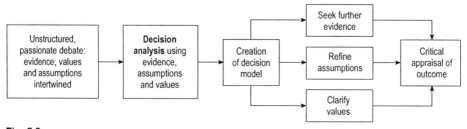

Fig. 5.8
The iterative process of decision analysis

5.11.4   Uses and abuses

The main use of decision analysis is to provide a decision-maker with an estimate of the impact an intervention may have on the population or group of patients for whom it is intended.

It should *not* be used to evaluate the effectiveness of an intervention

References

1. Lilford, R. and Royston, G. (1998) *Decision analysis in the selection, design and application of clinical and health services research.* J. Health Serv. Res. Policy 3: 159–66.
2. Thornton, J.G. and Lilford, R.J. (1995) *Decision analysis for medical managers.* Br. Med. J. 310: 791–4.
3. Fletcher, J., Hicks, N.R., Kay, J.D.S. (1995) *Using decision analysis to compare policies for antenatal screening for Down's syndrome.* Br. Med. J. 311: 351–6.
4. Murray, D. and Tennison, B. (1995) *'Decision analysis and screening for Down's syndrome.' Estimate of uptake of amniocentesis is overoptimistic. [Letter]* Lancet 311: 1371.
5. Spencer, K. (1995) *'Decision analysis and screening for Down's syndrome.' Not using age specific values invalidates study. [Letter]* Lancet 311: 1371–2.
6. Reynolds, T.M. (1995) *'Decision analysis and screening for Down's syndrome.' Costs were overestimated. [Letter]* Lancet 311: 1372.
7. Wald, N.J., Kennard, A., Watt, H. et al. (1995) *'Decision analysis and screening for Down's syndrome.' Testing should be in all women. [Letter]* Lancet 311: 1372.
8. Fletcher, J., Hicks, N.R., Kay, J.D.S. et al. (1995) *'Decision analysis and screening for Down's syndrome.' Authors' reply. [Letter]* Lancet 311: 1372–3.

Gentle Reader,

Empathise with the doctor. He turned his head to respond to the greeting, and was shocked to find himself looking at what appeared to be a statue carved in Carrara marble: sheets, cover, pillowslip, hair, face, all white.

'How are you, doctor?' the occupant of the bed asked cheerily.

The doctor struggled to recall the face, one of so many seen in a hectic year during the course of two busy surgical jobs.

'How are you?' said the doctor, dissembling well and still trying to recollect where he had seen the face before.

'I'm fine, doctor,' said the patient 'but it doesn't seem like 5 months since I was last admitted. I've had such good care throughout.'

Five months, last March, vascular surgery: the face came back, but not the name.

'That's a long time', said the doctor.

'Yes, but it's been wonderful whatever he's done, although I'm still trying to get used to this', replied the patient, waving his hand at the unnaturally narrow mound in the bed where two legs should have lain but now there was only one.

Back in the ward office, the doctor reviewed the case notes. The man had come in for a routine aortic graft. Although he had had symptoms of claudication, they were not very severe. No one had recommended the effective and safe therapy of exercise, which should be standard practice before the knife is considered. The patient's first operation had been uneventful, but 7 days later he had thrown off a clot that had blocked the artery to his left leg. After two more operations, the leg had been amputated. During his recovery from the amputation, he had developed a venous thrombosis in the remaining leg and suffered a severe pulmonary embolus. While he was still seriously ill from the pulmonary embolus, another clot had formed, this time in the artery leading to his intestine, and part of his intestine had been removed, leaving him with malabsorption.

He was now medically stable, waiting for a rehabilitation bed, and a place in the unit where amputees are helped to adjust to, and cope with, the loss of a limb.

Commentary

Perhaps it is unwise to speak of the outcome of care as if there is only one; there are frequently many outcomes, even though each clinician may see only one. The patient described in this prologue had thought that his initial operation was absolutely necessary, and he was tremendously grateful for what he considered to be a life-saving act. Each of the various clinicians who had seen the patient during his progress through the healthcare system had formed their own opinion about the effectiveness, appropriateness and cost-effectiveness of the care he had received, and the outcomes of that care, at each stage of the patient's perilous journey.

Assessing the outcomes found

6.1 Five key questions about outcomes

Once it has been established that the research is of sufficiently good quality for the outcomes of that research to be included within the framework of the decision, those outcomes must be assessed. There are five key questions about outcomes:

1. How many outcomes were studied?
2. How large were the effects found?
3. With what degree of confidence can the results of the research be applied to the whole population?
4. Does the intervention do more good than harm?
5. How relevant are the results to the local population or service about which the decision is being made?

For the clinician, there is also a sixth question:

6. How relevant is the research to this particular patient?

6.1.1 How many outcomes were studied?

The proposition that an intervention is 'effective' implies that there is only one outcome of care and only one objective in the design of that intervention. This is rarely the case. There are various outcomes of disease, and, if effective care is given, these outcomes may be ameliorated or improved (Table 6.1).

Although in Table 6.1 the beneficial outcomes of care have been presented, the possibility that adverse effects may also occur must always be considered. The balance between good and harmful effects of treatment should be weighed very carefully.

6.1.2 How large were the effects found?

There are two dimensions to the question 'How large were the effects found?':

1. What proportion of patients benefit?

Table 6.1 The outcomes of disease

Outcomes of untreated disease	Outcomes of effective care of disease
Death	Lower morbidity
Disability	Functional ability improved
Disease status deteriorates and risk of complications increases	Disease status improves and risk of complications decreases
Distress about effects of disease	Feeling better

2. What is the degree of benefit for the individual who does benefit?

- For a group of patients, magnitude of effect is usually expressed as the odds ratio (see Section 6.4.3.1).
- For individual patients, benefit is measured by the magnitude of the effect, which ranges from no effect to complete cure.

The odds ratio is the ratio of the frequency of the key event, such as mortality, in the group receiving treatment to the frequency of the key event in the control group.

6.1.2.1 Which yardstick?

In a situation where a condition was previously untreatable, any new treatment must be compared with a placebo in trials.

If a treatment for the condition is already available, it is important to compare the new treatment with that already in use to identify any differences in the effectiveness, safety, acceptability and cost between the two. This may seem self-evident, but sometimes a difference in any of these criteria does not exist.

Some trials, particularly those funded by the pharmaceutical industry, are designed to compare a new treatment with placebo irrespective of whether other therapies for that condition are already available; using this strategy, it is possible to give the impression that the new treatment may be more effective than it actually is.

6.1.3 With what degree of confidence can the results of the research be applied to the whole population?

Research studies produce results, but these results are not necessarily the answer to the decision faced by the decision-maker. Research is always conducted on a sample of the population of interest; for example, even in a mega-trial of myocardial infarction in which 46 000 patients are enrolled, those 46 000 comprise only a sample of the millions of people who will have a heart attack. Thus, a well-designed research study generates information about what happens only when the group of patients in that study is given a treatment; it must not be assumed that the results of the study can be applied automatically to the whole population.

The degree to which the results of any study are generalisable can be expressed as a probability, both numerically and diagrammatically, using confidence intervals. The results of individual research studies are shown as single points in Fig. 6.1. However, each of the results plotted is only an estimate of the true effect as each study was done on a sample of the population. Although each sample could represent the whole population perfectly, the method of sampling always introduces errors. It is possible, however, to estimate with a certain degree of assurance the range of values within which the true result actually lies; this range is known as the confidence interval.

It is usual practice to calculate the 95% confidence intervals, which indicate there is a 95% probability that the effect of treatment in the whole population would lie within the range of values. The larger the sample of the population studied, the narrower will be the range of values within the confidence intervals (Box 6.1).

An alternative way to express this is that there is a 1 in 20 chance that the effect in the whole population will lie outside this range. Although it is possible to calculate narrower confidence intervals, for example, 99%, these

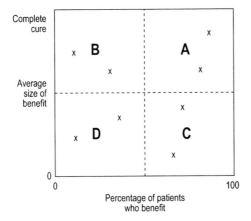

Fig. 6.1
Results of research studies. X represents the result for a single therapy; A represents good value, D poor value. If the effect is in either B or C, the judgement is more difficult

> **Box 6.1 Confidence intervals**
>
> - The larger the sample of patients, the narrower will be the confidence intervals.
> - The narrower the range of the confidence intervals, the greater will be the degree of confidence about the general applicability of the results.
> - If both ends of the range of confidence intervals lie on the side of the line which indicates that treatment does more good than harm, then we can be 95% confident that the true value lies within the interval.

often produce such a wide range of results that the preferred convention is to use 95% confidence intervals (Fig. 6.2).

It can be seen from Fig. 6.3 that, for high-risk patients, even if the result of the research is, by chance, more optimistic than the true effect in the whole population, the intervention is effective because there is a clear benefit at the lowest end of the confidence intervals – point B. For individuals at low risk, even if the result of the research is, by chance, more pessimistic than the true effect, the intervention is ineffective because there is no benefit at the highest end of the confidence intervals – point C. For those at medium risk, it would be unwise to generalise from these results because the range in which the true effect lies includes both ends of the confidence interval, indicating that the intervention might be either beneficial or harmful.

It is possible to estimate the number of patients required to ensure that a trial will be of sufficient size to produce a definite result. This is known as estimating the power of a trial (see Box 6.2 for the power rules).

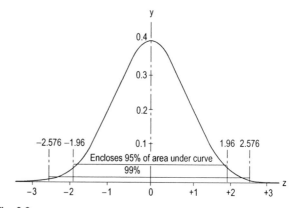

Fig. 6.2
A normal distribution curve

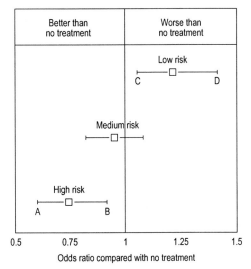

Fig. 6.3
Rate of coronary events in individuals receiving cholesterol-lowering
treatments divided by rate of coronary events in individuals not
receiving treatment, shown with 95% confidence intervals
(Source: adapted from Bandolier 1995; 5: 4)

Box 6.2 Power rules

- The smaller the effect predicted, the larger the trial required to produce a result.
- The larger the trial, the greater the power.
- The greater the power, the narrower the confidence intervals.
- If the power calculations are correct and the size of the beneficial effect is as predicted, both ends of the confidence interval will lie on the same side of the line as the result.

6.1.4   Does the intervention do more good than harm?

When an intervention has beneficial effects, it is
important not only to record their existence but also to
indicate the probability of both good and harm occurring.
Few treatments benefit every patient and the balance of
good and harm should always be estimated (Fig. 6.4).

One of the many ways in which Scottish law is better
fitted for purpose than English is the possibility of a verdict
in addition to those of 'guilty' and 'not guilty', that of 'not
proven' – a judgement of the strength of evidence. Similarly,
in evidence-based healthcare, rather than classifying

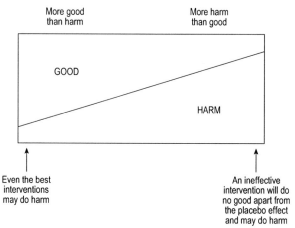

Fig. 6.4
The balance of good and harm

interventions as either 'effective' or 'ineffective', it is more accurate to classify them as:

- proven to do more good than harm – 'not guilty'
- proven to do more harm than good – 'guilty'
- of unproven effect – 'not proven'.

It must always be borne in mind that because an intervention has not been shown to be effective does not mean that it is ineffective, but neither can it be assumed to do more good than harm. Such an intervention should be evaluated in a well-designed research study.

6.1.5   How relevant are the results to the local population or service?

In protocols for research studies, especially trials, the criteria for the inclusion and exclusion of patients are stipulated. The use of these criteria ensures that a homogeneous group of patients is selected from which the intervention and control groups are randomised. However, this selection of a study population raises problems; for instance, how applicable are the results of a study of the treatment of heart failure in patients under the age of 75 years to patients who are over the age of 75 years? One way to increase the applicability of the findings would be to use less stringent inclusion criteria, thereby decreasing the proportion of patients excluded from the trial, but this strategy may also reduce the validity of the trial.

If certain results are considered to be applicable to the whole population, could they also be relevant to any local population that is the subject of a decision? Is a study of primary care in the Netherlands relevant to Northampton? Is the treatment given in a teaching hospital in Canada relevant to a district general hospital in Kent? A checklist of questions that can be used to assess the relevance of research findings to the local population is shown in Box 6.3.

6.2   Measuring outcomes

6.2.1   Problems and pitfalls of performance measurement

During the last decade of the 20th century, there was great enthusiasm for outcome measurement. However, there are many difficulties associated with the use of outcome measures. In an important article, David Eddy has identified the reasons why it is difficult to measure healthcare quality and outcome.[1] He divides the problems into two types: natural problems and man-made problems. It is possible to rectify the latter, whereas it is possible only to work around the former.

6.2.1.1 Natural problems

- *Probability factor*: almost all health outcomes are probabilistic, that is, it is not possible to guarantee a good

---

Box 6.3 Checklist for assessing the relevance of research findings to the local population

1. Does the population in the study differ from the local population in ways that are likely to be important, such as:
   - genetic composition?
   - health status, e.g. is there a higher or lower prevalence of risk factors of disease in the local population?
   - beliefs and attitudes, e.g. is the local population likely to be more or less compliant with invitations to attend for screening?
2. Does the local healthcare service have the potential to reproduce the service provided in the trial?
3. Could a similar level of resources as that available to the research workers be channelled into the local service?
4. Are the skills to deliver a service of adequate quality available locally? If not, is it possible to develop those skills at an affordable cost?

outcome for every patient, therefore measures of quality need to give some indication that probabilistic factors are being monitored, e.g. using probability or *P* values when expressing the difference between two services.

- *Low frequency*: many important health problems occur at a low frequency at the level of service management; for example, cervical cancer is rare at the level of the individual screening programme, although it is a major problem nationally.
- *Long delays*: it may take 5–10 years to detect and therefore measure a clinical outcome; this affects not only the feasibility of measurement but also its usefulness to the manager or clinician. For example, there will be a lapse of time before potential changes in the incidence of stroke become manifest following the introduction of a hypertension control programme.
- *Control over outcomes*: other factors may influence the outcome. For example, the prevalence of smoking is determined not only by the effectiveness of a health education programme but also by taxation policy.
- *Level of clinical detail*: this relates to the imprecision of clinical concepts; in order to derive an appropriate measure, it is necessary to have an operational definition of the disease under investigation, but this will differ among the various clinicians involved in any one service.
- *Comprehensibility*: some biological outcomes and process measures are not comprehensible in terms of the outcomes about which patients are concerned.

6.2.1.2 Man-made problems

Man-made problems are consequent upon the way in which a healthcare system has evolved:

- *Inadequate information systems*: systems that do not have the capacity to measure what they are intended to measure.
- *Too many measurers and measures*: for example, different sectors within the performance management system may request different measures of performance.

The two other man-made problems that Eddy identifies are *health plan complexity* and *funding*, both of which are specific to the US healthcare system.

It is also possible to add *inconsistency* or *lack of continuity* to Eddy's list of man-made problems, i.e. those responsible for measuring performance may change the measures to be used from year to year.

6.2.1.3 Resurgence of outcome measures in the measurement of quality

Despite the problems with outcome measures outlined above, a growing number of outcome measures relevant to patients has been developed. With the introduction of electronic patient records, the reporting and recording of patient-relevant outcomes is now feasible. In their book, *Redefining Health Care*,[2] Porter and Teisberg advocate the use of outcome measures as one of the essential contributions to better quality healthcare.

6.2.2   In praise of process

As the use of outcome measures for managing services is beset with many difficulties, many people prefer to use evidence-based process measures (Margin Fig. 6.1), i.e. measures of processes for which there is good evidence that if such processes were applied consistently the required outcome would be achieved. Indeed, in a recent paper by Peterson et al.[3] the authors describe a significant association between care process and outcomes.

The work conducted by the Institute of Healthcare Improvement (IHI) in the USA has underlined the need for process measurement to help realise quality improvement, and for taking action when process measures indicate cause for concern.[4]

For a more detailed discussion of the use of process measures in the assessment of quality, see Section 6.8.1.1.

Process

Chance

Outcome

Good process   ≠   Good outcome
(but it helps)

Margin Fig. 6.1

References

1. Eddy, D.M. (1998) *Performance measurement problems and solutions.* Health Aff. 17: 7–26.
2. Porter, M.E. and Teisberg, E.O. (2006) *Redefining Health Care. Creating Value-Based Competition on Results.* Harvard Business School Press, Boston, Massachusetts.
3. Peterson, E.D., Roe, M.T., Mulgung, J. et al. (2006) *Association between hospital process performance and outcomes among patients with acute coronary syndromes.* JAMA 295: 1912–20.
4. Berwick, D.M. and Nolan, T.W. (1998) *Physicians as leaders in improving health care: a new series in Annals of Internal Medicine.* Ann. Intern. Med. 128: 289–92.

6.3   Equity

Equity: 1. *The quality of being equal or fair; impartiality; even-handed dealing.* 2. *That which is fair and right …*
Shorter Oxford English Dictionary

To do equyte and justice.

William Caxton

Equity was my crowne.

Job, xxix.14

6.3.1   Dimensions and definitions

The definition of equity has occupied philosophers for many years; indeed, there is no simple definition. However, one of the objectives of the NHS, explicit at the time of its institution and still implicit in many of the decisions made, is to provide equity of care in relation to assessed need. Equity, therefore, is different to equality; no one would argue that different patient groups should have equal shares of NHS resources. Equity implies social justice, and fairness is one of the values on which NHS commissioning decisions are based.

The Cochrane Collaboration has now instituted a Cochrane Equity Field, which hosted a working session to develop guidelines for Cochrane review authors who assess equity issues as part of their systematic reviews. The Cochrane Equity Field based their definition on Whitehead's,[1] as 'unfair and avoidable differences in health'.

In the workshop, the acronym PROGRESS was used to identify factors that are a potential source of disadvantage (Box 6.4)[2] while recognising that other factors might also be important, e.g. age, sexual orientation, disability and HIV/AIDS status, but that it was not possible to fit them neatly into the framework of the chosen acronym. The Cochrane Collaboration Equity Field will work together with the Campbell Collaboration Equity Methods Group to assess the effect of interventions on health disparities and health equity.[3]

Box 6.4 Equity factors (Source: Robinson[2])

- Place of residence
- Race
- Occupation
- Gender
- Religion/culture
- Education
- Socio-economic status
- Social capital

The development of increasingly sophisticated healthcare interventions, such as those which depend on patient participation (e.g. cognitive behavioural therapy), have the potential to increase health inequality.

6.3.1.1 Measuring equity

Although social justice, or fairness, is felt keenly by everyone, can it be measured? Cost-utility analysis is a form of economic appraisal in which the quality-adjusted life year (QALY) is used as an outcome measure. It is theoretically possible to calculate the total number of QALYs provided for each patient group by a purchaser: *if* the QALY were a perfect measure of health benefit and *if* the purchaser had achieved perfect equity, the total number of QALYs for each patient group would be the same. Such an exercise might be impossible to undertake owing to the amount of effort it would require, and might be spurious given the imperfections inherent in the QALY as a measure.

6.3.1.2 Assessing equity: evidence-based cuts at the margin

There is one way in which evidence could be used to assess the equity of a purchaser's decisions: by analysing the effects of marginal changes. In the NHS, it is now possible to identify the total amount of money spent on different disease categories (using the WHO International Classification of Diseases version 10), which means that there is the capacity for commissioners or purchasers to determine the effects of either removing £1,000, 000 from, or adding £1,000, 000 to, each programme budget. The effects of reducing spending on any diseases category by £1,000, 000 could then be compared with the effect of increasing expenditure on another disease category by the same amount. This approach of programme budgeting and marginal analysis (see Section 1.5.1.1) should narrow the debate about cuts to a relatively limited set of service changes, and encourage decision-makers to seek evidence useful in the quantification of the effects of such marginal changes on the population served.

6.3.2   Searching

When searching for articles on equity, it is probably most useful to search using the text words "fairness" and "equity".

> **Box 6.5** Checklist for the appraisal of research information on equity
>
> * Is the definition of equity clearly set out in the article?
> * Is the definition of equity original or do the authors cite another source from which it was derived?
> * Do the authors identify or discuss how their own values could influence the interpretation of the findings?
> * Are there any data describing the opinions of individuals other than the authors about the equity of a particular decision or resource allocation?

6.3.3   Appraisal

When appraising articles on equity, the key issue is the definition of equity used by the authors. If the term is not clearly defined, it will be difficult to appraise the article. A checklist of questions for the appraisal of research information on equity is given in Box 6.5.

6.3.4   Applicability and relevance

Equity is an issue that inhabits the moral high ground; those who claim to argue in favour of equity put themselves in a strong moral position. Those who argue from this position should be treated with a high index of suspicion because they could be arguing, either consciously or unconsciously, for a change that will confer benefit on them rather than on society as a whole.

References

1. Whitehead, M. (2000) *The Concepts and Principles of Equity and Health*. World Health Organization, Geneva.
2. Robinson, V. (2007) *Addressing equity issues*. Cochrane News, issue 39, page 4.
3. Tugwell, P., Petticrew, M., Robinson, V. et al. for the Cochrane Equity Field Editorial Team (2006) *Cochrane and Campbell Collaborations, and health equity*. Lancet 367: 1128–30.

6.4   Effectiveness

London has seen the birth of many revolutionary ideas, one of the greatest of which was a national health service. This idea, first current in the 1930s,[1] was developed in many a draughty hall and lecture theatre. At one of these rallies, the young Archie Cochrane bore a banner carrying the slogan: 'All effective treatment must be free'.

The only reaction then, he reported,[2] was from someone who damned it for having Trotskyite tendencies. From this small beginning, the concept of effectiveness has become a major driving force for change in modern healthcare.

6.4.1 Dimensions and definitions

The effectiveness of an intervention, from single treatments through to services including the professionals within them, is the degree to which the desired health outcomes are achieved in clinical practice.

The quality of a service is the degree to which it conforms to pre-set standards of care (see Section 6.8.1).

Earlier definitions of effectiveness were broader and included efficiency;[3] today efficiency, or cost-effectiveness, is almost always used as a distinct criterion (Section 6.7.1.2), although it is not uncommon for the media to use the term 'efficient' when epidemiologists would use the term 'effective' (Margin Fig. 6.2).

The efficacy of an intervention is the degree to which the desired health outcomes are achieved *in the best possible circumstances.*

This distinction between efficacy and effectiveness is important and has implications for decision-makers who must apply the results of research:

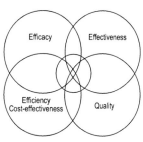

Margin Fig. 6.2

- the rigour necessary for the conduct of a research study design may give a biased picture of what could happen in real life (known as research bias) – an example showing the

	Use of NSAIDS in research trial	Use of NSAIDS in clinical practice
Condition treated	Joint pain in osteoarthritis	Joint pain in: • Osteoarthritis • Rheumatoid arthritis • Systemic lupus erythematosus
Co-prescribing present	None	Likely
Co-morbidities present	None	Likely
Patient coverage	Focused or specified	All comers
Risk for patients from adverse events	Low	Spectrum of risk but preponderance towards high

Matrix 6.1
Difference between the efficacy of a drug treatment in a research trial and its effectiveness in clinical practice (adapted from Dieppe et al.[4])

difference between the efficacy and effectiveness of non-steroidal anti-inflammatory drugs is shown in Matrix 6.1[4]

- research may be performed in an environment where the level of resourcing and/or the number of skilled staff are greater than those available to the local service.

For these reasons, it is vital to consider not only the results of research but also the relevance of those results to the particular population or group of patients about which the decision is being made: an intervention may be efficacious in an RCT at Massachusetts General Hospital, but will it be effective on a wet Thursday in Barchester District General Hospital?

6.4.1.1 Assessing effectiveness from the patient's perspective

It is essential to assess effectiveness not only from a clinical perspective, the focus of which is death, disease status and the functional ability of a patient, but also from the perspective of an individual patient.

The delivery of effective and safe healthcare by professionals who are sensitive to the needs of a patient can engender the following emotional responses in the patient:

- the patient feels better because intervention has brought about an improvement in his/her health
- the patient feels happy because s/he has been treated as an individual by a sensitive professional during the process of care.

Matrix 6.2

The various combinations of the relationship between a patient's state of health and their degree of happiness with the process of care are presented in Matrix 6.2.

As can be seen, it is possible for a patient not to improve, or indeed to deteriorate, during the process of care but still to be happy with the way in which care was given (outcome B). It is also possible for a patient to feel better because the disease causing the problem has been dealt with effectively while feeling unhappy about the process of care (outcome C). The ideal outcome is D. The worst outcome is A, in which a patient's health does not improve and the patient is unhappy about the process of care. In fact, outcome A is the least satisfactory for both patients and clinicians. Such patients are difficult to assess because their view about the process of care may be influenced by the poor outcome for health status.

6.4.1.2 Improving outcomes by providing emotional support

Not only may health outcome influence the patient's perception of the process of care, but the converse can also occur: the effectiveness of care may be increased if the patient's emotional needs are met by giving the patient support (Margin Fig. 6.3). This has been clearly demonstrated in an RCT of women in labour.[5] In comparison with the control group, the provision of emotional support by a professional or voluntary carer was found to:

- shorten the duration of labour
- reduce the rate of Caesarean section
- lessen the use of forceps
- decrease the length of stay of infant hospitalisation.

6.4.1.3 Improving outcomes through patient participation

The other important factor determining clinical outcome is the extent of participation the professional allows the patient in the process of care (Margin Fig. 6.4).

6.4.1.4 Improving outcomes through process: in the absence of an effective technical intervention

The process of care is of greater importance when treating patients in whom there is no apparent structural disease but who have distressing symptoms, such as headache.[6] In this type of health problem, the nature of the process of care is the main factor determining outcome.

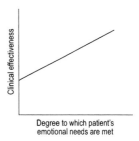

Margin Fig. 6.3

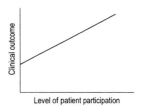

Margin Fig. 6.4

6.4.2   Searching

To search for evidence of effectiveness, consult the various databases in the sequence of steps as follows:

Step 1: The Cochrane Database of Systematic Reviews (CDSR).

Step 2: The Database of Abstracts of Reviews of Effectiveness (DARE).

Step 3: Medline and EMBASE for:

- systematic reviews
- RCTs
- other types of study.

Step 4: Specialist databases.

Search Medline, EMBASE and other specialist databases using the text word "effectiveness" in combination with your subject terms. Where a treatment is involved, the Medical Subject Heading (MeSH) Treatment Outcome/ can also be used in Medline.

6.4.3   Appraisal

Evidence of effectiveness can be generated by several different types of research study. In Box 6.6, the different research methods have been ranked in order of validity for obtaining evidence of effectiveness; for this ranking to hold, all the research must be of high quality.

A checklist of questions for the appraisal of research evidence on effectiveness is shown in Box 6.7.

Once evidence has been found and its quality appraised, it is necessary to address the implications of the research findings (see Box 6.8 and Table 6.2).[7–10]

Box 6.6   Research methods ranked in order of validity for obtaining evidence of effectiveness

1. Large RCTs (Section 5.4)
2. Systematic reviews of RCTs (Section 5.3)
3. Individual RCTs of inadequate size to detect adverse effects of treatment
4. Controlled trials without randomisation
5. Controlled before and after studies (Section 5.7)
6. Interrupted time series (Section 5.8)
7. Observational studies, such as cohort (Section 5.6) or case-control studies (Section 5.5), preferably from more than one research group
8. Reports of expert committees, the contents of which have been based on the sources of evidence cited and not simply the opinion of eminent committee members

---

Box 6.7 Checklist for the appraisal of research evidence of effectiveness

1. Does the research provide evidence about harmful or adverse effects (Section 6.5) and the patients' perspectives of outcome (Section 6.6)?
2. What is the magnitude of the beneficial effect?
3. With what degree of confidence can the findings in a research setting be reproduced in ordinary clinical settings?

Box 6.8 The possible implications of evidence of effectiveness for the provision of healthcare in a local service

- If the trial results are negative, that is, no effect is shown, and this treatment is being delivered within the 'local' service, search for other evidence because the treatment may not be effective.
- If the trial results are positive and this treatment is being delivered within the local service, ascertain how large the effect is at what risk and at what cost. (The NNT is of use in this assessment.)
- If the trial results are positive and this treatment is not being delivered within the local service, consider implementing the research findings but beware of the five positive biases (see Table 6.2).

Table 6.2 Five positive biases

Bias	Cause
Submission bias	Research workers and pharmaceutical companies are more strongly motivated to complete, and submit for publication, positive results
Publication bias	Editors are more likely to publish positive studies[7]
Methodological bias	Methodological errors such as flawed randomisation produce positive biases[8]
Abstracting bias	Abstracts emphasise positive results[9]
Framing bias	Relative risk data produce a positive bias[10]

6.4.3.1 Experimental studies of effectiveness

1. The odds ratio: the relative benefit
The magnitude of any beneficial effect is often expressed in relative terms as the odds ratio. In a controlled trial (refer to Fig. 6.3):

- if the odds ratio is equal to 1, the treatment probably has no effect
- if the odds ratio is less than 1, the treatment probably has a beneficial effect when compared with the intervention applied to the control group

- if the odds ratio is greater than 1, the treatment is probably less effective than the intervention applied to the control group.

For a lucid explanation of the odds ratio, follow the example given in the Cochrane Collaboration's *Reviewers' Handbook*, in the Cochrane Library.

The presentation of trial data in terms of relative risk introduces a bias: readers interpret the results as being more positive than they actually are – known as the framing effect (Section 5.4.4.1). It is therefore important to consider the absolute reduction in risk that a treatment will produce.

2. NNT: the absolute benefit

The number needed to treat (NNT) is a comprehensible measure of the absolute effects of treatment.[11] McQuay and Moore describe it as a clinically useful measure of the effort required to obtain a beneficial outcome with an intervention, and suggest it is particularly useful for expressing the relative effectiveness of several different interventions.[12] The NNTs for various interventions-to-outcomes calculated as a result of meta-analysis are set out in Table 6.3. The clarity gained by presenting data in this

Table 6.3   Results of meta-analyses providing NNTs (Source: Moore and McQuay, *Bandolier's Little Book of Making Sense of Medical Evidence, OUP*)

Intervention	Condition	Outcome	Number of patients	NNT
Statin	Secondary and primary prevention	Prevent fatal or non-fatal heart attack or stroke	44 748	19
Statin	Older people	Prevent major coronary event	25 499	23
Aspirin	Previous myocardial infarction	Prevent vascular event	20 006	28
Aspirin	Secondary prevention	Prevent any vascular event	6300	18
Ibuprofen 400 mg	Acute pain	At least half pain relief	4700	2.4
Finasteride for haematuria	Older men with BPH and haematuria	Prevent recurrence of haematuria	165	2.0
Finasteride for haematuria	Older men with BPH and haematuria	Prevent prostatic surgery	165	6.1
Anti-TNF antibodies	Spondylarthropathy	50% improvement in disease activity	150	2.0

way is striking. The same concept can be applied to adverse outcomes, in which case the measure is referred to as the number needed to harm (NNH).

6.4.3.2 Observational studies of effectiveness

One hope has been that health service data collected routinely on computer systems would enable the effectiveness of new technology to be evaluated within observational studies. The development of registers of hip replacements in Sweden[13] does demonstrate that this hope can be realised, and the increasing computerisation of health services will facilitate the realisation of this goal in future.

The potential of and pitfalls associated with observational studies are exemplified by the investigations of the safety of prostatic surgery. Transurethral resection of the prostate gland (TURP) for the condition benign prostatic hypertrophy became fashionable in the 1970s; by the mid-1980s, it was in common use. In 1989, the results of an observational study indicated that TURP was associated with a higher long-term mortality rate than the traditional operation of open prostatectomy (OP) – an increase of 45%.[14] Other evidence against the use of TURP was also published.[15,16] However, all the possible reasons for this difference in mortality had not been taken into account. In particular, during analysis of the results, no allowance had been made for the differences in selection criteria between those used for men undergoing OP and those used for men undergoing TURP. These differences pertain because there is an increase in short-term morbidity and mortality associated with OP. In an excellent study, Seagroatt[17] adjusted the data for differences in selection criteria and came to the opposite conclusion, as follows:

> The apparent excess in long-term mortality after TURP is unlikely to be caused by the operation itself. It is more likely to reflect relatively low long-term mortality in OP patients as a consequence of the OP patients having been relatively fitter than those having TURP.[17]

Thus, it is not possible to convict TURP of causing excess mortality; any previous convictions were made on the basis of flawed evidence. Seagroatt also concluded that any differences in long-term mortality can be 'answered only in a randomised clinical trial', but emphasised that such a trial may be impossible to organise.[17]

6.4.4   Applicability and relevance

Confidence intervals provide the best guide to the applicability of research results. The narrower the

> **Box 6.9** Checklist for assessing the applicability of research evidence of effectiveness to the local population and service
>
> - Is the study population similar to the local population:
>   - genetically?
>   - socio-economically?
>   - medically?
> - Is the service or treatment under investigation similar to that available locally in terms of:
>   - skills?
>   - resources?

confidence intervals, the more confident a decision-maker can be that the research evidence represents the effect it is possible to obtain in the whole population.

A checklist of questions for the assessment of the applicability and relevance of research evidence on effectiveness is shown in Box 6.9.

References

1. Webster, C. (1988) *The Health Services Since the War*, vol. 1. HMSO, London.
2. Cochrane, A. (1972) *Effectiveness and Efficiency*. Nuffield Provincial Hospitals Trust, London.
3. Doll, R. (1974) *Surveillance and monitoring*. Int J. Epidemiol. 3: 305–14.
4. Dieppe, P., Bartlett, C., Davey, P. et al. (2004) *Balancing benefits and harms: the example of non-steroidal anti-inflammatory drugs. [Clinical Review]* Br. Med. J. 329: 31–4.
5. Kennell, J., Klaus, M., McGrath, S. et al. (1991) *Continuous emotional support during labor in a US hospital.* JAMA 265: 2197–201.
6. Fitzpatrick, R. and Hopkins, A. (1981) *Referrals to neurologists for headaches not due to structural disease.* J. Neurol. Neurosurg. Psychiat. 44: 1061–7.
7. Easterbrook, P.J., Berlin, J.A., Gopalan, R. et al. (1991) *Publication bias in clinical research.* Lancet 337: 867–72.
8. Schulz, K.F., Chalmers, I., Grimes, D.A. et al. (1994) *Assessing the quality of randomization from reports of controlled trials published in obstetrics and gynecology journals.* JAMA 272: 125–8.
9. Gøtzsche, P.C. (1989) *Methodology and overt and hidden bias in reports of 196 double-blind trials of nonsteroidal anti-inflammatory drugs in rheumatoid arthritis.* Control. Clin. Trials 10: 31–56. [Published erratum: Gøtzsche, P.C. (1989) Control. Clin. Trials 10: 356.]
10. Fahey, T., Griffiths, S. and Peters, T.J. (1995) *Evidence-based purchasing: understanding results of clinical trials and systematic reviews.* Br. Med. J. 311: 1056–60.
11. Cook, R.J. and Sackett, D.L. (1995) *The number needed to treat: a clinically useful measure of treatment effect.* Br. Med. J. 310: 452–4.
12. McQuay, H.J. and Moore, A. (1997) *Using numerical results from systematic reviews in clinical practice.* Ann. Intern. Med. 126: 712–20.
13. Malchau, H., Herberts, P., Eisler, T. et al. (2002) *The Swedish Total Hip Replacement Register.* J. Bone Joint Surg. Am. 84(Suppl. 2): 2–20.

14. Roos, N.P., Wennberg. J.E., Malenka, D.J. et al. (1989) *Mortality and reoperation after open and transurethral resection of the prostate for benign prostatic hyperplasia.* N. Engl. J. Med. 320: 1120–4.

15. Andersen, T.F., Bronnum-Hansen, H., Sejr, T. et al. (1990) *Elevated mortality following transurethral resection of the prostate for benign hyperplasia! But why?* Med. Care 28: 870–81.

16. Sidney, S., Quesenberry, C.P., Sadler, M.C. et al. (1992) *Reoperation and mortality after surgical treatment of benign prostatic hypertrophy in a large prepaid medical care program.* Med. Care 30: 117–25.

17. Seagroatt, V. (1995) *Mortality after prostatectomy: selection and surgical approach.* Lancet 346: 1521–4.

6.5   Safety

Arthur Dent: *If I asked you where the hell we were, would I regret it?*

Ford Prefect: *We're safe.*

Arthur Dent: *Oh good.*

Ford Prefect: *We're in a small galley cabin in one of the space ships of the Vogon Constructor Fleet.*

Arthur Dent: *Ah, this is obviously some strange usage of the word safe that I wasn't previously aware of.*

> Douglas Adams, *The Hitch Hiker's Guide to the Galaxy*, 1979

In the Annual Report 2005[1] of the Chief Medical Officer (CMO) on the state of the public health in England, one of the main features covers patient safety in the NHS. The CMO takes the opportunity to draw parallels between safety in the aviation industry and patient safety to see what can be learnt from other high-risk situations. He concludes that a culture of safety needs to be created in healthcare, similar to that in aviation. In addition, he suggests that:

- clinical practice be standardised wherever there is an opportunity to do so
- clinical leaders be engaged with the issue of patient safety, in contrast to the prevailing perception that incident analysis is peripheral to clinical services
- patient safety should be a focus in healthcare training curricula.

6.5.1   Dimensions and definitions

Safety and risk are inversely related to one another, as follows:

> Safety=1-risk of adverse effects

Margin Note 6.1
Safety and risk in the aviation industry

In the aviation industry, risk is no longer defined in terms of poor outcomes, such as harm and adverse consequences. Safety is now viewed in terms of organisational 'risk resilience', which is defined as the organisational capacity to protect operations from the potential of minor mishaps, fluctuations or anomalies developing into major organisational breakdowns. Safety is reliance against minor incidents getting any worse. There are three main categories for judgements about risk and safety:

- acceptable risk resilience
- reduced risk resilience
- degraded risk resilience.

Margin Note 6.2
Ranking of probability phrases

(Source: Lichtenstein and Newman[2])

Most likely	1	Highly probable
	2	Very likely
	3	Very probable
	4	Quite likely
	5	Usually
	6	Good chance
	7	Predictable
	8	Likely
	9	Probable
	10	Rather likely
	11	Pretty good chance
	12	Fairly likely
	13	Somewhat likely
	14	Better than even
	15	Rather
	16	Slightly more than half the time
	17	Slight odds in favour
	18	Fair chance
	19	Toss-up
	20	Fighting chance
	21	Slightly less than half the time
	22	Slight odds against
	23	Not quite even
	24	Inconclusive
	25	Uncertain
	26	Possible
	27	Somewhat likely
	28	Fairly unlikely
	29	Rather unlikely*
	30	Rather unlikely*
	31	Not very probable
	32	Unlikely
	33	Not much chance
	34	Seldom
	35	Barely possible
	36	Faintly possible
	37	Improbable
	38	Quite unlikely
	39	Very unlikely
	40	Rare
Least likely	41	Highly improbable

* This probability phrase was scored differently in terms of the mean, median, σ, and range.

The risk associated with an intervention is the 'probability' that an adverse effect will occur.

The use of the word 'probability' is interesting: perhaps not surprisingly, most people use the 1576 definition, given in the *Shorter Oxford English Dictionary* as 'something which, judged by present evidence, is likely to happen', rather than the 1718 mathematical definition which is 'the amount of antecedent likelihood of a particular event as measured by the relative frequency of occurrence of events of the same kind in the whole course of experience'. Words used to describe frequency, such as 'likely', 'often', 'sometimes', 'possible' and 'frequently', can be interpreted by different individuals differently. This difference in interpretation is also evident in expressions of 'subjective possibility' (*SOED*); for example, 'Side-effects may occur'.

In an interesting study by Lichtenstein and Newman,[2] a questionnaire was sent to a random selection of 225 male employees at the System Development Corporation to determine the correspondence between numerical probabilities and a range of associated verbal phrases. Subjects were asked to give the probability number (from 0.01 to 0.99) that reflected the degree of probability implied by each phrase; 188 scorable replies were received. The results are shown in Margin Note 6.2.

Despite a few generally held distinctions, for instance, that 'probable' implies a higher frequency than 'possible', the variation in the weighting given to different words is so great that numbers have to be used, but which numbers?

Risk can be expressed in two ways:

1. relative risk
2. absolute risk.

Relative risk can be expressed using a numerical scale: for example, the relative risk of impotence in men who remain on the thiazide treatment for high blood pressure is 2.3, with 23% of men on thiazides being impotent after two years' treatment in comparison with only 10% of those receiving placebo.[3]

Absolute risk is used to express probability either as a simple percentage, for example, 'About 60% of patients will experience adverse effects', or as the number needed to harm (the NNH). Some patients may find the NNH more comprehensible than a percentage, i.e. the number of patients treated with thiazide diuretics that would result in one person being harmed over and above the risk in the general population is 8. To continue with the example, the number needed to cause an extra case of impotence (NNI) is calculated by converting the relative risk to an absolute figure using the following formula:

$$\text{Number needed to harm}/(\text{risk in treated population} - \text{risk in untreated population}) = 1$$

As for all other outcome estimates, confidence intervals should be given.

A new measure, which has been derived from the NNT and the NNH, is the likelihood of being helped and harmed (LHH) by a particular therapy.[4]

$$\text{LHH} = (1/\text{NNT}) : (1/\text{NNH})$$

The LHH was developed by Sharon Straus at the Centre for Evidence-Based Medicine in Oxford to give a patient-centred measure of the relative severities of being helped to being harmed; in the past, greater emphasis has been given to the potential benefits than to the potential harms of treatment.

6.5.2 Searching

To search for articles that contain information about the adverse effects of an intervention, combine the problem and intervention in question (e.g. a drug, test or operation), with a specific adverse effect or outcome – see Table 6.4 for an example of using the PICO (or PECO) formulation to conduct a search for adverse effects.

To search for articles on the unknown harms or adverse effects of an intervention, the best single Medline term to use is the text word "risk". Combine this with your problem and intervention terms.

Table 6.4 Components of a search for adverse effects

Component	Example
Problem (P)	High blood pressure
Intervention (I)	Thiazide
Adverse outcome (O)	Impotence

Margin Note 6.3
World Alliance for Patient Safety

In October 2004, the World Health Organization (WHO) launched the World Alliance for Patient Safety, see: http://www.qho.int/patientsafety/en/

Member states of the WHO are now setting up their own safety organisations. In England and Wales, the organisation is known as the National Patient Safety Agency (NPSA) (see Margin Note 6.4).

Margin Note 6.4
The National Patient Safety Agency

The National Patient Safety Agency (NPSA) is a special health authority in England and Wales and was established in 2001:

- to coordinate patient safety incidents
- to learn from these incidents in order to improve patient safety.

Since 2005, the NPSA is also responsible for:

- the National Clinical Assessment Service (NCAS), which supports local organisations in addressing their concerns about the performance of individual doctors and dentists
- the National Research Ethics Service (NRES), which ensures protection of the rights, dignity and welfare of those people participating in research through an ethics system
- the contracts for three confidential enquiries: Confidential Enquiry into Maternal and Child Health (CEMACH); National Confidential Enquiry into Patient Outcome and Death (NCEPOD); and National Confidential Enquiry into Suicide and Homicide by People with Mental Illness (NCISH).

It is not normally useful to stipulate a Publication Type. Although the best evidence is provided by a systematic review of RCTs, other methods of research can be helpful, therefore, it is important not to limit the boundaries of the search in this way.

6.5.3 Appraisal

The two main questions in the critical appraisal of research information about safety are:

1. Which is the best research method to give information about the risks of treatment?
2. How good is the quality of the research?

6.5.3.1 Which method?

The research methods that can generate information about safety, and the risk of adverse effects of treatment, are listed in order of quality of information provided:

- systematic review of RCTs (Section 5.3), which is generally better than an RCT for this purpose
- RCT (Section 5.4)
- survey (Section 5.9) and cohort study (Section 5.6)
- case-control study (Section 5.5).

Systematic reviews of any of these methods of research are better than single studies provided that the quality of the primary research is good.

It is relatively rare for the results of RCTs to generate useful evidence about the harmful effects of treatment, principally because adverse effects usually occur less frequently than beneficial effects. A trial designed with sufficient power to demonstrate the beneficial effects of treatment will probably not have sufficient power to detect any adverse effects (Section 5.5.1.2), and it is often necessary to perform a cohort study (see Section 5.6).

A cohort study is a research design in which one or more groups of patients are followed over time. For example, in the UK, thousands of women who were and were not taking oral contraceptives have been followed for years. However, those women not taking oral contraceptives cannot be compared directly with those who are; for instance, even though deep vein thrombosis may have been detected more often in pill users, it is possible that non-users may not have been prescribed the pill because they were considered to be at high risk of thrombosis.

Prospective cohort studies are less prone to bias and can be used when it is not possible to conduct an RCT. For example, most anaesthetists might refuse to participate in an RCT in which the hypothesis that epidural anaesthesia causes backache is tested. However, it did prove possible to follow 329 women for 6 weeks after delivery, 164 of whom had had epidural anaesthesia and 165 of whom had not. The results of this prospective study of these two cohorts did not show that backache was an adverse effect of epidural anaesthesia.[5]

The most appropriate study design to identify the adverse effects of drugs may be the case-control study, despite the fact that this research methodology may introduce a greater degree of bias than that introduced by cohort studies.

A major source of bias is introduced if data that were collected previously are reviewed. In an elegant experiment, 112 anaesthetists were asked to review 21 cases for which there had been adverse anaesthetic outcomes classified as either permanent or temporary.[6] In addition, the authors generated 21 matching alternate cases identical to the original except that in each case a plausible outcome of opposite severity was substituted. The original and the alternate cases were randomly assigned to two sets and presented to the anaesthetists. The results were startling:

- the proportion of cases in which care was deemed 'appropriate' *decreased* by 31% when the outcome was changed from temporary to permanent
- the proportion of cases in which care was deemed 'appropriate' *increased* by 28% when the outcome was changed from permanent to temporary.

From this study, it can be seen that foreknowledge of the outcome of care can alter the reviewer's perception of the safety of the procedure.[6]

6.5.3.2 Appraising the quality of studies on safety

Although the quality of each type of research study needs to be appraised against the criteria set out in the relevant sections of this book, there are also some general questions that should be used in the appraisal of any study designed to investigate adverse effects (Box 6.10).

6.5.4 Applicability and relevance

Evidence revealing risks associated with drug treatment can usually be applied to the whole population: the results will

---

Box 6.10 Checklist for appraising the quality of a study designed to investigate adverse effects

1. Was the assessment of outcomes free from bias?
2. Was there an adverse effect greater than that which would be expected by chance, taking into account the confidence intervals?
3. How important is the adverse effect clinically?
4. If more than one study is available, are the results consistent among them?

---

be relevant to all patients of exactly the same type as those described in the original trial. It is important to be aware that the harms observed in practice may be different from those reported in a trial on which the use of a drug has been based because drugs tend to be prescribed for a wider range of indications than those for which they are trialled[7] (see Matrix 6.1).

The risks associated with particular surgical operations or interventions, in which the skill of the professional is an important determining factor, may vary according to the professionals involved; therefore, the risk could be smaller or greater than that reported in the literature.

A checklist of questions for the assessment of the applicability and relevance of research findings on safety is shown in Box 6.11.

References

1. Donaldson, L. (2005) *The Chief Medical Officer on the state of the public health. Annual Report 2005.* Department of Health, London.
2. Lichtenstein, S. and Newman, R.J. (1967) *Empirical scaling of common verbal phrases associated with numerical probabilities.* Psychon. Sci. 9: 563–4.
3. Medical Research Council Working Party (1981) *Adverse reactions to bendrofluazide and propranolol for the treatment of mild hypertension.* Lancet ii: 539–43.
4. Straus, S.E., Richardson, W.S., Glasziou, P. et al. (2005) *Evidence-Based Medicine: How to Practice and Teach EBM,* 3rd edn. Churchill Livingstone, Edinburgh.
5. MacArthur, A., MacArthur, C. and Weeks, S. (1995) *Epidural anaesthesia and low back pain after delivery: a prospective cohort study.* Br. Med. J. 311: 1336–9.
6. Caplan, R.A., Posner, K.L. and Cheney, F.W. (1991) *Effect of outcome on physician judgements of appropriateness of care.* JAMA 265: 1957–60.
7. Dieppe, P., Bartlett, C., Davey, P. et al. (2004) *Balancing benefits and harms: the example of non-steroidal anti-inflammatory drugs.* [Clinical Review] Br. Med. J. 329: 31–4.

Box 6.11 Checklist for assessing the applicability and relevance of research evidence of safety

1. Were the professionals participating in the study more highly specialised or more experienced in this intervention than those who will be treating the local population?
2. Would the quality of training be important in determining the frequency of adverse effects?
3. Were the patients in the research study different from those in the local population, either by being fitter or by having more advanced disease?

6.6 Patient satisfaction and patients' experience of care

Gentle Reader

Empathise with Mr R. He spat accurately into the bucket that served as both spittoon and urinal. Disabled by a stroke and a gas lung sustained one afternoon during the First World War when the gas came 'rolling towards us', he was unable to climb the stairs to get to the bathroom of his damp council house. The room in which he lived was heated by only a small electric fire; mould had formed an opulent brocade on the walls. Although the young doctor and social worker were apologising for their inability to improve his health and environment, his views were clear. 'I'm grateful for all you're doing, but don't worry about me; I'm all right. Sixty years ago today I was up to my waist in mud and water.'

Commentary

Satisfied with his lot, satisfied with his services, this Old Contemptible would never have dreamed of complaining, even when the quality of care was manifestly poor. However, times have changed and patient satisfaction can no longer be taken for granted.

6.6.1 Dimensions and definitions

6.6.1.1 Acceptability of care

> *Finally, I will admit one thing: there is no way in which I would ever have a colonoscopy as a screening procedure.*
>
> Lecture given by a doctor about a pilot screening programme using colonoscopy to detect colorectal cancer

Acceptability is a theoretical construct used in service planning and technology assessment. It is often applied to interventions before they have been introduced into a service to test patients', or members' of the public, willingness to be treated in a particular way. Once an intervention has been introduced, acceptability as a concept becomes subsumed within the measurement of patient satisfaction and patients' experience of care.

6.6.1.2 Patient satisfaction

The assessment of patient satisfaction, although necessary, is not sufficient. Satisfaction is determined not only by the quality of the service but also by patient expectations. Patient satisfaction is an imperfect measure with which to assess the quality of any service: it is possible for patients to be delighted with healthcare in which the quality of clinical practice was poor if their expectations were low (Fig. 6.5).

6.6.1.3 Patients' experience of care

As patient satisfaction is an imperfect measure for the assessment of quality, it is necessary to investigate the patient's *experience* of care and make a judgement about the quality of that experience irrespective of whether the patient is satisfied. For instance, it is possible for a patient to be satisfied with the amount of information provided and the way in which it was provided, despite the fact that the information may have been wrong and misleading. It is essential, therefore, to complement the question 'Were you satisfied with the information you were given?' with the question 'What information were you given?'.

This novel approach of gathering patients' experiences was developed in the USA, where it has been used to improve medical care in hospitals.[1] Indeed, increasing use is being made of systems designed to assess patient experience, and the Picker Institute Europe, established in 1997 as a sister organisation to the Picker Institute in the USA, is now extending the use of this approach throughout Europe (see http://www.pickereurope.org/).

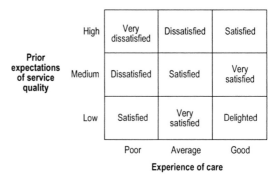

Fig. 6.5
The relationship between patient expectations and quality

A patient's experience is determined by three inter-related aspects of care (Margin Fig. 6.5):

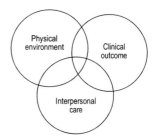

Margin Fig. 6.5

1. the clinical outcome
2. the physical environment in which care is received
3. the interpersonal relationships during care, namely, how patients are treated by the professionals giving care.

1. Clinical outcome: expectations and experience
Although a patient's expectations may be determined by many factors, the single most important factor is what the patient remembers the clinician said about clinical outcomes, such as:

- the magnitude of health improvement that could be expected, e.g. complete cure or alleviation of symptoms
- the probability that there would be a benefit
- the nature of side-effects that occur most commonly
- the probability that any of those side-effects would be suffered personally.

The optimal information exchange in a consultation is when the patient remembers all that the clinician said; however, this does not always occur (Margin Fig. 6.6). Thus, the most important factor is the quality of the clinician's communication.

The various reactions a patient might have are shown in Matrix 6.3.

Patients' reactions may also vary depending upon:

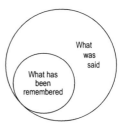

Margin Fig. 6.6

- factors over which the health service has no influence, e.g.
  - the patient's personality
  - the advice of ambulance-chasing lawyers
- factors over which the health service has influence, e.g.
  - the physical environment in which care is received
  - the quality of interpersonal care.

	Beneficial effect as predicted or expected	Beneficial effect absent or not as great as predicted or expected
No side-effects	Delighted	Disappointed
Side-effects as expected or predicted	Modified delight	Very disappointed
Side-effects worse than expected or predicted	Response dependent upon personality and other factors, e.g. satisfaction with interpersonal care	Desolate

Matrix 6.3

2. The physical environment: expectations and experience
Certain aspects of the physical environment in which care is delivered are of particular importance to patients:

- quality of food
- availability of parking
- the standard of cleanliness
- the comfort of the bed
- the 'external' environment (is it possible to see trees from the bed?)
- ease of access by public transport.

If the clinical outcome is satisfactory and the interpersonal care is good, satisfaction with the physical environment will be a bonus. If the patient is pleased with clinical outcome and interpersonal care, deficiencies in the physical environment are unlikely to lead to overall dissatisfaction and the registration of a complaint.

If there is dissatisfaction with the clinical outcome or interpersonal care, a high-quality physical environment is unlikely to compensate for deficiencies in these more important aspects of care. Furthermore, a low-quality environment may provide a focus for the discontent of a patient or their relatives if there is dissatisfaction with other aspects of care that are difficult to articulate.

3. Interpersonal skills: expectations and experience

Asking why his daughter needed further tests, a father was told: 'Your last child died of cancer. Draw your own conclusions.'

During a delivery, a junior doctor was told: 'Go slow, man, or you'll tear the baby's head off.'

A woman complaining of a 'congested' nose was told: 'Don't use long words. Use your own language, woman.'

Extracts from an article by William Evington entitled
'Physician, heal thyself' in the Thursday Review of
The Independent, 8 July 1999

Frank rudeness in healthcare professionals is an obvious cause of dissatisfaction and distress for both patients and their relatives. However, it is more common for failures in a professional's behaviour to be of a subtle non-verbal nature. It is important that any patient receives the impression that she or he:

- is an individual and not just a number

- does have a problem that the professional is taking seriously
- is the sole focus of that professional's attention during any interaction.

A healthcare professional may subscribe to this approach, but if it is not translated into appropriate behaviour the patient is unable to appreciate it: patients are not mind-readers.

6.6.1.4 The benefits of measuring patient experience

The measurement of patients' experience of care enables healthcare managers to identify ways to improve health services[2] which could lead to better outcomes. The Picker Institute has been involved in running the national patient survey programmes in England since the programme began in 1998.[3] The surveys are designed to ask patients about their experience of care using survey instruments that elicit detailed reports of recent experience. These reports give healthcare managers and clinicians information about what actually happened during the process of care, helping them to pinpoint any problems more precisely. In contrast, knowing the proportion of patients who rate their care as either 'fair' or 'poor', as in a patient satisfaction survey, does not give healthcare managers or clinicians any indication about where or how the quality of care needs to be improved.[2]

From the national NHS patient surveys in England, it appears that patients' experience of care has improved significantly in those service areas where coordinated action has been taken, such as hospital waiting times, cancer care, coronary heart disease and mental health, although there is still room for improvement with respect to the care of mental health patients in particular.[3] Improvement in the quality of care is possible when awareness of the patient's perspective is increased, and understanding and accommodating patients' needs can lead to improvements that patients notice.[4] It has been found that simply giving doctors patients' feedback is not enough to instigate a change in professional behaviour;[5,6] however, in some parts of the USA integrating patients' feedback into educational programmes (with the results made available to the public) can improve doctors' performance.[7,8]

Margin Note 6.5
Aspects of healthcare patients consider most important

From the national NHS patient survey programme in England,[2] there are eight aspects of healthcare that patients consider to be most important:

1. fast access to reliable health advice
2. effective treatment delivered by trusted professionals
3. involvement in decisions and respect for preferences
4. clear, comprehensible information and support for self-care
5. attention to physical and environmental needs
6. emotional support, empathy and respect
7. involvement of, and support for, family and carers
8. continuity of care and smooth transitions.

6.6.2   Searching

As patient satisfaction is determined to a great extent by the local characteristics of a particular service, as opposed to its effectiveness, studies of patient satisfaction may not be considered as research and therefore may not be indexed in Medline or EMBASE. However, it is still worth searching both databases using Medical Subject Headings (MeSH) such as Patient Satisfaction/ and Patient Acceptance of Health Care/, and the text phrases "patient perception" and "patient experience".

6.6.3   Appraisal

Critical skills are needed for two tasks:

1. the appraisal of an instrument for measuring satisfaction. There are many such instruments, usually a combination of a questionnaire and an interview, either face to face or by telephone. A checklist of questions for the appraisal of any instrument used to assess patient satisfaction is shown in Box 6.12
2. the appraisal of the study of patient satisfaction. Although the main focus of the appraisal is on the instrument used to measure satisfaction, it is also important to assess the overall study design (see Box 6.13).

6.6.4   Applicability and relevance

Surveys of patient satisfaction are primarily of use to the service about which they have been conducted. The degree to which any of the results are a function of patient expectations, which vary from one population to another, and the quality of the service those patients received, makes it difficult to apply findings about one service to others elsewhere. However, the reasons for complaint revealed

---

Box 6.12 Checklist for the appraisal of instruments used to assess patient satisftaction

1. How has the instrument been tested?
2. What is the inter-observer variability, i.e. how different are the answers if different people use the questionnaire on the same person?
3. How good is the instrument at measuring the three aspects of care that determine satisfaction: inter-personal care, the physical environment and clinical outcome?
4. How comprehensible are the questions to people of different reading abilities or different ethnic backgrounds?

Box 6.13 Checklist for the appraisal of study designs used to assess patient satisfaction

1. How well did the survey assess the experience of the patients as opposed to their reaction to that experience?
2. Was the sample interviewed a representative sample of the population served by the service or was it biased?
3. Are the results applicable to the population in general?
4. Are the results relevant to the local population?

by such surveys (e.g. noise), as opposed to the degree of patient dissatisfaction found, may be useful because they can indicate causes of dissatisfaction that could be relevant to any population.

References

1. Cleary, P.D., Edgman-Levitan, S., Walker, J.D. et al. (1993) *Using patient reports to improve medical care: a preliminary report from 10 hospitals.* Qual. Manage. Health Care 2: 31–8.
2. Coulter, A. (2006) *Can patients assess the quality of health care? [Editorial]* Br. Med. J. 333: 1–2.
3. Coulter, A. (2005) *Opinion and experience: do they concur?* In: Coulter, A., Nye, R. and Pollard, S. (eds) *What Patients Really Want.* Populus/Profile, London, pp. 33–58.
4. NHS Clinical Governance Support Team and Picker Institute Europe Patients Accelerating Change Programme. Available online at: http://www.pickereurope.org/page.php?id=13.
5. Vingerhoets, E., Wensing, M. and Grol, R. (2001) *Feedback of patients' evaluations of general practice care: a randomized trial.* Qual. Health Care 10: 224–8.
6. Wensing, M., Vingerhoets, E. and Grol, R. (2003) *Feedback based on patient evaluations: a tool for quality improvement?* Patient Educ. Couns. 51: 149–53.
7. Leeper, M.K., Veale, J.R., Westbrook, T.S. et al. (2003) *The effect of standardized patient feedback in teaching surgical residents informed consent: results of a pilot study.* Curr. Surg. 60: 615–22.
8. Leddy, K.M. and Woolsin, R.J. (2005) *Patient Satisfaction with Pain Control During Hospitalization. Improving Health Care Quality and Safety.* Joint Commission Resources, Oak Brook, Illinois.

6.7   Cost-effectiveness

Robert Evans, one of the world's leading health economists, wrote a leader for the *Annals of Internal Medicine*[1] about a report entitled *Economic Analysis of Health Care Technology.*[2] Evans points out that the work of the taskforce described in the report was funded entirely by the pharmaceutical industry, and asserts that the industry was giving a verisimilitude of objectivity to a technique that should be assumed to be biased. His criticisms are typically forthright; for example, he states that:

> A pseudodiscipline, 'pharmaco-economics', has been conjured into existence by the magic of money, with its own practitioners, conferences, and journals. There are a lot of drugs and there is a lot of money, so the 'field' is booming.

In response to two letters in which the original leader was criticised, he concludes:

> In the end, drug buyers and reimbursers will have to do their own evaluations and make their own purchasing decisions. Offers of participation and scientific co-operation from sellers always spring from the same underlying motive, to move the product. What else can they do?[3]

This may seem a cynical line to take but this issue must be faced, especially as studies of cost-effectiveness have an increasingly important role to play in the appraisal of new interventions.

6.7.1   Dimensions and definitions

The concept of cost-effectiveness has evolved from earlier conceptions of efficiency.

6.7.1.1 Productivity

As discussed in the section 'Defining our Terms', Wittgenstein proposed that when a word caused more confusion than clarification its use should be discontinued; this is now the case for the word 'efficiency'. The term is often used as if it were synonymous with productivity, and it is common in the NHS for efficiency to be calculated by relating the outputs of a service (i.e. episodes of care) to the inputs (i.e. costs), which is actually the method of calculating what is more accurately termed productivity (see Box 6.14 for examples of measures of productivity).

$$\text{Productivity} = \text{Outputs} / \text{Inputs}$$

Box 6.14 Examples of productivity measures (usually referred to as efficiency measures)

1. Episodes of care/Cost
2. No. episodes of care/No. beds

6.7.1.2 Efficiency and cost-effectiveness

The term efficiency relates inputs to the outcomes of care:

$$\text{Efficiency} = \text{Outcomes}/\text{Inputs}$$

Efficiency is a measure of the performance of a service that is being offered to patients. When estimates of the efficiency of a new service or treatment are being made, the term cost-effectiveness is used. Cost-effectiveness is calculated by relating the outcomes of a service (e.g. number of lives saved) to the inputs (i.e. costs):

$$\text{Cost-effectiveness} = \text{Outcomes}/\text{Cost}$$

However, when measuring cost-effectiveness, it is essential to remember that the outcomes of care may be harmful or adverse as well as beneficial:

$$\text{Cost-effectiveness} = \frac{\text{Beneficial outcomes} - \text{Adverse outcomes}}{\text{Cost}}$$

In a relatively recent editorial on healthcare 'productivity' in the NHS, Black[4] appears to have defined the term in several ways; the first is as we have defined it here and the second equates to our definition of 'cost-effectiveness'. Black mentions the term efficiency only once in relation to the delivery of health services, thus, there continues to be debate about the use and definition of all these terms.

6.7.1.3 The use of quality-adjusted outcome measures: QALYs and DALYs

Initially, the beneficial outcome of an intervention designed to prevent mortality was expressed only in terms of the number of extra years of life resulting from that intervention.

Subsequently, it was recognised that the quality of life during those extra years is an important consideration. In order to determine the quality of life during those extra years, various studies were undertaken to ascertain the value people attach to different states of health and illness. It was found that a consensus could be reached about the values people attach to certain states, ranging from a factor of 1, which represents excellent health, to 0, which represents the worst state of health. A method was then developed that enabled a combination of a patient's levels of disability and of distress to be assessed.[5] It was then possible to estimate the quality of life during the extra years as well as the quantity, and these two measures were combined to produce the quality-adjusted life-year (QALY):

> The number of extra years of life obtained
> ×
> the value of the quality of life during those extra years
> =
> quality-adjusted life-years(QALYs)

The concept of QALYs is now in fairly widespread use.

Another approach is described in *The Global Burden of Disease*, a text of tremendous importance.[6] In it, Murray and Lopez[6] introduce the concept of the disability-adjusted life-year (DALY), the focus of which is 'non-fatal health outcomes'. This type of approach emphasises the importance of neuropsychiatric conditions, principally depression. They describe a programme of work being undertaken by the World Health Organization to estimate the global burden of disease. To complete such an estimation, it was necessary to develop techniques to estimate the causes of death in the absence of robust data, and then to summarise the 'descriptive epidemiology of disability', namely:

- incidence, i.e. the number of new cases per year
- prevalence, i.e. the number of people living at any one time with a disability
- health expectancy, and the years of life lived with each type of disability.

In Fig. 6.6, where the rank order of DALYs for the 15 leading causes of disease in the world are shown for the year 1990 against the projection for the year 2020, it can be seen that as some of the traditional diseases of poor countries drop down the list, other diseases that appear to be consequent upon development, notably ischaemic heart disease and depression, move up.[6]

6.7.1.4 Marginal and opportunity costs

To determine the cost of an intervention, the cost of a health service unit, including all fixed costs, is divided by the number of interventions performed by that unit.

Marginal costs

A marginal cost is the cost of any *additional* interventions performed by a unit for which the cost of working at a particular rate has already been calculated. For instance, in a unit in which 1000 interventions are undertaken at a cost of £10 000 each, the fixed costs will be £9000 per intervention

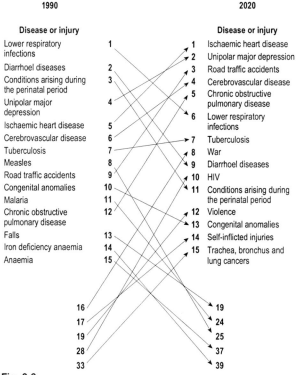

Fig. 6.6
Changes in the rank order of DALYs for leading causes of disease or injury in the world from 1990 to 2020 (Source: Murray and Lopez[6])

whereas the cost of the consumables per intervention will be £1000. Thus, the marginal cost of 100 extra interventions will be £100 000, i.e. the cost of the consumables at £1000 for each extra intervention.

Opportunity costs
Opportunity costs are defined as those uses, other than the one being resourced, on which the same amount of money could be spent. For example, the opportunity costs of the £100 000 that might be spent on 100 more cardiac operations could be expressed as the number of chiropody treatments or cataract operations that it is possible to purchase with the same amount of money.

6.7.1.5 Evaluations of cost-effectiveness

There are many different approaches to the evaluation of cost-effectiveness:

- cost–benefit analysis – an assessment of the return on investment in terms of money

- cost–utility analysis – an assessment of the return on investment in terms of QALYs, which is a more sophisticated form of cost–benefit analysis
- cost-effectiveness – an assessment of the relative merits of different methods of achieving the same objective.

Cost–benefit and cost–utility analyses enable decision-makers to assess the benefit that will be gained from investing resources in a particular type of health service, and then to compare the benefits of investing resources in services designed to treat different health problems. As an example, the results would allow the return on investment in an immunisation programme to be compared with the return that might be obtained from investment in another child health programme, or a different preventive programme for adults, or any other form of healthcare. Studies of cost-effectiveness enable decision-makers to compare the costs of different ways of tackling the same health problem.

- The results of a cost–benefit or cost–utility analysis would help a decision-maker to assess the returns on investing £100 000 additional resources in either a renal transplantation programme or a cardiac surgery programme; the decision-maker might then wish to carry out a cost-effectiveness study of the alternatives to renal transplantation.
- The results of a cost-effectiveness analysis would help the decision-maker assess the relative cost-effectiveness of dialysis and of transplantation as methods of treating end-stage renal failure.

Lilford et al.[7] point out that as assessments of cost-effectiveness are increasingly being used to derive the most benefit from limited healthcare resources it is important to be aware of a source of bias in the process of assessment. At present, in 'intention to treat' analyses, cost-effectiveness (an average QALY) is calculated for all candidates allocated to the new treatment irrespective of whether they accept it. This means that people allocated to the 'treatment arm' of a trial who refused the intervention, because of the balance between potential side-effects and potential benefits, are actually included in the assessment, which practice decreases the intervention's cost-effectiveness. Lilford et al. recommend that in future such patients be excluded from the calculation of cost-effectiveness. However, this recommendation does shift the evaluation towards a test of efficacy by excluding patients who withdraw or deviate from treatment. It could be argued that including such patients is a more accurate representation of what happens in routine clinical practice.

6.7.2 Searching

Specify the search term for the health problem and the intervention.

Step 1: Search the NHS Economic Evaluation Database (NHS EED) compiled by the Centre for Reviews and Dissemination (CRD) in York, a centre where cost-effectiveness studies and economic evaluations are systematically identified and described. Available at: http://www.york.ac.uk/inst/crd/crddatabases.htm

Step 2: Search Medline and EMBASE to identify papers that focus on the costs of the particular health problem and the cost-effectiveness of the intervention. These terms could include:

- Costs and Cost Analysis/
- Economics/
- cost
- costs
- economics.

6.7.3 Appraisal

In 1996, the Panel on Cost-Effectiveness in Health and Medicine published recommendations for reporting cost-effectiveness analyses[8] in order:

- to enhance the transparency of study methods
- to assist researchers in providing complete information
- to facilitate the presentation of comparable results across studies.

A checklist of questions for the appraisal of economic evaluations is shown in Box 6.15.[9]

However, for decision-makers to identify whether an intervention is cost-effective, they need to have timely and reliable information about both the clinical and the economic consequences of a treatment. Greenberg et al.[10] found that on average cost-utility analyses were published almost two years (range: 0–7.5 years) after the results of the corresponding trial, which suggests that economic data are usually not available in peer-reviewed journals when decisions on the adoption of a treatment need to be made.

6.7.4 Applicability and relevance

Cost–benefit and cost-effectiveness analyses are of most use to decision-makers; however, the results of research studies are of limited relevance to decision-makers who are responsible

---

Box 6.15 Checklist for the appraisal of economic evaluations of healthcare (Source: adapted from Drummond et al.[9])

1. Was a well-defined question posed in an answerable form?
2. Was a comprehensive description of the competing alternatives given (i.e. can you tell who did what to whom, where, and how often)?
3. Was there evidence that the programme's effectiveness had been established? [How strong was the evidence of effectiveness?]
4. Were all the important and relevant costs and consequences for each alternative identified?
5. Were costs and consequences measured accurately in appropriate physical units (e.g. hours of nursing time, number of physician visits, lost work-days, life-years gained)?
6. Were costs and consequences valued credibly?
7. Were costs and consequences adjusted for differential timing?
8. Was an incremental analysis of the costs and consequences of alternatives performed? [Were the additional (incremental) costs generated by one alternative over another compared to the additional effects, benefits, or utilities generated?]
9. Was allowance made for uncertainty in the estimates of costs and consequences?
10. Did the presentation and discussion of study results include all issues of concern to users?

---

for populations other than those in which the study was performed. Therefore, the findings of any research study must be carefully appraised for applicability and relevance to the local situation. This is because, although the effectiveness of a service is universal, a service's cost-effectiveness is influenced by local factors such as the incidence and prevalence of disease, and resource constraints.

A cost–benefit study of a coronary revascularisation programme is a function of the incidence and prevalence of coronary artery disease in the population served, and the prevailing resource constraints such as the availability of skilled cardiac surgeons. Similarly, if the opportunity costs are expressed in terms of tuberculosis control, they are influenced not only by the incidence and prevalence of tuberculosis in that population but also by the relevant resource constraints such as the availability of trained nursing staff.

In assessing whether an economic appraisal is relevant and can be applied to the local service, it is necessary to ask two questions:

- How similar is the study population to the local population?

- How similar are the healthcare costs and level of available resources in the research study to healthcare costs and resources available locally?

Although data showing the relative costs and benefits of different programmes are more useful than absolute data about a single programme, the results of all economic studies must be used with caution.

References

1. Evans, R.G. (1995) *Manufacturing consensus, marketing truth: guidelines for economic evaluation*. Ann. Intern. Med. 123: 59–60.
2. Task Force On Principles For Economic Analysis Of Health Care Technology (1995) *Economic analysis of health care technology. A report on principles*. Ann. Intern. Med. 123: 61–70.
3. Evans, R.G. (1996) *Principles of economic analysis of health care technology. [Response to letters]* Ann. Intern. Med. 124: 536.
4. Black, N. (2006) *Health care productivity. Is politically contentious but can it be measured accurately? [Editorial]* Br. Med. J. 333: 312–13.
5. Rosser, R. and Kind, P. (1978) *A scale of valuations of states of illness: is there a social consensus?* Int. J. Epidemiol. 7: 347–58.
6. Murray, C.J.L. and Lopez, A.D. (eds) (1996) *The Global Burden of Disease*. World Health Organization, Geneva.
7. Lilford, R., Girling, A., Stevens, A. et al. (2006) *Adjusting for treatment refusal in rationing decisions. [Analysis and comment]* Br. Med. J. 332: 542–3.
8. Siegel, J.E., Weinstein, M.C., Russell, L.B. et al. for the Panel on Cost-Effectiveness in Health and Medicine (1996) *Recommendations for reporting cost-effectiveness analyses*. JAMA 276: 1339–41.
9. Drummond, M.F., O'Brien, B., Stoddart, G.L. et al. (1997) *Methods for the Economic Evaluation of Health Care Programmes*, 2nd edn. Oxford University Press, New York.
10. Greenberg, D., Rosen, A.B., Olchanski, N.V. et al. (2004) *Delays in publication of cost utility analyses conducted alongside clinical trials: registry analysis*. Br. Med. J. 328: 1536–7.

6.8   Quality

6.8.1   Dimensions and definitions

Avedis Donabedian defined the quality of a service as the degree to which it conforms to pre-set standards of care.[1]

- The effectiveness of a professional or a service is the degree to which the objectives of care are achieved.
- The quality of a service is the degree to which the performance of that service meets or surpasses standards.

Standards are usually developed as part of a system of care, and each system of care comprises a set of activities that have common objectives. Whenever possible, the objectives for any service should be expressed in terms of the population served (see, for example, the original objectives for the NHS Breast Screening Programme shown in Box 6.16). For each objective, one or more criteria can be selected to measure progress towards quality improvement.

6.8.1.1 Quality assessment by measuring the process of care

The processes of care used to measure quality should be those for which there is good evidence. For example, for an assessment of the quality of a maternity service, the proportion of women going into labour prematurely who were given antenatal steroids[2] is an evidence-based process measure; in the assessment of the quality of care received by those suffering an acute myocardial infarction, the proportion of patients who receive streptokinase treatment within an hour of arriving at hospital is also an evidence-based process measure. By using such evidence-based process measures, the performance of an individual or service can be defined. This represents an objective assessment of what is being achieved.

Box 6.16 Original objectives of the NHS Breast Screening Programme

The aim of the programme is to reduce mortality from breast cancer in the population screened.
- To identify and invite eligible women for mammographic screening.
- To carry out mammography in a high proportion of those who were invited.
- To provide services that are acceptable to those who receive them.
- To follow up all women referred for further investigations.
- To minimise the adverse effects of screening – anxiety, radiation and unnecessary investigations.
- To diagnose cancers accurately.
- To support and carry out research.
- To make effective and efficient use of resources for the benefit of the whole population.
- To enable those working in the programme to develop their skills and find fulfilment in their work.
- To encourage the provision of effective acceptable treatment which has minimal psychological or functional side-effects.
- To evaluate the service regularly and provide feedback to the population served.

In an observational study of hospital care in 350 academic and non-academic centres in the USA for 64 775 patients with unstable angina enrolled in the CRUSADE National Quality Improvement Initiative between 1 January 2001 and 30 September 2003,[3] a significant association was found between the process of care and health outcomes. After risk adjustment, patients' likelihood of in-hospital mortality decreased by 10% for every 10% increase in adherence to treatments recommended in American College of Cardiology (ACC)/American Heart Association (AHA) Guidelines. The authors suggest that these results support the use of guideline-based performance measures as a way of assessing and helping to improve quality of care.

Nolan and Berwick[4] highlight the fact that all major quality measurement systems in the USA now use 'science-based indicators of proper processes of care', and point out that several individual performance measures are used to assess care for the same condition. This, however, presents a problem when calculating performance against multiple discrete process measures for the same condition because there is more than one way of doing this:

1. item-by-item measurement
2. composite measurement
3. all-or-none measurement.

Nolan and Berwick argue for all-or-none measurement because of the advantages it brings:

- all-or-none measurement more closely reflects the interests of patients, especially when process components interact synergistically or when partial completion of a series of steps of care is not sufficient to achieve a result
- all-or-none measurement fosters a system perspective, encouraging concern for a sequence of care and not just its parts
- all-or-none measurement provides a more sensitive scale for assessing improvement, and thereby may stimulate further improvement in quality.

As Nolan and Berwick point out, quality is often an all-or-none property.

Setting standards
A standard is a subjective judgement of a level of performance that *could* be achieved. Different levels of quality standard can be set (Fig. 6.7).

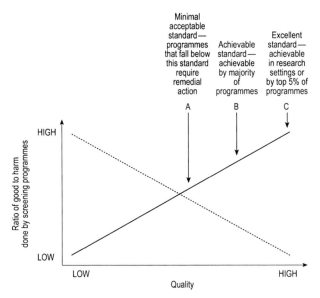

Fig. 6.7
Levels of quality standard set in the context of the ratio of
the amount of good (—) and harm (- - -) done by screening
programmes of different levels of quality

- The *minimal* acceptable standard below which no service
  should fall without urgent remedial action being taken.
- The *excellent* or *optimal* standard: the best level of
  service that can be achieved. Although this is a worthy
  standard, it is often achieved only by exceptional people
  and/or people working in exceptional circumstances.
  The excellent or optimal standard may be regarded by
  colleagues in other services as atypical and therefore
  it is of little use for motivating the majority of service
  providers.
- The *achievable* standard: the level of performance
  achieved by the top quartile of services. If one quartile
  of services can achieve a certain level of performance,
  almost all services have the potential to do so.

Setting targets
A comparison of actual performance with the standard
enables a target for quality improvement to be set. These
elements can be combined into a system of care as shown in
Fig. 6.8.

6.8.1.2 Quality assessment by measuring the outcome of care

The outcome of care is the result of undertaking healthcare
activities.

Objectives	Criteria	Standards		Present position	Targets
		Minimal	Achievable		
To cover the population who would benefit from cervical screening	Percentage of women who have **not** had a hysterectomy who have had a readable smear in the last 5 years	50%	80%	70 general practices less than 50% coverage 17 general practices greater than 80% coverage	By the end of year: 1 out of 70 general practices less than 50% 35 general practices greater than 80% coverage

Fig. 6.8
Standards incorporated into a system of care for cervical screening

When outcome measures were first proposed they were hailed as the ultimate measures that would enable the patient and purchaser to distinguish between a service of good quality and one of poor quality. Further experience with outcome-based measures of quality has stemmed this initial enthusiasm for two main reasons:[5]

1. The health status of an individual, a group of patients or a population receiving a service is determined by several factors other than the quality of that service, notably, severity of illness and state of health before treatment.
2. The collection of valid information about outcomes in ordinary service settings is difficult due to the problems of obtaining accurate data on what are known as confounding variables, namely, factors other than quality of care that could explain the variation in outcome.

Outcomes are rarely of use in measuring quality because it has not proved feasible to collect information on outcomes in large databases of sufficiently good quality to allow the adequate evaluation of existing services. However, there is still hope that such databases could be used to provide useful information on the quality of services delivered by individual institutions or clinicians.

Despite the numerous practical problems that must be resolved to ensure that databases contain accurate data on each and every case treated within a service, outcome measures, e.g. mortality rates for patients with specific conditions such as myocardial infarction, are being used to construct 'league tables' of hospital quality. Unless there is complete data coverage in a database, any conclusions drawn from database analysis may be misleading. However,

Margin Note 6.7
In a cervical screening programme, although mortality rates from cervical cancer are the only measures those responsible for evaluating national policy should use, for local decision-makers this outcome measure is not a good indicator of service quality for two reasons:

1. Changes in mortality rates are influenced by factors other than service quality, for example, changes in the incidence of cervical cancer.
2. Changes in mortality rate reflect the quality of the service pertaining several years ago, whereas the manager or purchaser needs information about the current state of quality.

completeness of data (in terms of quantity and quality) does not resolve all of the problems in using outcome measures because, in any comparison, factors such as co-morbidity and disease severity must be taken into account.

Co-morbidity is the presence of other conditions that may be relevant to a patient's outcome; *severity* describes the stage of disease a patient has reached. Those hospitals at which there are selective admission procedures – i.e. certain patients who have significant co-morbidity or a severe form of a disease are excluded – may appear to achieve better outcomes than those hospitals at which either all patients are admitted or more difficult cases are treated. The standard of care at hospitals with selective admission procedures may be no better than that in a hospital to which all cases are admitted; indeed, it may even be worse. Failure to correct for co-morbidity and/or disease severity is the most common reason why false conclusions are drawn from the analysis of such databases. Any league tables generated from databases for which co-morbidity and disease severity data are not routinely collected are of limited credibility, particularly with reference to those hospitals at which performance appears to be poor.

In addition to the need to collect robust data and to correct for co-morbidity and disease severity when assessing quality through outcome measures, it is also important to investigate the method used to calculate the outcome indicator (Casebook 6.1).[6]

Casebook 6.1 Importance of the method used to calculate an outcome indicator (Source: Iezzoni[6])

Even hospital mortality rates can be calculated in such a way as to distort perceptions of performance.

During the 19th century, William Farr and Florence Nightingale argued that urban hospitals, particularly those in London, were more dangerous than rural hospitals. They supported this contention with data showing the number of deaths ('mortality per cent on inmates') at the 106 principal hospitals in England, which were published in the *24th Annual Report of the Registrar-General*. According to this data, mortality at the 24 London hospitals was 90.84% compared with a mortality of 12.78% at the Royal Sea Bathing Infirmary in Margate. However, Farr had calculated the death rates as follows: total number of deaths at the hospital in 1861 divided by the number of patients at the hospital on 8 April 1861. As can be seen, the numerator reflected the figures for an entire year whereas the denominator reflected the figure for a single day in that year. Farr had actually calculated death rates per occupied hospital bed and not mortality rates per total number of hospitalised patients. Farr's methodology inflated the apparent mortality rates; when calculated as the annual number of deaths divided by the total number of inpatients treated during the year, the mortality rates for the general wards of 14 London hospitals averaged 9.7%.

6.8.1.3 Reporting outcomes in the public domain

The benefits and hazards of reporting medical outcomes in the public domain are set out in an excellent article[7] about the work of the New York (NY) State Department of Health to reduce mortality after coronary artery bypass grafting (CABG). In 1989, the NY State Cardiac Advisory Committee helped the NY Department of Health to set up a cardiac surgery reporting system in order to collect information about demographic variables, risk factors and complications, and mortality after operation. In 1990, the Department published the risk-adjusted mortality rates for each hospital. Using the freedom of information law, a newspaper then sued the Department to obtain the original data from which these rates had been calculated, and won. The data were published in December 1991 to a stormy reaction from the participating surgeons. Despite this, the NY Department of Health continued with the programme.

An analysis of the data showed that from the beginning of 1989 through to the end of 1992 there was a 41% decline in risk-adjusted operative mortality.[7] Although at that time no comparable data existed for other states, and many factors could explain the decline in mortality (e.g. improved surgical techniques), it is reasonable to assume that the reporting system was responsible for part of the improvement seen, which may have resulted from the ability to identify surgeons who had poor records, usually those performing only a small number of procedures. Between 1989 and 1992, 27 low-volume surgeons (those performing <50 operations/year) stopped performing CABG in New York State.

Although the cardiac surgery reporting system was bold and scientifically rigorous, it should be possible to use this type of approach elsewhere to improve performance for specific procedures that are relatively few in number but which have dramatic outcomes (e.g. death). It is not unrealistic to pursue an objective of making hospital- and operator-specific information publicly available for a small number of interventions.

6.8.2   Searching for and appraising evidence on standards of care

6.8.2.1 Searching for papers on quality standards

- Specify the intervention.
- Combine with terms that define the relevant parameters:

➡ Quality Assurance, Health Care/
➡ Quality Indicators, Health Care/
➡ "quality"
➡ "audit"
➡ "standards"
➡ "guidelines".

6.8.2.2 Appraising evidence on quality standards

The most appropriate form of study design is one in which a service is monitored over a period of time, not only to measure performance against agreed quality standards but also to assess the effects of the interventions designed to improve quality by measuring performance on at least two separate occasions. A checklist of questions for the appraisal of evidence on quality is shown in Box 6.17.

6.8.3   Searching for and appraising evidence on variations in healthcare outcome

The search for, and appraisal of, evidence about standards of care and means of quality improvement is often driven by the healthcare professionals or managers within a service. However, external forces, such as the publication of inter-hospital audit results or hospital mortality league tables, may also raise the issue. Although the identification of poor performance can provoke denial in those working within a service, it is possible to take a scientific approach to quality improvement.

6.8.3.1 Searching for papers on variations in healthcare outcome

Combine search terms for the disease/health problem with those for the intervention (e.g. an operation), and combine the results with terms for variations in care, such as the MeSH:

- Mortality/
- Unnecessary Procedures/

Box 6.17 Checklist for the appraisal of evidence on quality

1. Is there good evidence that the intervention used as the indicator of quality is an effective intervention?
2. Are there standards relating to acceptability and safety?
3. Is there clear information about the method used to develop the standards, e.g. are the standards set by taking the cut-off point for the top quartile of several services?
4. Is there only one measure of quality or are there several measures?

- Quality of Health Care/
- Appropriateness/.

6.8.3.2 *Appraising evidence on variations in healthcare outcome*

Large databases can also be manipulated to compare different types of institution, for example:

- teaching hospitals vs non-teaching hospitals
- services providing a high volume of care vs those providing a low volume.

For this type of comparison, it is not possible to perform an RCT; however, the 'natural experiment' created by the variety of health services provided presents an opportunity to identify the determinants of quality.

A checklist of questions for the appraisal of studies designed to investigate a possible managerial problem or to identify the determinants of service quality is shown in Box 6.18.[8]

6.8.4   Applicability and relevance

Is it possible to apply the results of studies on quality of care from one organisation, or population, to another? It has been argued that, because health service provision and methods of payment vary greatly from one population to another, work on quality is not generalisable but is specific to the population in which the study was done.

Although it is true that the *results* of studies of quality are not generalisable (poor quality of care in a service such as cervical screening in one population does not mean that the quality of cervical screening will be poor in all populations), the identification of criteria that can be used to set standards and measure quality, and the identification of the reasons for quality failure, are generally applicable. For example, in the study of CABG in New York State,[7] the identification of the high risk of mortality associated with low-volume surgeons is a generalisable finding. It is immaterial whether the high mortality rate arose because those surgeons were less practised in the operation or because fewer patients were referred to those surgeons by physicians who were aware of their colleagues' performance (a common quality standard used within the profession); the association was demonstrated and is relevant to all the parties involved – patients, physicians, providers and purchasers.

Box 6.18 Checklist for the appraisal of studies of quality in the provision of healthcare (Source: adapted from Naylor and Guyatt[8])

1. Are the outcome measures accurate and comprehensive?

Large databases tend to include only simple outcome measures, such as death, and rarely hold data on measures such as disability or quality of life.)

2. Were there clearly identified and appropriate comparison groups?
3. Were the comparison groups similar with respect to important determinants of outcome other than the one of interest?

For example, when comparing teaching hospitals with non-teaching hospitals, the question must be asked: 'Are the two groups of patients similar from the point of view, for example, of the prognosis?' Useful appraisal questions to ask include:

- Did the investigators measure all known important prognostic factors?
- Were measures of patients' prognostic factors reproducible and accurate?
- Did the investigators show the extent to which patients differ on these factors?
- Did the researchers use some form of multivariate analysis to adjust for all the important prognostic factors?
- Did additional analysis (particularly in low-risk subgroups) demonstrate the same results as the primary analysis?

4. Were all possible hypotheses examined?

Often the report of an observational study has as a focus the most dramatic finding, e.g. a difference between teaching and non-teaching hospitals, but when comparing services in which there are differences in the same outcome measure more than one explanation is possible.

- Who did the operation, e.g. specialist or generalist?
- When was it done, e.g. day or night, weekday or weekend?
- Where was it done, e.g. in a large-volume or small-volume service?
- How was it done?
- Which operation was done?

References

1. Donabedian, A. (1980) *The definition of quality: a conceptual exploration*. In: *Explorations in Quality Assessment and Monitoring. Volume 1: The Definition of Quality and Approaches to its Assessment*. Health Administration Press, Ann Arbor.
2. Crowley, P.A. (1995) *Antenatal corticosteroid therapy: a meta-analysis of the randomized trials, 1972 to 1994*. Am. J. Obstet. Gynecol. 173: 322–5.
3. Peterson, E.D., Roe, M.T., Mulgand, Y. et al. (2006) *Association between hospital process performance and outcomes among patients with acute coronary syndromes*. JAMA 295: 1912–20.
4. Nolan, T. and Berwick, D.M. (2006) *All-or-none measurement raises the bar on performance*. JAMA 295: 1168–70.
5. Schroeder, S.A. and Kabcenell, A.I. (1991) *Do bad outcomes mean substandard care?* JAMA 265: 1995.

6. Iezzoni, L.I. (1996) *100 apples divided by 15 red herrings: a cautionary tale from the mid-19th century on comparing hospital mortality rates*. Ann. Intern. Med. 124: 1079–85.
7. Chassin, M.R., Hannan, R.L. and DeBuono, B.A. (1996) *Benefits and hazards of reporting medical outcomes publicly*. New Eng. J. Med. 334: 394–8.
8. Naylor, C.D. and Guyatt, G.H. (1996) *User's guides to the medical literature. X. How to use an article reporting variations in the outcomes of health services.* JAMA 275: 554–8.

6.9   Appropriateness

6.9.1   Dimensions and definitions

Appropriateness is a measure of the way in which an intervention is used in clinical practice. It is based on a subjective judgement about whether it is right to give a particular intervention to:

- an individual
- a group of patients
- a population.

It is assessed on a balance of probabilities: the probability of doing good against the probability of doing harm; however, the judgement must also take into account the resources available – what is appropriate at the Mayo Clinic may not be appropriate in Chelyabinsk.

The appropriateness of care provided to an individual patient or group of patients can be determined in several different ways:

- by asking an independent clinician or group of clinicians and patients to pass judgement on the intervention given
- by comparing the intervention given to a patient with clinical guidelines indicating which patients are most likely to benefit, or least likely to be harmed, by that intervention.

As the distinction between appropriateness and inappropriateness is a matter of judgement, there is a spectrum of potential categories. In many studies of appropriateness, three categories are identified (Fig. 6.9):

- clearly appropriate
- clearly inappropriate

Unequivocally appropriate	The grey zone	Unequivocally inappropriate

Fig. 6.9
The spectrum of judgements about appropriateness

- a category in-between, where clinicians, experts and patients disagree about appropriateness depending on their values – a grey zone.

The concept of appropriateness is particularly useful when making decisions about what Naylor has called the 'grey zones of clinical practice', namely, aspects of care for which the evidence is scarce or the evidence available is not relevant to the patient or the service under consideration.[1]

6.9.1.1 Appropriateness for individual patients

In clinical practice, any judgement of appropriateness should take into account the needs, values and expressed wishes of the individual patient. Chemotherapy with agents that carry a high probability of side-effects may be appropriate for a patient who has potentially curable cancer but may be inappropriate for a patient who has incurable cancer, depending upon the relative values the patient attaches to a few more months of life on the one hand and to suffering from side-effects on the other. Hitherto, financial cost has not been a factor in clinical decisions about appropriateness relating to individual patients, but it has become a factor as demand on resources increases.

6.9.1.2 Appropriateness for groups of patients or populations

For groups of patients and populations, the concept of appropriateness relates not only to the benefits and risks but also to the costs of intervention. Furthermore, the appropriateness of providing an intervention or a service for any population may change with the volume of service provided.

If resources are limited, a service is usually given only to those who are most likely to benefit. As resources increase, the threshold for intervention changes and the intervention may be offered to people who are at lower risk or less severely affected. The benefit obtained decreases with each unit of increase in resources with a flattening of the cost–benefit curve – known as the law of diminishing returns (Fig. 6.10).[2]

However, interventions have adverse as well as beneficial effects. Donabedian, who invented the concept of 'structure, process and outcome' in healthcare evaluation, also introduced the benefit-to-harm graph.[2]

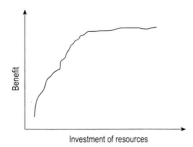

Fig. 6.10
The law of diminishing returns – the decrease in the amount of
benefit obtained for each unit of increase in resources
(Source: Donabedian[2])

He argued that when the volume of healthcare offered
is increased, the cost–benefit curve flattens but the
cost–harm curve does not; that is, side-effects may be
as common in individuals at low risk or who have mild
disease as in those at high risk or who have severe
disease. For each unit increase in resources or volume of
care, there is a concomitant increase in harmful or adverse
effects (Fig. 6.11).[2]

Thus, as the proportion of a population covered
by a health service increases, the balance of good to
harm changes. This can be expressed most simply by
subtracting harm from good and showing the net benefit
graphically (Fig. 6.12). As coverage increases, a point
is reached, referred to by Donabedian as the point of
optimality, where the difference between benefit and harm
starts to diminish (see Fig. 6.12).

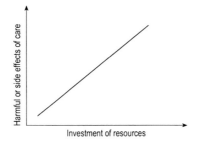

Fig. 6.11
The balance of benefit to harm – for each unit of increase in
resources, or volume of healthcare, there is an increase in harmful
or adverse effects (Source: Donabedian[2])

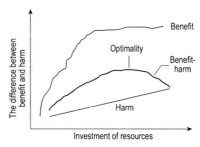

Fig. 6.12
The balance of benefit to harm – the net benefit to the population
as the proportion receiving healthcare increases (Source:
Donabedian[2])

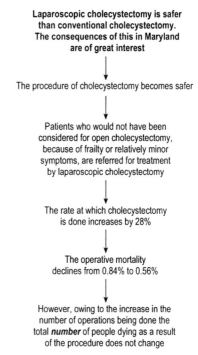

Fig. 6.13
The epidemic of cholecystectomies (Source: Steiner et al.[3])

For an example of the benefit-to-harm phenomenon in
the treatment of gallstone disease, see Fig. 6.13.[3]

6.9.1.3 Identifying concerns about appropriateness

There are several ways in which the appropriateness of use
of a particular intervention may be identified as being a
matter of concern, notably:

- as part of an audit project
- following the publication of an article on appropriateness

Table 6.5 The underlying problems indicated by variation

Variation:	Possible problem:
– in outcome	Quality
– in rates of intervention, i.e. in process	Appropriateness

- following the publication of a league table showing variations in the rate of use of a particular intervention by different clinicians or services; in such situations, pressure to change will fall on the professional or service deemed to be the least appropriate, i.e. at the end of the league table that denotes poor performance.

Evidence-based analysis of variations in levels of use may indicate variations in appropriateness of use (variations in outcome may indicate variations in quality) (Table 6.5).

During the 1990s, the results of an increasing number of studies demonstrated wide variations in rates of care provided. Some of the variations observed are far greater than can be explained by variations in the incidence and prevalence of disease. In one of the classic studies of this phenomenon, Wennberg et al. compared the provision of hospital services in Boston and in New Haven.[4]. The two communities receiving hospital care were similar demographically (in terms of percentages of those who were below the poverty line, black, and aged 65 years or over). In both Boston and New Haven, a large proportion of the resident population was admitted to major teaching hospitals. Excluding any beds occupied by non-residents, it was found that people in Boston occupied 4.5 beds per 1000 population, whereas people in New Haven occupied only 2.9. The overall rates of admission in Boston were found to be nearly 50% higher than those in New Haven, with the average length of stay being 7% longer. Since this classic study in the late 1980s, Wennberg's work on variations in the level of use of interventions has been recognised as describing an important phenomenon and highlights clinical services in which interventions are either over- or under-used.

Wennberg has identified the obstacles to remediating unwarranted variations in healthcare[5] as follows:

- a quality agenda that has yet to be given a focus on improving the quality of patient decision-making
- economic incentives that do not reward exemplary practice
- the poor state of clinical science.

In addition, Wennberg believes it is necessary to challenge two cultural biases, namely, that:

- more care is better
- physicians must know best.

Wennberg and co-workers[6] investigated the Medicare rates for surgery to treat degenerative diseases of the hip, knee and spine among hospital referral regions (HRRs) in the USA and found:

- the rates to be highly variable among the HRRs
- the relative risk for surgery to be constant within an HRR from year to year, a large part of the variation in surgery in 2000/01 being explained by the variation in rates in 1992/93.

The authors suggest that there are two strategies which may have promise for reducing unwarranted regional variation and local constancy surgery risk:

1. shared decision-making
2. outcomes research.

The results of other studies of the phenomenon of variation have also disclosed its occurrence in the provision of care for almost every condition in which clinical judgement plays a part. A consideration of the results of all these studies highlights the need for detailed study of clinicians' behaviour and in particular the ways in which their interpretation of the evidence, influenced by local custom, culture and practice, result in one population receiving a different level of care, and thereby consuming a different amount of resources, to a similar population living elsewhere.

Unfortunately, there is no evidence as yet to show that these variations in clinical practice are decreasing in England. The Annual Report 2005 of the Chief Medical Officer (CMO) contains as one of its main features a chapter on variation in clinical practice,[7] which highlights four examples:

- tonsillectomy rates
- coronary revascularisation rates
- statin prescription rates
- hysterectomy rates in young women.

Although some variations in clinical practice can be explained by the health needs of patients, the behaviour of pathological processes and the scientific evidence base, the CMO concludes that the healthcare in the NHS at present is inequitable:

> to some extent, the inequity arising in part as a result of the influence of one or more of the following factors:
> - the preference of clinicians
> - the socio-economic status of patients
> - the empowerment of patients
> - decisions regarding specific local resource allocation.[7]

According to the CMO, variability in the delivery of specific interventions across the NHS that cannot be explained would suggest one of several problems:

- inappropriate resource allocation
- poor spread of new knowledge to the consulting room
- insufficiently robust and ineffective appraisal processes and decisions (with respect to subject matter, conduct, dissemination or implementation).

6.9.1.4 It may be appropriate but is it necessary?

Once all ineffective interventions and services have been excluded, if resources are limited, it may not be possible to provide all of the *effective* and appropriate services. The team from the RAND Health Sciences Program has developed a further criterion to evaluate appropriate interventions: necessity.[8] Their definition of appropriateness is that the benefits should sufficiently outweigh the risks to make the procedure worth performing, and they extend this definition by proposing criteria that can be used to decide whether a procedure is necessary (Box 6.19).[8]

A high necessity rating indicates that it is improper clinical judgement not to recommend the procedure; a low

Margin Note 6.8
Both under-use and over-use of treatments are rife in this and most other countries and are enemies of effective healthcare.
Sir Liam Donaldson, Chief Medical Officer for England[7]

Box 6.19 Criteria for identifying necessary interventions (all four must be met) (Source: adapted from Kahan et al.[8])

- The procedure must be appropriate, as defined above.
- It would be improper care in the judgement of most clinicians not to recommend this service.
- There is a reasonable chance that the procedure will benefit the patient. Procedures with a low likelihood of benefit but few risks are not considered necessary.
- The benefit to the patient is not small. Procedures that provide only minor benefits are not necessary.

necessity rating indicates that there are alternative courses of action (including no action) that are equally or almost equally appropriate. This is an important and novel way of thinking about procedures being used by the RAND team.

Necessity can be measured by asking a panel of clinicians to rate a set of cases. Although there is, as would be expected, variation in rating, there is sufficient consistency for the measure of necessity to be useful. One obvious use is to determine which procedures are not necessary to the well-being of patients. However, the RAND team points out that the converse is also possible, namely, that patients do not receive necessary treatment either because of costs or because of the judgement of the clinicians. The RAND team reviewed 243 patients with angina who had positive exercise stress tests. They found that patients who were under the care of a cardiologist were more likely to receive a 'necessary' exercise stress test than those who were under the care of a generalist or primary care physician.[9]

6.9.1.5 Who defines necessity?

Hitherto, the definition of necessity has been made by doctors (Fig. 6.14).

However, dramatic changes to the conception of appropriateness are taking place, and two of the other stakeholders in medical decision-making – patients on the one hand, and payers on the other – are becoming much more influential.

Rosenbaum et al.[10] have identified three issues in the definition of necessity:

1. Who has the power to decide what is meant by necessity?
2. What evidence can and must be used to justify the decision?
3. Who bears the burden of proof: must the insurer demonstrate with acceptable evidence that a recommended treatment is unnecessary, or does the patient bear the burden of demonstrating that the treatment in question is necessary?

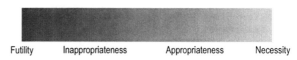

| Futility | Inappropriateness | Appropriateness | Necessity |

Fig. 6.14
The spectrum of appropriateness for healthcare interventions from futility to necessity

It is interesting to note there is no mention of the clinician in this discussion – a portent of things to come?

6.9.1.6 Medical futility

A consideration of what constitutes appropriate care has led to the identification of some interventions as not only inappropriate but also futile.[11]

The definition of futility is problematic, but a useful definition has been developed by the Council on Ethical and Judicial Affairs of the American Medical Association (AMA).

> *In the course of caring for a critically ill patient it may become apparent that further intervention will only prolong the final stages of the dying process. At this point, further intervention is often described as futile.*[12]

The Council recognises there has been controversy in both the literature and clinical practice about what comprises a futile intervention. It has been suggested that futile interventions are those which sustain life for patients in a persistent vegetative state, or which continue 'aggressive' therapy, such as chemotherapy, for people with advanced terminal cancer who have no realistic expectation of cure or symptom relief. Owing to the difficult position that many clinicians find themselves in when dealing with patients at the end of life, the Council on Ethical and Judicial Affairs reviewed the problems they had to face and proposed a 'fair process' for managing futility cases. The process comprises seven steps: four aimed at deliberation and resolution; two aimed at securing alternatives in case of irresolvable differences; and a final step designed to achieve 'closure' when other alternatives have been exhausted (Fig. 6.15; see also Section 10.6).[12]

Burt[13] points out that there is no clear general principle available to resolve conflicts between patient self-determination and physician autonomy, and argues that although extended negotiation is the only way to reach a satisfactory resolution it may not always be possible to arrive at an agreement. Therefore, Burt recommends that the legal system provides both patients and clinicians with some authority and power to exert over each other to maximise engagement in the negotiating process.

Schneiderman et al. conducted a randomised controlled trial on the effects of ethics consultations on non-beneficial (i.e. futile) life-sustaining treatments in an intensive care

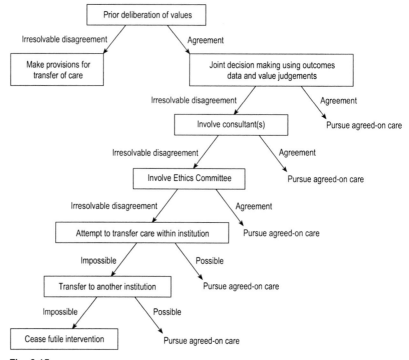

Fig. 6.15
The process for considering futility cases devised by the American Medical
Association Council on Ethical and Judicial Affairs[12]

unit,[14] and found that ethics consultations resulted in less
time spent on ventilators for patients who eventually died
and patients' families being satisfied with the process of
care.

In making decisions about the futility of further
intervention, the AMA model outlined in Fig. 6.15
emphasises the need for a decision-making process and
structure within a healthcare organisation, supported by an
institutional committee. Such committees are usually called
clinical ethics committees, to distinguish them from research
ethics committees, which consider the ethical implications
of research protocols. The role of clinical ethics committees
is evolving, and different types of ethics committees have
developed in different kinds of healthcare organisation and
in various countries.

In 1997, Herb and Lazar[15] identified three main themes of
work for ethics committees:

1. education
2. policy review and evaluation
3. case review.

However, they emphasise that these functions become interwoven because the consideration of individual cases tends to reveal problems that may require the development of new policies and/or necessitate individual, team or organisational learning.

There is an increasing number of clinical ethics committees at hospital trusts in the UK:[16] by 2003, 60 of the 315 acute NHS trusts had a clinical ethics committee.[17] The areas of work of these committees follow the themes identified by Herb and Lazar:[15]

- providing ethics input into hospital trust policy and guidelines around patient care
- facilitating ethics education of health professionals in the trust
- giving advice to clinicians on individual cases.

In 2001, a UK Clinical Ethics Network was established,[16] the principal aims of which are:

- to promote the development of clinical ethics support in the UK
- to encourage a high level of ethical debate in clinical practice
- to facilitate sharing of best practice between clinical ethics committees.

In a Commentary on ethics committees in Croatia,[18] Ashcroft reflects on how some of the issues relevant to this eastern European country could resonate across all countries in Europe. He poses the suggestion that, as many health systems in Europe are under pressure – from inadequate resourcing, high direct costs for patients, inequalities in access, corruption and formal or informal rationing – these issues are as real subjects to address as the traditional clinical ethical issues ethics committees address about decision-making at the end of life and conflict resolution between family members and healthcare staff. In addition, he remarks on the migration of clinical research into health systems which means that hospitals may be under pressure to take on research projects that may not be in the best interests of patients or the institution as a whole. He concludes that to be useful to both clinicians and patients, and to maintain moral legitimacy, ethics committees need to have not only a clear sense of purpose but also a clear sense of how best to achieve that purpose.

During the consideration of ethical issues, it is important for clinical ethics committees to base their decisions on evidence. Studies of evidence and ethical-based decision-making in the treatment of patients who have a poor prognosis are now being published. In an important study of the 'aggressive surgical management' of patients with penetrating brain injuries, usually from gunshot wounds, the relatives of patients were given evidence about the probable outcome of surgical management. Levy et al.[19] found that it was possible to make evidence-based decisions about aggressive surgical treatment that were satisfactory to the relatives, but that also limited the number of pointless new surgical procedures while still 'liberally' favouring those patients who had even a small chance of surviving to live independently. The authors emphasised the need to see the role of the physician as being not only a surgical interventionist but also 'a provider of information and co-decision-maker' (see Sections 10.2, 10.3 and 10.4.3).

6.9.2   Searching

We make the following suggestions to help you find articles on appropriateness:

Step 1: Specify the intervention for which there are different rates of utilisation. The relevant Medical Subject Heading (MeSH) is Utilization Review/, an American term similar to clinical audit.

Step 2: Limit this to a Publication Type of Guideline [pt] or Practice Guideline [pt].

Step 3: The MeSH Guidelines/ can also be used – this should be exploded to include Practice Guidelines/.

Step 4: The text words "guideline" and "appropriateness" can also be included. The MeSH for appropriateness is Regional Health Planning/, which it may be necessary to explode.

6.9.3   Appraisal

Most of the research published on appropriateness is a review of data about patients that were collected previously. A checklist of three sets of questions useful for the appraisal of evidence of appropriateness is shown in Box 6.20.[20]

6.9.4   Applicability and relevance

Appropriateness is a subjective measure of whether an intervention, or level of intervention, is right; this judgement of 'rightness' is influenced by the incidence or prevalence of the disease in the population and by the resources available.

Box 6.20   Checklist for the appraisal of evidence of appropriateness (Source: adapted from Naylor and Guyatt[20])

1. Are the criteria evidence based?
* Is there evidence to support the judgements about:
   - right patient?
   - right place?
   - right time?
   - right intervention?
   - right professional?
* What is the quality of the evidence on which the judgements have been made and the criteria chosen?
* How good was the agreement between experts on the panel?
* Were patients' views on outcomes taken into account?
2. How scientifically was the study done?
* Were steps taken to minimise bias, for example, by using more than one auditor or by using explicit criteria to audit notes?
* Was the sample of patients representative and large enough to produce valid results?
3. Are the criteria relevant to the local service?
* How similar is the local population to the population studied?
* Were the clinicians on the panel similar to the local professionals?
* How different from the local facility was the facility studied?

Although the results of studies of appropriateness may not be generalisable, they may be of relevance to different populations because they can reveal areas of clinical uncertainty. Thus, a study of appropriateness could indicate an interesting area to investigate in the local health service; if validated, the methods used in the study can probably be transposed to the local service, with modification. However, the levels of intervention judged to be 'right' for the local population must be determined according to local circumstances.

References

1. Naylor, C.D. (1995) *The grey zones of clinical practice*. Lancet 345: 840–2.
2. Donabedian, A. (1980) *Explorations in Quality Assessment and Monitoring. Volume 1: The Definition of Quality and Approaches to its Assessment.* Health Administration Press, Ann Arbor.
3. Steiner, C.A., Bass, E.B., Talamini, M.A. et al. (1994) *Surgical rates and operative mortality for open and laparoscopic cholecystectomy in Maryland*. N. Engl. J. Med. 330: 403–8.

4. Wennberg, J.E., Freeman, J.L. and Culp, W.J. (1987) *Are hospital services rationed in New Haven or over-utilised in Boston?* Lancet i: 1185–8.

5. Wennberg, J.E. (2004) Perspective: *Practice variations and health care reform: connecting the dots.* Health Aff. (Millwood) (Suppl. Web Exclusives): var140–4.

6. Weinstein, J.N., Bronner, K.K., Morgan, T.S. et al. (2004) Trends: *Trends and geographic variations in major surgery for degenerative diseases of the hip, knee and spine.* Health Aff. (Millwood) (Suppl. Web Exclusives): var81–9.

7. Donaldson, L. (2005) *The Chief Medical Officer on the State of the Public Health. Annual Report 2005.* Department of Health, London.

8. Kahan, J.P., Bernstein, S.J., Leape, L.L. et al. (1994) *Measuring the necessity of medical procedures.* Med. Care 32: 357–65.

9. Borowsky, S.J., Kravitz, R.L., Laouri, M. et al. (1995) *Effect of physician specialty on use of necessary coronary angiography.* J. Am. Coll. Cardiol. 26: 1484–91.

10. Rosenbaum, S., Frankford, D.M., Moore, B. et al. (1999) *Who should determine when health care is medically necessary?* N. Engl. J. Med. 340: 229–32.

11. Zucker, M.B. and Zucker, H.D. (eds) (1997) *Medical Futility and the Evaluation of Life-Sustaining Interventions.* Cambridge University Press, Cambridge.

12. Council On Ethical And Judicial Affairs, American Medical Association (1999) *Medical futility in end-of-life care. Report of the Council on Ethical and Judicial Affairs.* JAMA 281: 937–41.

13. Burt, R.A. (2002) *The medical futility debate: patient choice, physician obligation, and end-of-life care.* J. Palliat. Med. 5: 249–54.

14. Schneiderman, L.J., Gilmer, T., Teetzel, H.D. et al. (2003) Effects of ethics consultations on non-beneficial life-sustaining treatments in the intensive care setting: a randomized controlled trial. JAMA 290: 1166–72.

15. Herb, A. and Lazar, E.J. (1997) *Ethics committees and end-of-life decision making.* In: Zucker, M.B. and Zucker, H.D. (eds) *Medical Futility and the Evaluation of Life-Sustaining Interventions.* Cambridge University Press, Cambridge.

16. Slowther, A., Johnston, C., Goodall, J. et al. (2004) *Development of clinical ethics committees. [Education and debate]* Br. Med. J. 328: 950–2.

17. UK Clinical Ethics Network. *What are clinical ethics committees?* http://www.ethics-network.org.uk/what.htm

18. Ashcrfoft, R. (2005) *Ethics committees and countries in transition: a figleaf for structural violence? [Commentary]* Br. Med. J. 331: 229–30.

19. Levy, M.L., Davis, S.E., McComb, G. et al. (1996) *Economic, ethical, and outcome-based decisions regarding aggressive surgical management in patients with penetrating craniocerebral injury.* J. Health Commun. 1: 301–8.

20. Naylor, C.D. and Guyatt, G.H. (1996) *User's guides to the medical literature. XI. How to use an article about a clinical utilization review.* JAMA 275: 1435–40.

Gentle Reader,

Empathise with the secretary of the Faculty of Public Health Screening Committee. He was musing on the particular lightness of green that makes the leaves of early summer stand out sharply against the blue sky of May. The movement of the leaves was a comfort to him. He looked at them for at least 3 minutes before letting his eyes drop for a second time to the letter from another public health professional that lay on the desk before him, which had been written in all innocence but was so disturbing in content.

> *Dear Colleague,*
>
> *I would be grateful to know the evidence to support the introduction of screening for abdominal aortic aneurysm which we are currently considering. The proposal is strongly supported. It would have a very beneficial impact on our efficiency index because many more people would be referred to hospital, but I would also be interested to know what health benefits we can describe to the health authority.*

Commentary

Organisations take on a life of their own. The culture of an organisation imbues any decision-making with the prevailing preoccupation, in this case a preoccupation with productivity. To counteract this, a different hierarchy within the decision-making process is vital, one in which it is possible to ask the following questions:

1. *Will the proposal have a beneficial effect on health?*

2. *Is there a harmful effect, and what is the balance between benefit and harm?*

3. *What is the cost of the innovation?*

4. *How does this proposal compare with other proposals currently under consideration?*

5. *Is it possible to deliver the new service at acceptable levels of quality and cost?*

Evidence-based health service management

7.1 Creating the context for an evidence-based organisation

The key components in an evidence-based health service are:

1. healthcare organisations designed with the capability to generate, and the flexibility to incorporate, evidence
2. healthcare professionals who, as individuals and teams, are able to find, appraise, and use knowledge from research as evidence (see Chapter 9).

These two components are inter-related (Fig. 7.1).

For any healthcare organisation to increase the degree to which decisions taken within it are evidence-based, it is important to develop the appropriate *systems* and *culture*; it may also be necessary to change the *structure* of the organisation (Margin Fig. 7.1). Individuals and organisations need to be supported by systems that provide the best knowledge currently available when and where it is required, and to exist in an evaluative culture.

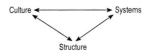

Margin Fig. 7.1

- The culture of an evidence-based healthcare organisation is evaluative – there is an obsession with finding, appraising, and using research-based knowledge as evidence in decision-making.
- In every system of an evidence-based healthcare organisation, research-based knowledge must be sought, appraised, and used as evidence when making decisions. Within that organisation, there must also be systems for managing knowledge, and for developing the skills of individuals who work in the organisation.
- The structure of an evidence-based healthcare organisation should promote and facilitate evidence-based decision-making.

The culture, systems and structure for evidence-based healthcare organisations are discussed in Sections 7.2, 7.3 and 7.4, respectively.

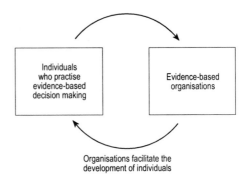

Fig. 7.1
The relationship between individuals and organisations within an evidence-based paradigm

7.1.1   Tacit and explicit knowledge management

Organisations, particularly those that consist of large numbers of individuals, should have the capacity to manage all the knowledge that they need. Indeed, knowledge management has become one of the dominant management trends of the last decade.

Of fundamental importance in thinking about knowledge management is the distinction between two types of knowledge:

- tacit knowledge is practical and subjective, for example, knowing what other people in the organisation are doing
- explicit knowledge is theoretical and objective, for example, the published results of formal research.

Tacit knowledge can be converted into an explicit form in two ways:

- concepts and models are combined into new forms
- knowledge is externalised, e.g. the interpretation of a strategy into recommendations.

Explicit knowledge can be absorbed into the tacit knowledge base by a process closely related to learning by doing.

Evidence-based decision-making has largely been based on the use of explicit knowledge, but it is possible to use knowledge that is tacit.

The characteristics of tacit and explicit knowledge are shown in Table 7.1.

External to an organisation, a clinical network is a forum in which tacit and explicit knowledge can be brought together and shared. Although senior management

Table 7.1 The characteristics of tacit and explicit knowledge

Tacit knowledge	Explicit knowledge
Created by clinicians, patients and managers	Created by researchers
Rarely published; sometimes not even written down	Published in scientific journals
States how to do it	States what to do
May be only locally applicable	Generalisable
Traditionally of low value	Traditionally highly valued

at hospitals which may be in competition with one another might resist the advantages of belonging to a clinical network, there is growing evidence that the volume, complexity and demands for quality involved in modern healthcare mean that clinicians are increasingly nervous about working in isolation. The evolution of multidisciplinary teams and clinical networks offer the individual clinician access to some of the knowledge resources that she or he needs.[1–4]

7.1.1.1 Knowledge from experience

As indicated above, the results of formal research are not the only source of knowledge that is useful to organisations. Experience, particularly in the context of learning from adverse events, can be a valuable form of knowledge if it is used to improve or remedy organisational performance. However, in the past, learning from experience was perceived as ineffective, and potentially harmful in that it might be a way of replicating 'errors'. One of the fields in which learning from adverse events has been successful is aviation, where the primary aim has been to improve safety measures and practices (see Section 6.5).

7.1.2   The learning organisation

The introduction of evidence-based decision-making into an organisation requires cultural change, but in order to integrate an evidence-based approach to decision-making the entire organisation must focus on learning. The characteristics of a learning organisation have been most elegantly described by Peter Senge in his influential book *The Fifth Discipline – the Art and Practice of the Learning Organization*.[5] He has identified five disciplines that are necessary for any organisation to become a learning organisation:

1. personal mastery – the discipline of continually clarifying and deepening one's personal vision and objectivity

Margin Note 7.1
Images of organisations

Organisations can be described in many different ways using a variety of images and metaphors. In his book *Images of Organisation*,[6] Morgan discussed the way in which images are used to characterise an organisation. The images employed are often dictated by the predominant management theorists of the time, for example, Taylor created the concept of the organisation as machine.[7] Organisations have also been likened to:

- families
- brains
- neural networks.

2. making mental models – the discipline of creating with metaphors and language a mental model of what the organisation is, what it stands for, and how it works (Margin Note 7.1[6,7])

3. building shared visions – the discipline of translating the vision of an organisation's leader or leaders from the objectives shared by a few to a vision for everyone in that organisation

4. team learning – the discipline of ensuring that the collective intelligence of a team is greater than the sum of the individual intelligence; if a team is dysfunctional, the intelligence of a team will be less than the summed intelligence of the individuals

5. systems thinking, in which individual elements are linked together into a coherent set of activities with a common set of objectives.

7.1.3 Hypertext organisations

Knowledge-creating organisations, i.e. organisations that produce new knowledge and new ways of working in addition to managing the knowledge produced by others, have been described as hypertext organisations.

In his study of successful Japanese companies, Professor Nonaka describes the need for successful organisations to have:

a non-hierarchical self-organising structure working in tandem with its hierarchical formal structure ... as business organisations grow in scale and complexity they should simultaneously maximise both corporate level efficiency and local flexibility ... the most appropriate name is the hypertext organisation[8] (Fig. 7.2)

In the hypertext organisation:

- each individual belongs to a team, which is usually composed of people who have similar skills
- the organisation is in the process of undertaking several projects
- a leader is assigned to each project, together with various individuals who will be working on it, who are almost always drawn from more than one team
- each individual usually works on more than one project.

Although it is not possible to represent the structure of a hypertext organisation as a matrix, this non-hierarchical self-organising structure is shown in the left-hand side of

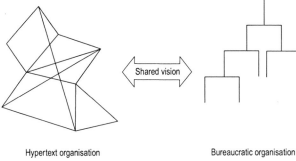

Hypertext organisation   Bureaucratic organisation

Fig. 7.2
Diagrammatic representation of a hypertext organisation, showing
the non-hierarchical self-organising structure in tandem with the
hierarchical formal structure united by a shared vision (Source: Nonaka
and Takeuchi[8])

Fig. 7.2. The use of browsers within such an organisation
would enable each project and each team, and even each
individual, to have their own page on the World Wide Web.
However, what unites the two complementary structures is
a shared vision within the organisation.

7.1.4   The evidence-based knowledge-rich learning organisation

Is it possible to encompass all these theories into a vision
for the 21st century organisation? Perhaps the most
appropriate metaphor to use is that of the organisation as
a human being, an entity that is greater than a series of
neural networks, because human beings have hopes, fears,
and morale. The characteristic of an organisation that I, as
author of a book about evidence-based healthcare, would
most like to see developed is the capacity to create, find,
appraise, use, and retrieve evidence in order to inform
decision-making.

An evidence-based knowledge-rich learning organisation
is one in which:

- the creation and use of knowledge is valued and the
  availability of knowledge is assured
- there is a commitment to knowledge management to
  ensure that systems and skills for finding, appraising,
  and using evidence, i.e. knowledge derived from
  research, are developed and supported (see Chapter 9)
- both tacit and explicit knowledge are readily available
  when and where needed.

References

1. Bushby, J. and Ayiku, L. (2005) *Managed clinical networks.* NLH Health Management Specialist Library October 2005. Available online at: http://www.library.nhs.uk/healthmanagement/ViewResource.aspx?resID=29543&tabID=290.

2. Moir, D., Campbell, H., Wrench, J. et al. (2001) *First steps in developing a managed clinical network for vascular services in Lanarkshire.* Health Bull. (Edinb.) 59: 405–11.

3. Hamilton, K.E., Sullivan, F.M., Donnan, P.T. et al. (2005) *A managed clinical network for cardiac services: set-up, operation and impact on patient care.* Int. J. Integr. Care 5:e10. Epub 2005 Sep 9.

4. Tolson, D., McIntosh, J., Loftus, L. et al. (2007) *Developing a managed clinical network in palliative care: a realistic evaluation.* Int. J. Nurs. Stud. 44: 183–95. Epub 2006 Jan 19.

5. Senge, P.M. (1990) *The Fifth Discipline. The Art and Practice of the Learning Organisation.* Century Business, London.

6. Morgan, G. (1998) *Images of Organisation.* Sage Publications, London.

7. Taylor, F. (1947) *Scientific Management.* Harper & Row, New York (originally published in 1911).

8. Nonaka, T. and Takeuchi, H. (1995) *The Knowledge-Creating Company. How Japanese Companies Create the Dynamics of Innovation.* Oxford University Press, USA.

7.2   Culture

Gentle Reader,

Marvel at Ernest Schneider, responsible for one of the major sporting breakthroughs of the 20th century: the change in downhill skiing from reliance on the Nordic telemark technique to the fixed heel approach of the European Alps. In the Foreword to his book published in 1936, he said 'more than 29 years of experience as a teacher are behind the assertions I make here'.

Commentary

In general, there are two types of statement in decision-making:

1. propositions supported by evidence
2. unsubstantiated assertions, which tend to be subjective.

Ernest Schneider made the basis for his statement absolutely clear. How many healthcare decision-makers do the same?

Culture in an organisation is created through language and behaviour. The behaviour of the chief executive and of the board are of particular importance.

7.2.1   The evidence-based chief executive

It is vital that the promotion of evidence-based decision-making is not a task assigned solely to the

medical director or the director responsible for R&D or
clinical development, although such personnel do have a
central role in this activity; the chief executive must also be
committed to evidence-based decision-making. S/he must
be able, and be seen:

- to search for evidence, alone if necessary
- to appraise evidence, having participated in a critical
  appraisal skills workshop
- to store important evidence in a way that allows it to be
  retrieved, for example, using bibliographic management
  software, Internet 'favourites' or appropriate file
  management
- to use evidence to make decisions
- to help those individuals accountable to the chief
  executive to develop evidence management skills and
  to change the systems for which they are responsible
  such that evidence can be incorporated into
  decision-making.

7.2.2　The evidence-based board

Gentle Reader,

*Empathise with the medical director. He ground his teeth and bit his tongue: 'That's the third
financial ledger system being introduced in less than 5 years, and there's no evidence to suggest
that this system will be any better than the last two. They've spent hundreds of thousands of
pounds, and no one asked for evidence of effectiveness when the decisions were taken about
which information systems to buy, particularly the financial information systems. All they kept
banging on about was clinical effectiveness. What about some evidence-based management in
this organisation!'*

Commentary

*There has been much emphasis on the need to improve clinical effectiveness and to promote
evidence-based clinical practice. In this book, the need to be more scientific and to use evidence
when making purchasing and managerial decisions about clinical services has been promoted,
but what of the need to use evidence in managerial decisions about management?*

*1. What was the strength of the evidence on which the decision to introduce resource
   management was based?*
2. How good is the evidence used to justify investment in new IT?

In this book, I have focused primarily on decisions
about clinical services, mainly because there is a paucity
of evidence on the effectiveness, or cost-effectiveness,

Casebook 7.1 Effects of small changes in clinical practice on expenditure

Barchester District General Hospital employs 140 consultants and has a turnover of £80 million – an expenditure of £570 000 per consultant per year. Over a year, about 3 million clinical decisions are taken that will affect resource use. If each consultant were to change their clinical practice by increasing the volume or intensity of care at the cost of about £3000 (an increase of 0.52%), due to an increase in clinical and support costs, which may not fall within their clinical directorate, the NHS Trust and its commissioners would face an increased cost of £420 000 a year. This would cause a major problem, yet which clinician would recognise a change of 0.52% in their practice?

of different management arrangements. It is important, however, to ensure that a scientific approach is taken to all aspects of the work of a health service provider because cost pressures may be generated by the accumulation of many small changes, as the example in Casebook 7.1 illustrates.

To ensure that a scientific approach is taken to the management of the provision and delivery of health services, it is advisable to embed evidence-based decision-making at the level of the board in any organisation. The operating objectives of an evidence-based board should be as follows:

- To make decisions based on papers containing explicit references to the evidence
- To include in the minutes of board meetings references to the evidence accepted in support of (or against) any decisions taken
- To nominate one of the board members to be the Chief Knowledge Officer (CKO) (for the role and responsibilities of the CKO, see Section 7.4 and Box 7.6, and Section 2.5.1.1 and Box 2.4)

7.3 Systems

The evidence-based organisation should comprise systems that are capable of:

- providing evidence
- promoting the use of evidence
- consuming and using evidence.

7.3.1 Systems that provide evidence

7.3.1.1 The 'evidence centre'

An evidence-based organisation needs an 'evidence centre', which has:

- access to the World Wide Web
- access (or subscriptions) to the most relevant sources of data, such as Medline and the Cochrane Library
- a limited number of appropriate books and journals
- arrangements in place for obtaining documents or photocopies, e.g. reprints of articles
- personnel who can manage these resources, provide training in and promote their use, and keep up to date with changes in their field, such as a librarian or information professional.

The evidence centre should not simply be a location that decision-makers can visit, but viewed as a resource that can be accessed to provide evidence when it is needed. To fulfil the latter function, it is important to consider not only what evidence is needed but also when it is needed, in what situations and in what form.

The commonest situations in which evidence is needed are:

- in a meeting
- on a ward round/in a clinic.

At present, most decision-makers would have to walk to the library – or, in the case of general practitioners, drive to the hospital, park the car (often a nightmare), then walk to the library, find the evidence and drive back to the health centre. The barriers to accessing evidence are often too great.

A series of systems for accessing evidence is shown in Table 7.2.

7.3.1.2 The National Library for Health

In 1998, the UK Government published an Information Strategy[1] in which the National Library for Health (NLH; previously known as the National electronic Library for Health – NeLH) was introduced. The overall aims for the establishment of NLH were:

- to link all existing libraries or evidence centres
- to provide easy access to best current knowledge.

Table 7.2 Systems for gaining access to evidence and their associated drawbacks and advantages

System	Drawbacks	Advantages
Walk or drive to the library	Time	Break from work
Exit from patient record computer system and access the 'evidence centre'	Time	Possible within hospitals at present; no technology required
Consult 'evidence centre' through a parallel system while patient record is still running	Expensive; two systems needed	Possible at present; needs separate telephone line for primary care
Consult evidence base on laptop or PDA	Expensive (but getting cheaper)	Portable system
Prompts appear on screen with evidence and guidelines when diagnosis, patient's name or test result is entered	None	Minimises time and facilitates incorporation of evidence

The intention was to contribute to improving health and healthcare, clinical practice, and patient choice.

7.3.2   Systems that promote the use of evidence

7.3.2.1 Evidence-based clinical audit

The use of evidence should be incorporated into the audit cycle (Fig. 7.3). There are two ways in which this can be done:

1. by ensuring that the evidence of effectiveness or safety for the intervention subject to audit is of good quality
2. by ensuring that the standards applied within the audit process are scientific and based on the best evidence available.

It is possible to select subjects for audit and suitable services for purchasing by analysing the research evidence. In the UK, the North Thames Regional Health Authority commissioned the London School of Hygiene and Tropical Medicine to undertake such an exercise; 10 topics were identified in a review of opportunities for evidence-based audit and purchasing (Box 7.1).[2]

For each service or type of treatment, it is also possible to identify those interventions that are necessary in order to achieve a good outcome. This approach allows the identification of criteria that can be used to measure quality. A list of evidence-based criteria for the management of elderly patients with fractured neck of femur is shown in Box 7.2.[3-6]

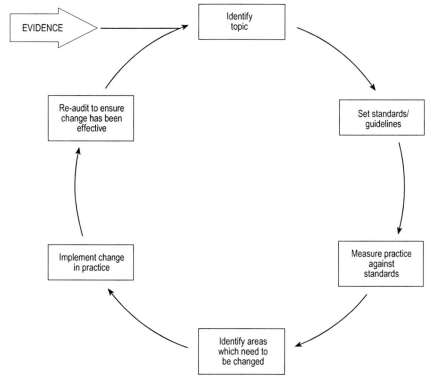

Fig. 7.3
The evidence-driven audit cycle

7.3.2.2 Training for evidence-based decision-making

Within the training and development programme of any
organisation, there must be strategies to develop the skills
of all personnel such that they can practise evidence-based
decision-making and thereby:

Box 7.1 Evidence-based opportunities for audit (Source: Sanderson[2])

1. Prenatal steroids to prevent respiratory distress syndrome
2. Vacuum extraction vs forceps for obstetric delivery
3. Diagnostic D&C in young women
4. Systemic adjuvant therapy for breast cancer
5. Treatment of *Helicobacter pylori* to prevent recurrence of ulcer
6. Thromboprophylaxis for orthopaedic and general surgery
7. Management of mild hypertension
8. Cholesterol screening and use of cholesterol-lowering drugs
9. Aspirin, thrombolysis and anticoagulation after myocardial infarction
10. ACE inhibitors for chronic heart failure

Box 7.2 Evidence-based criteria for the management of elderly patients with fractured neck of femur (Source: References[3-6])

1. Spending less than 1 hour in casualty
2. Receiving prophylactic antibiotics
3. Receiving pharmaceutical thrombo-embolic prophylaxis
4. Having surgery within 24 hours
5. Recording the grade of surgeon and anaesthetist performing the operation
6. Number of days after surgery by which 50% of patients were mobilised
7. Occurrence of pressure sores, urinary tract infection and pneumonia
8. Provision of a thorough medical and social assessment
9. Degree and effectiveness of joint working between orthopaedic surgeons and consultants in medicine for the elderly
10. Adequacy of discharge planning and implementation

- search for and retrieve evidence (Section 9.4.2)
- appraise evidence (Section 9.4.3)
- apply and use evidence (Section 9.4.4).

Previously, health service managers were responsible for the organisation and the systems within it; it was the responsibility of the professions and the educational establishments related to the health service to influence individual clinicians. This division of responsibilities has now changed for two reasons:

1. the professions and the educational establishments are considered to have been too slow in promoting evidence-based clinical practice
2. it has been recognised that the development of systems and of individuals are inter-related (see Fig. 7.1).

Moreover, as those who pay for and manage health services must identify the resources to invest in audit and continuing professional development, they are interested in which types of intervention are effective in bringing about change in professional practice. Although certain interventions have already been shown to be effective, more detailed work is being done, as part of the Cochrane Collaboration, to review the effectiveness of the interventions.[7] A selection of Cochrane Collaboration reviews of specific interventions is shown in Box 7.3.[8]

Box 7.3 Cochrane Collaboration topics under the Effective Practice and Organisation of Care – a selection of the reviews of specific interventions (Source: Cochrane Collaboration[8])

Continuing education and quality assurance

Educational meetings (including lectures, workshops and traineeships)

Continuing education meetings and workshops: effects on professional practice and healthcare outcomes

Local opinion leaders

Local opinion leaders: effects on professional practice and healthcare outcomes

Patient-mediated interventions

Audit and feedback: effects on professional practice and healthcare outcomes

Financial interventions

Provider oriented

Fee-for-service

Capitation, salary, fee-for-service and mixed systems of payment: effects on professional practice and healthcare outcomes

Organisational interventions

Provider oriented

Revision of professional roles, and clinical multidisciplinary teams
Interventions to promote collaboration between nurses and doctors

7.3.3 Systems that consume and use evidence

7.3.3.1 Systems that should be more evidence-based

Although evidence should be used to inform every decision, there are some aspects of healthcare for which the evidence is scanty. However, there are other aspects of healthcare to which evidence could and should be applied to a much greater extent than at present to ensure that the best value is obtained from the resources available, for example:

• drugs and therapeutics decision-making
• equipment purchasing.

As decision-making about drugs is usually centralised within a hospital or primary care team, it should be possible to exercise control over it. There are also good sources of information about the costs, safety and effectiveness of new drugs, which form the foundations of a sound evidence base. In a study of the drivers for the increase in spending on prescription drugs in the province of British Columbia,

Canada,[9] Morgan et al. classified newly patented drugs (including derivatives of existing medicines), which had been appraised by the Canadian Patented Medicines Prices Review Board (CPMPRB) between 1990 and 2003, into one of three categories:

1. breakthrough drugs, defined as the first drug to treat effectively a particular illness, a drug that provides a substantial improvement over existing drug products, subsequent formulations and dosages of a classified breakthrough drug, and competing drugs that enter the clinical subgroup established by a classified breakthrough drug
2. 'me-too' drugs, defined as a drug that does not provide a substantial improvement over existing drug products
3. 'vintage brand' or 'vintage generic' drugs, defined as drugs first marketed before 1990 for which there is no appraisal by the CPMPRB.

Of the 1147 drugs entered into the study, only 142 (12.4%) were classified as breakthrough drugs; 1005 (87.6%) were classified as 'me-too' drugs. When spending on prescription drugs in British Columbia between 1996 and 2003 was analysed, they found that per-capita expenditure more than doubled (from $141 to $316) during this time period, and that most of the increase (80%) was explained by the use of 'me-too' drugs, which did not offer substantial improvements on less expensive alternatives that were available before 1990 (for a breakdown of results, see Table 7.3).[9]

Morgan et al. point out that as the top 20 drugs in terms of global sales include newly patented versions of drugs in long-established categories (i.e. marketed before 1990), 'me-too' drugs 'probably dominate spending trends in most developed countries'.

Table 7.3 Patterns of expenditure and use of different categories of prescription drugs in British Columbia, Canada, between 1996 and 2003 (Source: Morgan et al.[9])

Category of drug	Expenditure (% of total)		Use (% of total)	
	1996	2003	1996	2003
Breakthrough	6%	10%	1%	2%
'Me-too'	41%	63%	24%	44%
Vintage brand and vintage generic	53%	27%	75%	54%

Decision-making about the purchase of equipment, however, is more problematic: there is less evidence available, and the evidence that is available is of poor quality, partly because RCTs of equipment are more difficult to organise and partly because there is no requirement to demonstrate efficacy before introducing new equipment, as is the case for the introduction of new drugs. The introduction of new equipment usually follows one of two routes. The first is via the hospital 'equipment bank' or similar budget, the disbursement of which has to be undertaken with some degree of equity among different departments. A possible consequence of this arrangement is that a particular department may request a new piece of equipment because it is 'their turn', even if good evidence cannot be presented to support the application. The second is via public subscription and charitable appeals due to the constraints imposed on equipment budgets. In this situation, equipment is bought using money obtained directly from the public, for example, through a 'scanner appeal', the consequence of which is that the purchase often bypasses any form of evaluation (Fig. 7.4).

A checklist of questions useful when appraising the evidence base for any proposals to change clinical practice is shown in Box 7.4; these questions can be applied to the introduction of new drugs or of new equipment, and should be incorporated into the system in which information is assimilated for decision-making. In cases where there is uncertainty about the introduction of new equipment, it is advisable to approve any such introduction *only when* there is definitive evidence of efficacy from a research study.

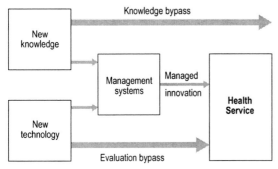

Fig. 7.4
The two main bypass routes for innovations in healthcare

Box 7.4 Checklist for the appraisal of proposals to change clinical practice

1. How did you search for evidence to support this proposal? (Please append the search strategy to this application.)
2. What is the best quality evidence supporting the proposal?
3. What will be the magnitude of the benefit compared with present practice? (Please give estimates based on the most optimistic and the most pessimistic estimate of the effect – the upper and lower confidence intervals.)
4. Compared with present practice, will there be any changes in:
   - patient safety?
   - acceptability and patient satisfaction?
   - cost:
     a) to your directorate?
     b) to any other directorate?
     c) to any other part of the health service?

In 1999, the National Institute for Clinical Excellence (NICE – now known as the National Institute for Health and Clinical Excellence) was set up as a special health authority in the NHS for England and Wales.[†] Its role was to provide patients, healthcare professionals and the public with authoritative, robust and reliable guidance on:

- health technologies, including new and existing medicines, treatments and procedures within the NHS
- clinical practice, including appropriate treatment and care of people with specific diseases and conditions within the NHS.

NICE uses a cost-utility approach to economic evaluation to help judge the value of new technologies that provide additional benefit but at an increased cost.[10] The key measure used to assess the marginal value of new technology for different patient groups is the additional cost per quality-adjusted life-year (QALY) gained. In the absence of data on quality of life, an alternative, such as cost per

---

[†]In 2005, NICE became the National Institute for Health and Clinical Excellence when it was given additional responsibility for public health, providing those working in the NHS, local authorities and the wider public and voluntary sector with guidance on the promotion of good health and the prevention of ill health.

life-year gained, is used to assess cost-effectiveness. Thus, the growing number of NICE assessments will provide a source of evidence about new technologies. However, it is important to note that NICE does not make a judgement about whether a new technology is affordable, and states that this is a government responsibility.[10,11]

However, in 2006, NICE announced a new programme of work to help the NHS make better use of its resources by reducing spending on ineffective treatments, i.e.:

- treatments that do not improve patient care
- treatments that do not represent 'good' value for money.

The three new types of product to be generated under this programme are:

1. technology appraisals and clinical guidelines aimed at reducing ineffective practice
2. recommendation reminders – documents that highlight recommendations from existing NICE guidance that advise the NHS to stop an intervention that is ineffective or poor value for money
3. commissioning guides providing practical advice for commissioners on how to commission routine services in line with NICE recommendations.

7.3.3.2 Systems for managing innovation

A single issue of any journal might contain material that could prompt a clinician to make changes to his/her clinical practice; for example, take the issue of the *Annals of Internal Medicine* published on 22 January 2007 (Box 7.5) in which there are as many as four innovations in knowledge and technology suitable. Extrapolating from this figure, there may be more than 100 innovations a year in one

---

Box 7.5 Innovations in knowledge and technology that appeared in the *Annals of Internal Medicine* of 22 January 2007

- Combined aspirin–oral anticoagulant therapy compared with oral anticoagulant therapy alone among patients at risk for cardiovascular disease: a meta-analysis of randomised trials
- Magnetic resonance imaging for diagnosing foot osteomyelitis: a meta-analysis
- Suppression of human immunodeficiency virus type 1 viral load with selenium supplementation: a randomised controlled trial
- Evaluating the value of repeat bone mineral density measurement and prediction of fractures in older women: the study of osteoporotic fractures

journal alone. Given the large number of innovations being developed and published, it is essential to institute a system whereby the introduction of any innovation is managed.

There are two types of innovation: new knowledge and new technology. At present, new technology may enter directly into the service without evaluation, whereas new knowledge is not assimilated into clinical practice rapidly or systematically (see Fig. 7.4), hence the need on both counts for a Chief Knowledge Officer (CKO) (see Sections 7.4 and 2.5.1.1 and Box 2.4).

Those who pay for or provide healthcare must introduce systems to manage the introduction of innovation by deciding:

- what action, if any, is needed in the light of new knowledge
- what new technology should be introduced
- what new technology should be prevented from entering the service, or removed from the service if it is currently being offered and yet known to be ineffective (Sections 2.5.1.2 and 7.6.3.2).

References

1. Department of Health, NHS Executive (1998) *Information for Health: an Information Strategy for the Modern NHS 1998–2005 – a National Strategy for Local Implementation.* Department of Health, London. Available from: DH Distribution Centre, PO Box 410, Wetherby LS23 7LN, UK.

2. Sanderson, C. (1996) *Evidence-based Candidates for the Audit and Purchasing Agenda. [Report]* North Thames Regional Health Authority, London. Cited in: Bandolier 25(3): 5.

3. Royal College of Physicians (1989) *Fractured neck of femur, prevention and management: summary and recommendations of a report of the Royal College of Physicians.* J. Roy. Coll. Phys. 23: 8–12.

4. Audit Commission (1995) *United They Stand: Co-ordinating Care for Elderly Patients with Hip Fracture.* HMSO, London.

5. Todd, C.J., Freeman, C.J., Camilleri-Ferrante, C. et al. (1995) *Differences in mortality after fracture of the hip: the East Anglian audit.* Br. Med. J. 310: 904–8.

6. Bedford, M. (1996) *Broken hips – measuring performance.* Bandolier 25(3): 4.

7. Freemantle, N., Grilli, R., Grimshaw, J.M. et al. (1995) *Implementing the findings of medical research: the Cochrane Collaboration and effective professional practice.* Qual. Health Care 4: 45–7.

8. Cochrane Collaboration. Cochrane review topics. *Effective Practice and Organisation of Care.* Available online at: http://www.cochrane.org/reviews/en/topics/61.html Accessed 19 September 2006.

9. Morgan, S.G., Bassett, K.L., Wright, J.M., et al. (2005) *'Breakthrough' drugs and growth in expenditure on prescription drugs in Canada.* Br. Med. J. 331: 815–16.

10. Pearson, S.D. and Rawlins, M.D. (2005) *Quality, innovation, and value for money. NICE and the British National Health Service.* JAMA 294: 2618–22.

11. Rawlins, M.D. and Culyer, A.J. (2004) *National Institute for Clinical Excellence and its value judgements. [Education and debate]* Br. Med. J. 329: 224–7.

7.4   Change management

The term and role of 'knowledge broker' was developed in Canada to describe an intermediary between research and action (Fig. 7.5).

Knowledge brokering is defined by the Canadian Health Services Research Foundation as follows:

> *all the activity that links decision-makers with researchers, facilitating their interaction so that they are able to better understand each other's goals and professional cultures, influence each other's work, forge new partnerships, and promote the use of research-based evidence in decision-making.*[1]

Many commercial organisations now have a Chief Knowledge Officer (CKO), which is a responsibility rather than a job.[2] In a healthcare setting, the CKO is a responsibility that should be given to a board member, for example, the medical director. With this responsibility, the CKO in a healthcare setting should ensure, and be able to assure the chief executive and the board, that knowledge in the organisation is being managed to best effect. To do this effectively, the CKO needs the support of a librarian or information scientist. A list of suggestions covering the responsibilities and priority tasks of the CKO is shown in Box 7.6,[3] which can be used as the basis of a job description.

7.4.1   Evidence-based re-organisation?

As discussed in Section 7.2.2 , many management decisions are not based on evidence. Re-organisation, a relatively common management practice directly affecting organisational structure, has been lampooned in a 'spoof' review by Oxman et al.,[4] and the lack of evidence for this practice was highlighted.

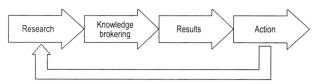

Fig. 7.5
Getting research into action: role of the knowledge broker

Box 7.6 Responsibilities and priorities of a chief knowledge officer (CKO)

Responsibilities

To control the flow of knowledge:

- into the organisation, for example, by reporting to the board on a monthly basis on significant new knowledge requiring action
- throughout the organisation, for example, by ensuring that all significant innovation such as the introduction of a new diagnostic test is based on best current evidence
- out of the organisation, for example, by ensuring that patient leaflets remain evidence based and up to date and are replaced as they become outmoded.

Priority tasks (Source: Kelleher and Levene[3])

- Sponsoring the development of a knowledge management strategy
- Taking steps to improve the management of knowledge
- Collaborating with human resources to ensure that those who manage knowledge are appropriately recognised and rewarded
- Working with information technology to ensure that documents and knowledge are managed well to complement the traditional focus on the management of data
- Developing criteria that the organisation can use to see how well it is doing
- Developing systems within the organisation for importing, storing, distributing and exporting knowledge
- Leading the changes required to create both culture and systems

---

We identified several overlapping reasons for reorganizations, including money, revenge, money, elections, money, newly appointed leaders, money, unemployment, money, power-hunger, money, simple greed, money, boredom and no apparent reason at all. ... Internal justifications for reorganizing identified in our mega-analysis include:

- *You need to hide the fact that an organization has no reason to continue to exist;*
- *It has been 3 years since your last reorganization;*
- *A video conferencing system has just been purchased out of your employees' retirement fund;*
- *Your CEO's brother is an organizational consultant;*
- *The auditor general's report on your organization is about to be released.[4]*

References

1. Lomas, J. (2007) *The in-between world of knowledge brokering*. Br. Med. J. 334: 129–31.

2. Gray, J.A.M. (1998) *Where's the Chief Knowledge Officer?* Br. Med. J. 317: 832–40.

3. Kelleher, D. and Levene, S. (2001) *Guide to Good Practice in Knowledge Management*. British Standards Institution, London.

4. Oxman, A.D., Sackett, D.L., Chalmers, I. et al. (2005) *A surrealistic mega-analysis of redisorganization theories.* J. R. Soc. Med. 98; 563–8.

7.5   Evidence-based primary care

Primary care is care to which a patient can gain access directly. It comprises primary medical care, community nursing and those aspects of mental health and learning disability services that are delivered to people at home.

There are several important differences between the provision of primary care and that of hospital-based care (Table 7.4).

In primary care, the provision of healthcare is undertaken over a large area at many scattered sites, and decision-making covers a wide range of health problems, sometimes in situations where it is not possible to access support. For these reasons, evidence-based decision-making is more difficult to organise in primary care. However, it is possible to distil the introduction of evidence-based decision-making in primary care to manageable proportions. Although the range of health problems encountered is wide, only a small number commonly occur and the organisation of evidence for these common problems is feasible.

In a retrospective review of case notes at a suburban training general practice in the UK,[1] it was found that effective treatment for the health problems suffered by

Table 7.4   Differences in the provision of primary care and hospital-based care

Feature	Primary care	Hospital-based care
No. sites for healthcare provision per million population (UK)	250	3–4
No. work sites for individual professionals	100–200	1–2
No clinical decisions per million population (UK)	30 million	10 million
Health problems seen by individual professionals	Wide spectrum across numerous specialties	Narrow spectrum within one specialty
Site(s) of decision-making about patients	Primary care premises; patients' homes	Hospital
Access to a library/support of a librarian	Difficult	Available

a large proportion of patients was based on evidence. Consecutive doctor–patient consultations ($n = 122$) conducted over 2 days were assessed to determine the proportion of interventions based on evidence from clinical trials; 21 were excluded because of insufficient data while the remaining 101 were assigned to one of three categories:

1. interventions substantiated by evidence from RCTs (Type I)
2. interventions substantiated by convincing non-experimental evidence, e.g. incision and drainage of an abscess (Type II)
3. interventions without substantial evidence.

The results are shown in Table 7.5.[1-3] It can be seen that for almost one-third of consultations, the intervention was based on evidence from RCTs, and for half of the consultations it was based on convincing non-experimental evidence. However, it can also be seen from Table 7.5 that the proportion of consultations in general practice based on evidence from an RCT can differ from country to country: in Japan,[2] the proportion was lower than that in the UK at 21% (although the study included only drug interventions, and the sample size was smaller), and in Spain[3] the proportion was higher at 38% (although the sample size was much larger and covered 34 primary health care centres). Tsuruoka et al.[2] point out that one of the problems in Japan is a lack of evidence in the Japanese language.

Similarly, when making decisions about the provision of mental health and learning disability services, or about individuals who require such services, a small number of common problems recur, and therefore the relevant evidence base is of a manageable size.[4,5]

Table 7.5   The nature of the supporting evidence for interventions undertaken in general practice (Source: Gill et al., Tsuruoka et al., and Suarez-Varela et al.[1-3])

	Evidence from an RCT (Type I)	Non-experimental evidence (Type II)	Not supported by substantial evidence	No. interventions/ patients
England – Gill et al.[1]	30%	51%	19%	101/122
Japan – Tsuruoka et al.[2]	21%	60%	19%	53/49
Suarez-Varela et al.[3]	38%	4%	58%	2341/1990

7.5.1 Improving access: promoting finding

Those whose job it is to provide evidence to decision-makers must:

- ensure easy access to information
- provide relevant information, i.e. minimise the amount disseminated to the busy primary care professional.

7.5.1.1 Ease of access to information
(Margin Fig. 7.2)

It can take hours for a primary care professional to reach and use a library and then return to base but, provided the service of a good librarian is available, access to that same information can be achieved by:

- phone
- fax
- Wide Area Network
- the Internet.

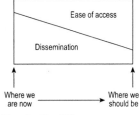

Margin Fig. 7.2

Access to information can be facilitated by:

- using computer resources designated for management and administration to provide evidence to decision-makers
- using a Web page, with access by a separate telephone line to protect the confidentiality of primary care information systems
- regularly downloading information for storage on the primary care hard disks to minimise the dependence on slow Internet connections.

To be of use, information must be stored in convenient systems. Access to information can be promoted by:

- offering primary care professionals bibliographic management software
- providing information in various media, e.g.:
  - in Filofax size on paper
  - in a form that can be downloaded to a personal organiser or other palm-top
  - in hypertext files for a PC or Macintosh
  - as cue card software that will appear on screen when the primary care system is running patient record software
  - as an MP3 file.

7.5.1.2 Provision of relevant information

Although Medline and EMBASE are excellent resources, they can generate a large volume of detailed information inappropriate to decision-making in primary and community care, principally because most of the articles indexed have been written by researchers for researchers. Primary care and community professionals need summaries of primary research that relate to the clinical problems they encounter, such as evidence-based guidelines, supported by the facility to access the evidence directly if necessary (Table 7.6). In a primary care setting, however, the 'Types of Evidence' model (Fig. 7.6) is helpful because clinicians need both systems and summaries of evidence.

Table 7.6   Need for, and accessibility of, different types of clinical information in primary care

Type of clinical information	Frequency of need	Accessibility
Evidence-based guidelines	++++	+
Written abstract of the systematic review on which the guideline is based	+++	++
Data from the systematic review	++	+++
Primary research on which the systematic review is based	+	++++

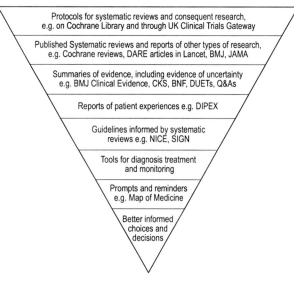

Fig. 7.6
'Types of Evidence' model of knowledge

Other ways in which relevant information can be made available to primary care professionals include:

- providing every primary and community care site with access to the Cochrane Library – at the time of writing, the NLH has a UK-wide subscription to the Cochrane Library thereby allowing free access
- ensuring on-line access to Medline
- disseminating in a systematic way, for instance, in a newsletter, new information of high quality needed by primary care decision-makers
- ensuring that each professional has the support of a librarian for the development of searching and retrieval skills.

7.5.2   Improving appraisal skills

As primary care professionals have to deal with a wide range of health problems, they need to search a broad evidence base and must be taught the skills of appraisal (see Chapter 9, particularly Sections 9.4.2 and 9.4.3). Although the approach that needs to be taken is no different from that for decision-makers in a hospital, primary care professionals may benefit from different examples during training.

References

1. Gill, P., Dowell, A.C., Neal, R.D. et al. (1996) *Evidence based general practice: a retrospective study of interventions in one training practice.* Br. Med. J. 312: 819–21.
2. Tsuruoka, K., Tsuruoka, Y., Yoshimura, M. et al. (1996) *Evidence based general practice: drug treatment in general practice in Japan is evidence based.* [Letter] Br. Med. J. 313: 114.
3. Suarez-Varela, M.M., Llopis-Gonzalez, A., Bell, J. et al. (1999) *Evidence based general practice.* Eur. J. Epidemiol. 15: 815–19.
4. Geddes, J.R., Game, D., Jenkins, N.E. et al. (1996) *What proportion of primary psychiatric interventions are based on evidence from randomised controlled trials?* Qual. Health Care 5: 215–17.
5. Summers, A. and Kehoe, R.F. (1996) *Is psychiatric treatment evidence-based?* [Letter to the Editor] Lancet 347: 409–10.

7.6   Paying for or commissioning healthcare using the evidence base

In health services world-wide, there is a trend to separate the function of paying for or commissioning healthcare from that of providing healthcare. Those who pay for healthcare make decisions about which health services to buy;

providers deliver healthcare to individual patients within the resources available. This separation of functions enables those who pay for healthcare to focus on how best to use finite resources with respect to:

- particular groups of patients
- particular diseases, such as heart disease
- particular interventions, such as hip replacement.

The aim of those who pay for healthcare for different groups of people with, or at risk of, different diseases is to maximise the value obtained from the resources available by ensuring that:

- the resources are allocated to the groups in amounts that maximise value, i.e. after allocation it is not possible to achieve further health gain for the population by redistribution of resources
- the healthcare professional responsible for managing each of these groups achieves maximum value from the resources allocated to the group by:
  - offering only those interventions that do more good than harm at reasonable cost
  - ensuring that these interventions are offered to those who are most likely to be helped rather than harmed
  - ensuring that the interventions are given as well and as cheaply as possible.

Those who pay for healthcare can use their purchasing power to accomplish five evidence-based tasks:

1. resource re-allocation among disease management systems (Section 7.6.1)
2. resource re-allocation within a single disease management system (Section 7.6.2)
3. managing innovation (Section 7.6.3)
4. improving the quality of care (Section 7.6.4)
5. controlling increases in healthcare costs without affecting the health of the population.

However, in the current context of increasing involvement of patients and the general public in healthcare decision-making, those who pay for health services should bear in mind that the aims of the public for resource allocation may be different to those of healthcare professionals.

- The aim of an individual patient is to ensure the maximum allocation of resources to treat his/her case.
- The aim of a group of patients or carers who have the same problem is to obtain more resources for the particular patient group, and openness and equity in the distribution of healthcare resources for that group.
- The aim of representatives of the general public is to ensure openness and equity in the distribution of resources across the entire range of patient groups.

Those who pay for healthcare in the UK experience certain advantages and disadvantages in comparison with those who pay for healthcare elsewhere in the world. A major disadvantage is that in many parts of the UK there is no, or only limited, choice of providers when compared with, for example, the USA. However, a major advantage is coverage of discrete populations; in the USA and in some European countries, the population of a single city may be covered by three or more nationwide insurers.

The advantage of being able to focus on a discrete population has two important consequences:

1. it facilitates the process of population needs assessment
2. it enables the organisation paying for healthcare to undertake the broader role of health 'commissioner', that is, being able to integrate the health services that are pur-chased with a broad range of public health measures to prevent disease, promote health, and reduce inequalities in a defined population.

1. Population needs assessment
A definition of health need that can be used when paying for healthcare on the basis of evidence is as follows:

> a health problem for which there is an intervention about which there is strong evidence, based on good-quality research, that it does more good than harm.

Population needs assessment comprises:

- the estimation of the frequency of various health problems in a population
- the appraisal of the evidence for the beneficial and harmful effects of the interventions used to treat each health problem, which is the focus of this book.

2. Commissioning
Commissioners have the ability to supplement what has been achieved by negotiation with providers during the contracting process with the following functions:

- the promotion of health in general
- public and patient education
- professional education, thereby exerting an influence through the resources invested in education
- commissioning research where evidence is lacking.

7.6.1   Resource re-allocation among disease management systems

A disease management system consists of all those services and interventions designed to improve the health of individuals who have a particular disease (e.g. diabetes) or a group of diseases (e.g. cardiac disease). Such systems can be managed by the use of guidelines, for both the referral and discharge of patients (see 1–3 in Fig. 7.7), and for the treatment of patients (see A–D in Fig. 7.7). If all the elements of a system are governed by the use of guidelines, the care provided is often referred to as 'managed care' (see Section 1.7.1).

In the NHS, disease management systems are rudimentary because the service is still dominated by broad distinctions between primary and secondary care, or between hospital and community care. It is not possible to make an evidence-based decision about the balance of expenditure between primary and secondary care as a whole; it is possible only to make evidence-based decisions about the balance of expenditure between primary and secondary care for a particular disease. A comparison of the health outcomes arising from investment in different disease management systems requires information from studies of safety, effectiveness, and cost, for example, by comparing the cost per QALY.

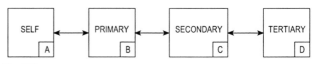

Fig. 7.7
Schematic representation of a disease management system showing routes for the care of patients

However, those who pay for healthcare are not usually asked to re-allocate resources on the basis of specific diseases; paying for healthcare is usually founded on contracts for particular patient groups, and payers face demands to increase the amount of investment in the ENT, the oral surgery or the gynaecology contract (sometimes all three). If payers are able to address only the secondary care sector of these systems, it is worth asking the following questions:

- What would be the beneficial health effects of adding £500000 to each of these three contracts?
- What would be the health effects of subtracting £500000 from each of these three contracts?

In both cases, it is wise to elicit the evidence upon which any answers have been based.

7.6.2   Resource re-allocation within a single disease management system

Any decision-maker trying to re-allocate resources within a disease management system on the basis of evidence that resources could be better spent faces several problems:

- increased expenditure in budget A, such as the drug budget, is required before there can be savings in budget B, the inpatient budget
- the budgets may be in different compartments
- the potential savings may appear to be large when calculated nationally; for instance, increasing the prescription of ACE inhibitors in general practice will reduce hospital costs for the treatment of heart failure, but for an individual hospital the actual reduction in the amount of resources used may not be sufficient to allow a facility, such as a ward, to be closed and 'real' cash to be released for re-allocation into another part of the system.

These problems are particularly difficult for those who pay for healthcare to address because:

- they may not be able to reduce expenditure on hospital care and redirect it into primary care drug budgets
- they may not have access to diagnostic service costs, which are not subject to external contract but allocated internally within a provider unit
- professionals in any service in which savings from better management of one disease could be made can

usually identify needs among a different group of patients under their care which they believe should be met with these savings; for example, professionals in a respiratory unit would argue that any savings on hospital care of asthma should be spent on sleep apnoea or cystic fibrosis.

Although the main opportunities for better disease management within a hospital are open to the managers at that hospital, it is possible for health 'commissioners' to promote investment in disease management systems by focusing on specific points at the primary/secondary care interface, rather than making broad generalisations about need for closer cooperation between the two sectors. Within a single disease management system, those who pay for healthcare will attempt to promote cost containment on the basis of research evidence and to minimise any adverse effects on the health of the population (Fig. 7.8).

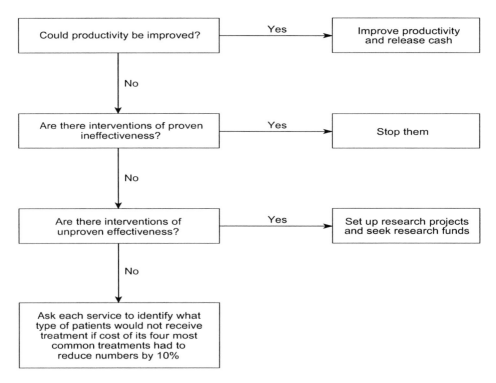

Fig. 7.8
Evidence-based cost containment or cutting

7.6.3 Managing innovation

Innovation occurs continually. Those who pay for healthcare must try to manage the introduction of innovation in the following ways:

- *starting starting right* – promoting innovation, i.e. introducing those innovations that do more good than harm, and which are *affordable*, at a defined standard of quality (Section 7.6.3.1)
- *starting stopping* – no longer offering those innovations that have already entered the service but do more harm than good (Section 7.6.3.2)
- *stopping starting* – not introducing those innovations that do more harm than good (Section 7.6.3.3)
- *promoting trials* – investigating innovations of unknown effect during trials. (Section 7.6.3.4)

7.6.3.1 Promoting innovation: starting starting right

Part of the management of innovation is to identify interventions that do more good than harm at affordable cost and drive them into the service quickly and effectively – starting starting right. It is no longer acceptable to allow important innovations to drift into practice in a piecemeal fashion.

When promoting a novel intervention, for example, thrombolysis after acute myocardial infarction (AMI), it is possible for purchasers to be explicit about their requirements. The development of better systems of care is particularly important in situations in which a change in professional practice is not sufficient to ensure a better outcome for patients. As an example, for thrombolysis after AMI to be delivered effectively, a reconfiguration of the system of care is necessary to change the way in which patients with chest pain are managed:

- when they contact their GP
- when they are in transit in the ambulance
- and when they arrive at the A&E department.

Further means of promoting change can also be used to supplement the specifications of those who pay for healthcare, namely:

- changing individual behaviour through professional education and audit, and public and patient education
- the development of better systems of care.

Greenhalgh et al.[1] conducted a systematic review of the diffusion and implementation of innovations in health service delivery and organisation. On the basis of their findings, they have developed a conceptual model for considering the determinants of the diffusion of innovations in health services (Fig. 7.9).[1] To apply this conceptual model in a service context, Greenhalgh et al. have also developed a two-stage framework or process to guide managers. The fundamental questions to ask in Stages 1 and 2 are shown in Box 7.7.[1]

7.6.3.2 Stopping starting

When there is no evidence from good-quality research that an intervention does more good than harm, it should not be introduced – stopping starting (see Section 2.5.1.2). In such situations, it is vital for those who pay for healthcare to be clear about innovations they do not want to purchase for a particular population because of lack of evidence of effectiveness. The logic is easy for the media and the general public to understand: all interventions are associated with risk; some people will suffer if any intervention is introduced; if there is no evidence of a beneficial effect, the harm done by the intervention will be greater than the good.

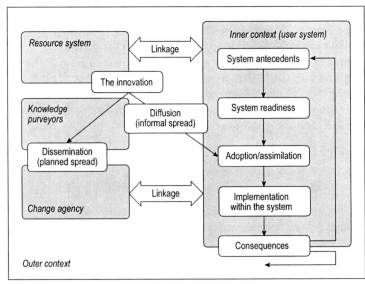

Fig. 7.9
A conceptual model of diffusion and implementation of innovations in health service delivery and organisation (Source: Greenhalgh et al.[1])

> **Box 7.7 Two-stage framework for the diffusion and implementation of innovations in health service delivery and organisation (Source: Greenhalgh et al.[1])**
>
> **Stage 1**
> - What are the attributes of the innovation as perceived and evaluated by the intended users?
> - What are the characteristics of the intended adopters and the adoption process?
> - What is the nature of communication and influence about the innovation?
> - What is the nature of the organisational context and how conducive is this to the assimilation of innovations in general?
> - What is the organisation's level of readiness for this innovation in particular?
> - What is the nature of the outer (environmental) context and how will this impact on the assimilation process?
> - Is the implementation and maintenance process (as opposed to the adoption by individuals) adequately planned, resourced and managed?
> - What (if any) is the nature, capacity and activities of external agencies?
>
> **Stage 2**
> Consider the complex interaction between the variables in the conceptual model in relation to the specific local context and setting. Although the number of possible interactions is high, managers must use situational judgement to prioritise the key questions in a particular initiative. For example:
> - Interaction between adopter and the innovation: How does this particular adopter perceive the attributes of this particular innovation (and can he/she be supported to change these perceptions)?
> - Interaction between opinion leadership and the nature of innovation: What is the overall perceived potential of this particular innovation by the more influential members of this particular social group, and what impact is this likely to have on the behaviour and choices of the 'rank and file'?
> - Interaction between the task (innovation-in-use) and the boundary role: What impact does the nature of the task(s) associated with the innovation have on the preferred boundary-spanning role (linking the organisation with the external world)?
> - Interaction between organisational structure and stage of assimilation: For this particular innovation, what is the balance between high structural complexity (hence promoting innovativeness and hence adoption) and low structural complexity (hence facilitating diffusion of the innovation within the organisation)?

Interventions of proven ineffectiveness and unproven effectiveness should be clearly identified. If any intervention in the latter group is introduced, it must be only as part of a properly designed and ethically approved trial (see Section 7.6.3.4).

7.6.3.3 Starting stopping

There are interventions that are already in routine use for which there is either no evidence of effectiveness, or evidence of ineffectiveness. The strategy in such cases is to discontinue their use by starting stopping (see Section 2.5.1.2). However, it is more problematic when trying to change established professional practice, for instance, persuading gynaecologists to stop performing dilatation and curettage (D&C) operations in women under the age of 40 years, or to perform fewer Caesarean sections.

7.6.3.4 Promoting trials

Interventions of unproven effectiveness should be tested within an RCT; purchasers should promote and support the performance of RCTs. One benefit of promoting trials is that it enables those who pay for healthcare to be categorical about which services/interventions will be supported.

7.6.4   Improving the quality of care

It is possible for those who pay for healthcare to influence not only the distribution of resources (see Sections 7.6.1 and 7.6.2) and the introduction of innovations (Section 7.6.3), but also the quality of care by ensuring that the right things are done right (Section 2.2.5). Although there are several strategies available to help people who pay for or commission healthcare achieve quality improvement – which can be described under the broad heading of 'pay for performance' – this approach is in its infancy in developed countries.

McNamara[2] identified three potentially overlapping strategies that could enable those who pay for healthcare to improve quality:

- quality-based selective contracting
- payment differentials based on quality
- public domain information on comparative provider performance.

In each of these strategies, providers of healthcare are rewarded directly, through higher payment rates, or indirectly, with a greater volume of patients. McNamara points out that the strategy employed will depend on context, but none of them are mutually exclusive. However, there is little published research evidence on the effectiveness of paying for performance, particularly with respect to contracting and to payment innovations.

In a systematic review of studies to assess the effect of explicit financial incentives for improved performance on measures of healthcare quality, Petersen et al.[3] noted how few studies were available for review. They concluded that ongoing monitoring of incentive programmes was critical in order to determine the effectiveness of financial incentives, and in particular whether this type of strategy would have unintended effects on the quality of care through 'gaming behaviour,' whereby the incentive produces improvements in documentation rather than in the quality of care given to patients. As such, Petersen et al. suggest a future research agenda including RCTs and observational studies with concurrent control groups to guide the implementation of strategies using explicit financial incentives and to assess their cost-effectiveness. However, it should be borne in mind that financial incentives and payment systems in healthcare are not the only drivers for quality improvement.

Thomson and Berwick[4] have identified several ways in which the NHS in the UK can learn from the US healthcare system in order to improve the quality and safety of healthcare:

- a fully integrated system of care, which for the NHS means vertical integration between community-based and hospital-based care supported by investment in electronic medical records and decision support systems
- a system for collaborative improvement, which could be achieved through models such as that initially developed by the Institute for Healthcare Improvement (IHI), whereby healthcare organisations learn from each other more efficiently and quickly than learning on their own, particularly with respect to changes in systems for healthcare delivery – see Casebook 7.2 for an example of collaborative improvement led by the IHI[5,6]
- a patient-centred approach over and above the conduct of surveys of patient satisfaction, including patient representatives on hospital boards and committees, and transforming the language and culture of healthcare
- controlling the demand for services created by hospitals and specialists – in the USA, specialist supply is positively correlated with mortality;[7] this is especially pertinent, given the move towards independence for foundation trusts and privately run diagnostic and treatment centres in England.

Casebook 7.2   The 100 000 Lives Campaign in the USA (Adapted from Berwick et al.[5] and McCannon et al.[6])

To quicken the pace of quality improvement in healthcare, the Institute of Healthcare Improvement (IHI) in the USA launched the 100 000 Lives Campaign in December 2004.[5] The campaign was a national initiative in which the goal was to save 100 000 lives among hospital patients over 18 months through improvements in the safety and effectiveness of care. A life saved was defined as 'a patient successfully discharged from a hospital who, absent the changes achieved during the campaign, would not have survived'. To save these lives, IHI proposed that at the hospitals which enrolled as many as possible of six 'highly feasible' interventions (for which 'efficacy' is documented in the peer-reviewed literature and reflected in standards set by relevant US specialty societies and government agencies) are implemented.

1. Rapid response teams to prevent potential cardiac arrest by initiating changes in care that prevent arrest or by facilitating transfer to an intensive care unit where fast resuscitation efforts are likely to be more successful.

2. Reliable evidence-based care for acute myocardial infarction – early administration of aspirin, aspirin at discharge, early administration of a beta-blocker, beta-blocker at discharge, angiotensin-converting enzyme (ACE) inhibitor or angiotensin-receptor blockers at discharge for patients with systolic dysfunction, timely initiation of perfusion, and smoking cessation counselling.

3. Medication reconciliation to prevent adverse drug events – clinicians to review patients' medicine from orders and track the drugs administered before and after a transition of care to identify and correct any discrepancies between the drug regimen intended and that received.

4. Prevention of central-line infections – hand hygiene, maximal barrier precautions, chlorhexidine skin antisepsis, optimal catheter site selection (subclavian vein as the preferred site for non-tunnelled patients) and daily review of necessity with prompt removal of unnecessary lines.

5. Prevention of surgical site infections – guideline-based use of prophylactic antibiotics, appropriate hair removal (avoidance of shaving), peri-operative glucose control (for patients who had undergone major cardiac surgery and are being cared for in an intensive care unit) and peri-operative normothermia (for patients who had undergone colorectal surgery).

6. Prevention of ventilator-associated pneumonia – elevation of the head of the bed to between 30° and 45°, daily 'sedation vacation' and daily assessment of readiness for extubation, peptic ulcer disease prophylaxis, and deep vein thrombosis prophylaxis.

The calculation of how many lives were saved involved:

• tracking hospital mortality rates and comparing a hospital's mortality data for each month of the campaign with the corresponding data from the same month in 2004
• aggregating monthly 'lives saved' across all months and all participant hospitals
• applying a national case-mix adjustment to account for the overall change in patient acuity between 2004 and the campaign period.

As of April 2006, after 15 months of the campaign, it was estimated that over 84 000 lives had been saved (based on 83% of participant hospitals having submitted mortality data)[6] and in June 2006 it was announced at a press conference that an estimated 122 342 lives had been saved.

Since then, the IHI has announced a further national campaign to reduce medical harm in US hospitals: The 5 Million Lives Campaign, in which will be promoted 12 interventions, the six featured in the 100 000 Lives Campaign and six new interventions:

- prevention of MRSA infection
- reducing harm from high-alert drugs (focusing on anticoagulants, sedatives, narcotics and insulin)
- reducing surgical complications
- prevention of pressure ulcers
- reliable evidence-based care for congestive heart failure
- getting boards on board to accelerate the improvement of care.

Thomson and Berwick[4] conclude that on the basis of examples from the American healthcare system to improve quality and safety of care in the NHS, it is advisable to develop:

- well-articulated, nationally endorsed aims based on high-quality research
- a measurement system for quality and safety
- strategies to encourage and support the translation of the best knowledge into reliable uniform everyday clinical practice.

7.6.4.1 Competition as a way of improving healthcare

Porter and Teisberg[8] identified what they believed to be one of the most important reasons why competition in American healthcare was failing to improve quality, which is the 'wrong' type of competition. In their book *Redefining Healthcare*,[8] they identified hospital vs hospital or HMO vs HMO competition as irrelevant at best and confusing at worst. They advocated competition at the level of the 'integrated patient unit', namely one heart service competing against another heart service, or one cystic fibrosis service competing against another cystic fibrosis service. This type of competition would be effective at improving quality only if each system undertook monitoring and evaluation using the same domains for data collection, including outcomes of importance to patients.

7.6.5   Evidence-based insurance

In the past, the source of finance has dictated the system of healthcare introduced. In countries in which systems of paying for healthcare develop, there are two main sources of finance:

1. insurance
2. taxation.

In some countries, there may be complicated permutations of these two systems, for instance, government underwriting of insurance schemes. Insurance-based systems derive revenue from customers; in tax-based systems, health services are paid for directly from funds raised through taxation. The distinction between the two systems has changed dramatically in recent years. Some insurance companies provide their own healthcare, for example, in health maintenance organisations such as Kaiser Permanente. In tax-based systems, such as the NHS, the opposite trend is taking place, as demonstrated by the division between paying for and providing healthcare.

Insurance schemes operate in a different way to commissioning or paying for healthcare in the NHS. Instead of negotiating contracts for services for geographical populations, insurance companies develop health plans that cover those people (sometimes called the 'members') who pay premiums to the company. The contents of the health plan describe the interventions or benefits for which the company will pay.

Insurance schemes have two dimensions to consider:

- breadth
- depth.

Breadth refers to the coverage decision: who should be included and who should be excluded from the scheme. Governments, of course, cannot exclude any citizen.

Depth refers to the extent of interventions and services covered, and having achieved universal coverage the insurance scheme will have to manage costs by limiting the services for which those covered are eligible.

However, Palmer has highlighted the limited role of evidence in making decisions about improving health status and meeting efficiency and equity objectives in private health-insurance initiatives.[9]

In developing countries, the most important issue is protecting people from what the World Bank has called 'health shocks,' namely massive costs from severe health problems that can bankrupt families and ruin small businesses.[10] Indeed, this is still a problem in the USA where universal coverage does not exist. There is constant negotiation at the margin of any health scheme, whether it be in the NHS or Medicare, with debates about the added value of certain procedures such as cosmetic surgery or complementary medicine.

7.6.6 'Black belt' decision-making

The approach described hitherto is relatively simple, but detailed flow charts can be used to describe a framework for more complex decision-making, an example of which is shown in Fig. 7.10.[11]

7.6.7 The limits of structural reform

Faced by soaring healthcare costs, most governments took steps in the last decade of the 20th century to control the rate of increase of expenditure. The principal means of doing this, supported by the World Bank, has been the introduction of structural reform. The key components of structural reform are shown in Box 7.8.

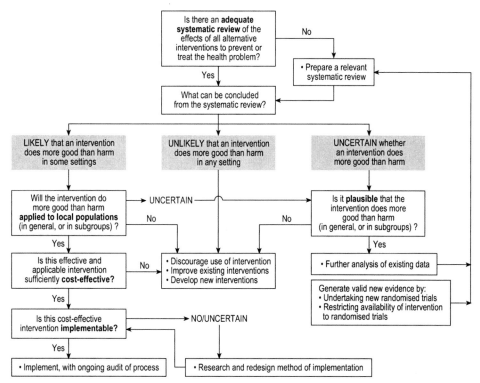

Fig. 7.10
Flow diagram of decision-making based on research synthesis (Source: Irwig et al.[11])

> **Box 7.8 Key components of structural reform**
>
> - Imposition of a limit to the amount of gross national product (GNP) or public expenditure allocated to health services
> - Separation of the functions of paying for (or commissioning) and providing healthcare
> - Introduction of managed care
> - Shift to insurance-based funding of care

The double burden of disease experienced in middle-to-low income countries, the persistence of infectious diseases, child and maternal mortality and undernutrition, and the emergence of diabetes, obesity, cardiovascular disease, stroke, cancer, mental ill health and injuries requires a response involving health-system reforms. However, this response requires more than a liaison among agencies, such as the World Bank and the World Health Organization (WHO), and individuals; it requires a commitment to evidence-informed health-system development at the country level.[12]

Since 2000, Mexico has been a 'global laboratory for health-system reforms'[12] and two of the solutions developed in that country are shown in Casebook 7.3.[12]

Frenk and Horton[12] call for more evidence-informed and less ideological strategies for health-system development, and believe that country experiences of health-system reform have relevance for all policy-makers adapting to transitions in their country's patterns of development, demography and disease.

Casebook 7.3 Health-system reforms in Mexico (Source: Frenk and Horton[12])

In 1997, a programme of conditional cash transfers, now called Oportunidades, was established to help improve health, nutrition and educational outcomes for people living in severe poverty and break the trans-generational cycle of poverty. In 2006, the coverage of this programme was 5 million families.

In 2001, a national health-insurance programme, called Seguro Popular, was established to improve the welfare and well-being of Mexicans, to ensure financial protection against illness and to provide equity of not only access to, but also uptake of, high-quality health services. The aim is to realise universal health insurance by the year 2010. A comprehensive information system has been set up as part of Seguro Popular to support the health-policy reforms. Furthermore, Seguro Popular is being evaluated as part of a cluster-randomised trial.

Structural reform is essential for the control of costs. Some aspects of quality can also be improved by structural reform. It is possible to use structural reform to control the introduction of expensive innovations, for example, breast cancer screening for women under the age of 50 years, by instructing providers that there will be no reimbursement for such a service. It is also possible to tackle specific issues within a context of structural reform by using the appropriate levers in the system, e.g.:

- centralisation of services
- improving patient experience and thereby the level of satisfaction with care, for example, by reducing waiting lists
- increasing productivity
- enabling decisions to be made in a more open and explicit way.

However, it is difficult to ensure that maximum value is obtained from the resources invested in healthcare through structural reform because an increase in value is determined not only by a small number of big changes but also by a large number of small changes, as Eddy has identified (see Sections 1.2 and 2.6). For every million population, there may be a thousand healthcare professionals, each of them changing their practice in many small ways, most of which will be too small for managers to identify and control.

Thus, structural reform cannot be used in isolation to improve the value obtained from resources invested; cultural reform is also necessary with the aim that every professional is asking the following questions:

- 'Does this intervention do more good than harm?'
- 'What is the evidence on which I should base this change in my practice?'

References

1. Greenhalgh, T., Robert, G., Bate, P. et al. (2005) *Diffusion of Innovations in Health Service Organisations: A Systematic Literature Review*. BMJ Books and Blackwell Publishing, Malden, Massachusetts.
2. McNamara, P. (2006) *Purchaser strategies to influence quality of care: from rhetoric to global applications*. Qual. Safe. Health Care 15: 171–3.
3. Petersen, L.A., Woodward, L.D., Urech, T. et al. (2006) *Does pay-for-performance improve the quality of health care?* Ann. Intern. Med. 145: 265–72.
4. Thomson, C.R.V. and Berwick, D.M. (2006) *What can the UK learn from the USA about improving the quality and safety of healthcare?* Clin Med. 6: 551–8.
5. Berwick, D.M., Calkins, D.C., McCannon, C.J. et al. (2006) *The 100,000 lives campaign: setting a goal and a deadline for improving health care quality*. JAMA 295: 324–7.

6. McCannon, C.J., Schall, M.W., Calkins, D.R. et al. (2006) *Saving 100,000 lives in US hospitals. [Analysis and comment]* Br. Med. J. 332: 1328–30.

7. Starfield, B., Shi, L., Grover, A. et al. (2005) *The effects of specialist supply on populations' health: assessing the evidence.* Health Aff. (Millwood) (Suppl. Web Exclusives): W5.97-W5.107.

8. Porter, M.E. and Teisberg, E.O. (2006) *Redefining Health Care. Creating Value-Based Competition on Results.* Harvard Business School Press, Boston, Massachusetts.

9. Palmer, G.R. (2000) *Evidence-based health policy-making, hospital funding and health insurance.* Med. J. Aust. 172: 130–3.

10. Baeza, C.C. and Packard, T.G. (2006) *Beyond survival: protecting households from health shocks in Latin America.* World Bank, Stanford, California.

11. Irwig, L., Zwarenstein, M., Zwi, A. et al. (1998) *A flow diagram to facilitate selection of interventions and research for health care.* Bull. World Health Organ. 76: 17–24.

12. Frenk, J. and Horton, R. (2006) *Evidence for health-system reform: a call to action. [Comment]* Lancet 368: 3–4.

7.7   The ethics of prioritisation

Rationing is the inevitable corollary of prioritisation, and is ubiquitous in all healthcare systems.[1]

7.7.1   Prioritising the good of the individual or that of society?

Any robust interrogation of the individual who wishes to do good for society highlights the problems of utilitarianism, the ethical system devised by John Stuart Mill in which the concept of 'the greatest good for the greatest number' was promoted.

Those who have to make decisions about groups or populations often adopt a utilitarian approach, but the utilitarian approach can lead to what Mill, in his famous essay *On Liberty*, called 'the tyranny of the majority'. In a health service, the application of the greatest good for the greatest number will always result in the provision of treatment for people who have common diseases, thus aggravating the problems of those who suffer from rare diseases. Moreover, although such patients certainly benefit from attracting the interest of their medical advisers, it is likely that therapies are few in number and expensive because the pharmaceutical industry is generally less likely to invest in R&D to find a therapy for a disease from which a thousand people suffer than for a disease from which a million people suffer.

During prioritisation, therefore, it is important to recognise that at the end of each decision there is an individual. This is an unpleasant and difficult fact to accept, but those who make decisions about groups and populations must remain continually aware of it.

7.7.2   Decision-making in the context of prioritisation

Although the process of decision-making is poorly understood, especially in the context of rationing or the need to prioritise, evidence is beginning to emerge about the factors that influence the decision taken at both a local and a regional level.

A priorities panel forum was established at a primary care trust in England to debate the merits of competing priorities for limited resources within a structured framework.[2] A structured scoring tool was used to give each of 66 proposals an agreed priority score, and then the proposals were ranked in ascending order of priority. Although the authors of the paper identify shortcomings in the process and the vulnerability to bias from a range of influences, it was found that proposals involving 'locally driven priorities', i.e. those likely to relieve local pressures, took precedence over some nationally driven priorities such as funding of specific NICE guidance.

In a study of funding priorities assigned by health ministry officials in Ontario, Canada,[3] officials were asked to allocate a fixed sum of money to one of two programmes in a pair. It was found that 23% of healthcare decision-makers found it difficult to choose between programmes that had similar overall gains and distributional differences. As the authors point out, this finding is consistent with the utilitarian assumptions of cost-effectiveness analysis. However, in cases where the distributional differences were large, the decision-makers 'clearly favoured' large gains for a few people rather than small gains for many people.

The results of these studies serve to highlight a research priority, that is, to develop and evaluate tools for those who pay for healthcare to help them make decisions in the context of limited resources and a growing demand for healthcare. Empirical studies are needed of the following tools:

- the Disease Impact Number[4]
- the Population Impact Number of eliminating a risk factor, which can be defined as the potential number of disease events prevented in a population over a defined period of time by eliminating a risk factor.[4-7]

However, tools by themselves are only of limited use. In a systematic review of studies of policy-makers' perceptions of their use of evidence,[8] the most commonly reported facilitators to the use of evidence were:

- personal contact
- timely relevance
- inclusion of summaries with policy recommendations.

From the results of this study, it can be seen that, for policy-makers, although the evidence is important, timeliness and personal contact are slightly more influential. Thus, evidence has to be delivered when and where it is needed, and it is not enough simply to rely on publication and hope that the evidence will be found.

References

1. Maynard, A., Bloor, K. and Freemantle, N. (2004) *Challenges for the National Institute of Clinical Excellence.* Br. Med. J. 329: 227–9.
2. Iqbal, Z., Pryce, A. and Afza, M. (2006) *Rationalizing rationing in health care: experience of two primary care trusts.* J. Pub. Health 28: 125–32.
3. Choudhry, N., Slaughter, P., Sykora, K. et al. (1997) *Distributional dilemmas in health policy: large benefits for a few or smaller benefits for many?* J. Health Serv. Res. Policy 2: 212–16.
4. Heller, R.F. and Dobson, A.J. (2000) *Disease impact number and population impact number: population perspectives to measure risk and benefit.* Br. Med. J. 321: 950–2.
5. Heller, R. F. and Page, J. (2002) *A population perspective to evidence based medicine: 'evidence for population health'.* J. Epidemiol. Community Health 56: 45–7.
6. Heller, R.F., Buchan, I., Edwards, R. et al. (2003) *Communicating risks at the population level: application of population impact numbers. [Education and debate]* Br. Med. J. 327: 1162–5.
7. Heller, R.F. (2005) *Evidence for Population Health.* Oxford University Press, Oxford.
8. Innvaer, S., Vist, G., Trommald, M. et al. (2002) *Health policy-makers' perceptions of their use of evidence: a systematic review.* J. Health Serv. Res. Policy 7: 239–44.

7.8   Evidence-based policy-making

Policy: *5. a course of action adopted and pursued by a government, party, ruler, statesman, etc.; any course of action adopted as advantageous or expedient. (The chief living sense.)*

Shorter Oxford English Dictionary

To govern is to make choices.

Duc de Lévis, *Politique*

You can't do it all by sums, Adrian. We're not academics,
we're civil servants. We have to deal with things as they
are. We have to deal with people, with events.

John le Carré, *The Looking Glass War*, 1965

7.8.1   The dominance of values in policy-making

There is nothing a politician likes so little as to be well
informed; it makes decision making so complex and difficult.

John Maynard Keynes

Politics tends to be driven by values, and it is the values
politicians believe to be important that dominate decision-
making about policy. Although such decisions will be
tempered by the availability of resources in relation to the
needs of the population, resource allocation can also be
based on beliefs and values. Evidence can be used during
policy-making, but some policies are formulated without
consideration of the available evidence (see Casebook 8.1).
The factors that affect choice during decision-making about
policy are shown in Margin Fig. 7.3.

Margin Fig. 7.3

7.8.2   The influence of budgetary pressures

However, a shortage of resources can force policy-makers
to consider the evidence and alter policy as a result. This is
illustrated by an eloquent letter written by Danial Patrick
Moynihan, Chairman of the US Senate Finance Committee.[1]

Dear Dr Tyson,

You will recall that last Thursday when you so kindly
joined us at a meeting of the Democratic Policy Committee
you and I discussed the President's family preservation
proposal. You indicated how much he supports the
measure. I assured you I, too, support it, but went on to ask
what evidence was there that it would have any effect. You
assured me there was such data. Just for fun. I asked for
two citations.

The next day we received a fax from Sharon Glied of your
staff with a number of citations and a paper, 'Evaluating
the Results', that appears to have been written by Frank
Farrow of the Center for the Study of Social Policy here
in Washington and Harold Richman at the Chapin Hall
Center at the University of Chicago. The paper is quite
direct: '… solid proof that family preservation services can
affect a state's overall placement rates is still lacking.'

Just yesterday, the same Chapin Hall Center released an 'Evaluation of the Illinois Family First Placement Prevention Program: Final Report'. This was a large-scale study of the Illinois Family First initiative authorized by the Illinois Family Preservation Act of 1987. It was 'designed to test effects of this program on out-of-home placements of children and other outcomes, such as subsequent child maltreatment.' Data on case and service characteristics were provided by Family First caseworkers on approximately 4,500 cases; approximately 1,600 families participated in the randomized experiment. The findings are clear enough. 'Overall, the Family First placement prevention program results in a slight increase in placement rates (when data from all experimental sites are combined). This effect disappears once case and site variations are taken into account.' In other words, there are either negative effects or no effects.

7.8.3　The growing influence of evidence in policy-making

Experts advise, ministers decide.

Traditional policy-making proverb

Margin Note 7.2
Scientific knowledge and public policy
The project on Scientific Knowledge and Public Policy (SKAPP) investigates how science is used and misused in government decision-making and legal proceedings. The aim of SKAPP is to enhance understanding of how knowledge is generated and interpreted. The intention behind the project is to promote transparent decision-making based on the best available science to protect the public health. Available online at: http://www.defendingscience. org/About-Us.cfm

Policy-making has changed over the last 20 years. The use of political advisers and the influence of lobby groups have transformed the traditional function of the departmental expert. For instance, Washington DC is now a city in which lobby firms have significant, and some would say too great an influence.

In the UK, this phenomenon is not so marked, and the traditional function of the departmental expert remains relatively strong, as evidenced by two books in which the influence of policy-making in England has been anatomised.

In *Speak Truth to Power*, Clive Smee, Chief Economic Adviser to the Department of Health, praised three Secretaries of State for: 'their recognition of the virtues of the 'challenge' function – of the value of alternative evidence-based views'.[2] Smee writes that this: 'was essential for ensuring that analysts were able to "speak truth to power" during the period'.

However, it should be borne in mind that the process of evidence-based policy-making generates policy that is *based* on evidence and that values and a consideration of the other uses to which the resources could be put are also important to decision-taking. Thus, although economic advisers give advice to ministers on the costs and benefits of various policy approaches, they are relatively remote from the political process, during which these other considerations are taken into account. In contrast, the heads of government departments are close to the process of political decision-making and the values brought to bear upon it. One of the policy debates that created most concern during the 1990s was about the control of bovine spongiform encephalomyelitis (BSE). In a book about the politics of this issue,[3] the permanent secretary at the Ministry of Agriculture during the crisis exposes in considerable detail the way in which decisions were made, the political pressure exerted at the time and its effects.

7.8.4 Evidence-based healthcare policy-making

Healthcare policies relate to the financing and organisation of health services. At the highest level, government takes decisions about the level of investment that will be made in a country's health services. Policy-makers also make decisions about the organisation of those health services, which are usually related to service financing. Organisational change may be instigated to fulfil one or more central government objectives, such as:

- to decentralise power
- to involve more people in decision-making
- to encourage cost control
- to reduce the number of managerial staff
- to encourage competition as a stimulus to reduce costs and increase quality.

Although the idea underpinning the introduction of any organisational change may reflect the ideology of the political party in power, or that of an individual, pressure group or think tank, the decision taken can be based on evidence (Fig. 7.11). The nature of the evidence may be:

- the experience of what happened since the last change in service financing and organisation
- derived from research findings.

However, the amount of research evidence available on which to base healthcare policy is often limited, and politicians may argue that the introduction of a particular policy is supported by common sense (Fig. 7.11).

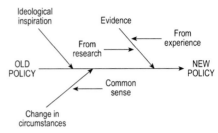

Fig. 7.11
Factors underlying healthcare policy changes

7.8.5   Evidence-based policy-making in the developing world

Although most of the work referred to in Section 7.8 has been undertaken in developed countries, evidence-based policy-making is of paramount importance in developing countries. However, the availability of research evidence may be limited because the performance of RCTs in countries with limited resources can be problematic. Despite this, it is possible to carry out high-quality controlled trials in poor countries but it does require considerable commitment and skill as shown by the examples that follow.

The Collaborative Eclampsia Trial,[4] in which the effects of different anticonvulsant regimens on recurrent convulsions and maternal mortality in women suffering from eclampsia were investigated, was designed such that:

- the results could be applicable to areas where maternal mortality is highest
- it could be conducted within existing health services
- treating women within the trial would be easier and faster for clinicians than treating women outside it, to ensure that clinicians were not burdened and large numbers of women could be included. The authors point to the low attrition, high compliance, and completeness of data collection in this study as indicators of the achievement of these aims.

In a study of the introduction of a community-based maternity-care delivery system in Matlab, Bangladesh,[5] it appeared that the new service had significantly reduced direct obstetric mortality when compared with the three years prior to the introduction of the programme. However, Ronsmans et al.[5] investigated whether this effect was sustained over time. They found that although the introduction of the maternity-care programme coincided with a declining trend in direct obstetric mortality in the areas covered by the programme, a decline also occurred in one of the areas not covered by the programme. Therefore, it is necessary to exercise caution in the interpretation of a short-term trend in only one indicator in studies that have been designed without random allocation of the intervention to a treatment and a control group.

References

1. Moynihan, D.P. (1995) The Congressional Record, 12 December 1995. Reproduced as: *Congress builds a coffin*. New York Review of Books, January 11, 1996, pp 33–6.
2. Smee, C. (2005) *Speaking Truth to Power: Two Decades of Analysis in the Department of Health*. Radcliffe Publishing, in association with the Nuffield Trust, Abingdon.
3. Packer, R. (2006) *The Politics of BSE*. Palgrave Macmillan.
4. Eclampsia Trial Collaborative Group (1995) *Which anticonvulsant for women with eclampsia? Evidence from the Collaborative Eclampsia Trial*. Lancet 345: 1455–63.
5. Ronsmans, C., Vanneste, A.M., Chakraborty, J. et al. (1997) *Decline in maternal mortality in Matlab, Bangladesh: a cautionary tale*. Lancet 350: 1810–14.

7.9   Evidence-based litigation°

7.9.1   'Evidence' in court

Although the word 'evidence' is much used in court, the nature of the evidence that is presented and appraised in that setting, and upon which judgements are made, differs in quality to the nature of the evidence discussed in this book (Table 7.7).

In the judicial system of some countries, e.g. the UK and the USA, expert witnesses can be called to give 'evidence'. However, this evidence may merely reflect the expert's opinion rather than be based on evidence derived from research. Indeed, both the prosecution and the defence try to find an expert whose opinion will support their case. In the USA, an 'expert' industry has developed, in which big companies maintain and support experts in research institutions and ensure that their work is publicised (as opposed to published) in the media.

Table 7.7   The qualities of evidence in two different contexts

Evidence in court	Evidence used in an evidence-based approach
Opinion of experts	Evidence based on research
All or nothing	Probabilistic

Furthermore, after an expert has given an opinion, its generalisability and relevance to the individual case under judgement appears to be treated with remarkable naivety.

Probabilistic thinking is inimical to a system in which the outcome is either 'guilty' or 'not guilty', and its potential contribution in this situation has been emphatically ruled out in the UK by the bench of the Court of Appeal, as one president of the Royal Statistical Society described in his presidential address:[1]

> *Evidence of the Bayes Theorem or any similar statistical method of analysis in a criminal trial plunged the jury into inappropriate and unnecessary realms of theory and complexity, deflecting them from their proper task ... Their Lordships ... had very grave doubts as to whether that evidence was properly admissible because it trespassed on an area peculiarly and exclusively within the jury's province, namely the way in which they evaluated the relationship between one piece of evidence and another. The Bayes Theorem might be an appropriate and useful tool for statisticians, but it was not appropriate for use in jury trials or as a means to assist the jury in its task.*

The sometimes dramatic consequences of exploiting the potential of accepting 'expert' opinion as evidence in court in the USA are described by Marcia Angell in *Science on Trial*,[2] a brilliant book about the legal handling of the purported harmful effects of breast implants. Despite the lack of research-based evidence that breast implants increase the risk of auto-immune disease, a class action totalling $4.25 billion evolved in which more than 400 000 women believed themselves to have been harmed by implants. This belief was fired by media and legal hyperbole, supported by the opinion of 'experts' who had published nothing of note on the subject. Apart from the fact that many lawyers have become fabulously rich working on such cases, the most dispiriting aspect of this saga is the lack of impact the type of evidence that readers of this book might accept actually had on the judges or the jurors. Prosecution lawyers even subpoenaed, and accused of conspiracy, the *New England Journal of Medicine*, of which Dr Angell is the Executive Editor, when it published the Food and Drug Administration's statement on breast implants[3] in conjunction with Dr Angell's editorial.[4]

In the UK, the matter of breast implants was dealt with somewhat differently. The Departments of Health commissioned an Independent Review Group to conduct a systematic review of the evidence. The conclusion was that silicone gel breast implants 'are not associated with any greater health risk than other surgical implants' and there is 'no evidence of an association with an abnormal immune response or typical or atypical connective tissue disease or syndromes'.[5] An interesting and important focus in the report of the independent review group is the need for evidence-based patient choice. In the chapter entitled 'Consent to medical treatment', the need to give patients full, clear and written information is emphasised. This is the first time the need for patients to be given 'full knowledge' has been made explicit in a document of this type, and, as knowledge becomes a dominant commodity in society, the provision of best current knowledge to patients must become standard practice.[6]

However, the consequences of being an expert witness can be serious, as recent cases in the UK involving child protection legislation have demonstrated.[7] In an accompanying editorial, Chadwick[8] outlines the medical evidence base on child abuse, concluding that it is 'robust and thriving' but far from perfect and incomplete. He points out that in order to develop this evidence base and use it in court to protect children, doctors need:

- the support of the public
- the type of protection provided by laws on child abuse reporting and witness immunity current in the USA.

In the USA, where the welfare safety net is gossamer thin, plaintiff lawyers *can* use expert witnesses to help the poor and disadvantaged obtain the resources they need to cope with the effects of disease. Such a situation is described by Peter Pringle in his book *Dirty Business*,[9] the story of the legal battle to hold American tobacco companies to account for the damage tobacco caused to the public health.

7.9.2   Death of an expert witness

The death of the expert witness may now be imminent. In a famous case brought to trial in America, *Daubert et al. v. Merrell Dow Pharmaceuticals*, concerning the role of Bendectin in causing birth defects, the judgment held that federal trial judges have the responsibility to ensure that an expert's testimony is reliable and relevant.[10] Judges are now required to undertake: 'a preliminary assessment of whether the testimony's underlying reasoning or methodology is scientifically valid and properly can be applied to the facts at issue.'[10]

To fulfil this expanded responsibility for determining the validity of scientific evidence, the judiciary has made greater use of a long-held responsibility to appoint any expert witness agreed upon by the parties, and of its own selection. These panels are known as 'Daubert panels' and their functions are:

- to assess the qualifications of expert witnesses
- to evaluate the evidence
- to assess the nature of the issues.

Thus, there is a requirement for experts to provide relevant opinions grounded in reliable methodology, which some authorities have hailed as a way of reducing the volume of 'junk science' in court.

Hulka et al.[11] report on their experiences as members of the National Science Panel appointed by Judge Pointer, who was responsible for overseeing all federal cases involving silicone gel-filled breast implants (see Section 7.9.1). The Panel was charged with providing the federal judiciary with unbiased scientific evidence on the relation between silicone breast implants and connective tissue diseases and auto-immune dysfunction. They believe that such panels should be used more frequently because they can bring unbiased information about complex scientific and medical matters into the courtroom.

This move has not been popular, particularly with those who make a good living as expert witnesses, but it could mark the beginning of the end of opinion masquerading as evidence in court. In a RAND study,[12] it was found that since the introduction of the Daubert standard the percentage of expert testimony excluded from the courtroom significantly rose. However, apart from this study, there is little empirical evidence of the impact of Daubert. Thus, the case for or against such an approach is, in the words of Scottish legal judgement, 'not proven'.

7.9.3 The influence of clinical guidelines in malpractice litigation

The application of medical practice guidelines in courts may also accelerate the decline of the use of expert witnesses.

In a survey of 960 randomly selected medical malpractice attorneys in the USA, Hyams et al.[13] investigated the lawyers' awareness of medical practice guidelines and the use of guidelines in malpractice litigation. The authors also conducted a computerised search to find cases in the US courts in which medical practice guidelines and standards had been used from January 1980 to 31 May 1994.

There was a 60% response rate to the survey. One half of the attorneys who responded were 'very' or 'somewhat' aware of the concept of medical practice guidelines. The search of the US courts' practice yielded 28 cases in which guidelines were used successfully: in 22 of these, the guidelines were used to support the plaintiff's case; in the remaining six, they were used to support the defendant, i.e. the clinician. The search also disclosed seven cases in which plaintiffs were unsuccessful in using guidelines and two cases in which defendants were unsuccessful in using guidelines.

In reviewing the different perspectives on medical practice guidelines – professionals and those who pay for healthcare see them as a 'one-way street' designed to favour clinicians, whereas the courts and attorneys for the plaintiff see them as a one-way street in favour of the plaintiff – the authors conclude that guidelines have been applied as two-way streets, i.e. as evidence to support either side's case. Hurwitz also recognised that guidelines could be used by the clinician's defence lawyer as well as by the plaintiff's.[14]

However, it would appear that attorneys for the plaintiff are more active in finding and using guidelines than those for the defendant. Hyams et al. believe that 'on the whole practice guidelines are a rationalizing force in malpractice litigation'.[13]

7.9.4   Failure to act on the evidence

There is the possibility that failure of a health professional to act on evidence of effective forms of care might *ipso facto* be grounds for litigation brought by patients. In a debate about the importance of research and development conducted in the *Health Service Journal*, one correspondent urged patients and patients' organisations to consider using this strategy as an option for the future.

> *Five years ago I wrote to The Lancet speculating that parents might begin to sue the Royal College of Obstetricians and Gynaecologists because it had taken so long to pro-*

mote use of prenatal steroids, which research had shown reduced the risk that premature babies would die or survive handicapped. I might have added that there would be a case for suing the health authorities and trusts which were acquiescing in under-use of prenatal steroids, particularly as they also reduce health service costs.

Both as a potential patient and a taxpayer, I was prompted by parts of Barbara Millar's article to ask when patients will begin to sue HAs and trusts for ignoring research. A mass of research evidence relevant to the wellbeing of NHS users is available, much of it through the NHS R&D Programme. Over two years ago, in the NHS Executive's paper Promoting Clinical Effectiveness, it was made clear that 'every NHS trust should have access to up-to-date sources of information such as the Cochrane and Centre for Reviews and Dissemination databases'. Yet last year an article in the Journal ('Who's acting on the evidence?', 3 April 1997) made it clear that this advice was being widely ignored by trusts.

I urge patients and patients' organisations to consider suing HAs and trusts which are ignoring the important information available through the NHS R&D programme. As a potential patient, I will certainly consider suing if I am not offered forms of care which have been shown to be effective for people experiencing heart attacks, strokes and trauma.[15]

References

1. Smith, A. (1996) *Mad cows and ecstasy: chance and choice in an evidence-based society.* J. R. Stat. Assoc. A 159: 367–83.
2. Angell, M. (1996) *Science on Trial.* W.W. Norton, New York.
3. Kessler, D. (1992) *The basis for the FDA's decision on breast implants.* N. Engl. J. Med. 326: 1713–15.
4. Angell, M. (1992) *Breast implants: protection or paternalism? [Editorial]* N. Engl. J. Med. 326: 1695–6.
5. Independent Review Group (1998) *Silicone Gel Breast Implants. The Report of the Independent Review Group.* Prepared for publication by Jill Rogers Associates, Cambridge. Available online at: http://www.silicone-review. gov.uk/silicone_implants.pdf.
6. Gray, J.A.M. (1999) *Breast implants: evidence based patient choice and litigation. The only safety lies in providing patients with full information.* Br. Med. J. 318: 414.
7. Gornall, J. (2006) *Child abuse. Royal College rewrites child protection history. [Analysis and comment]* Br. Med. J. 333: 194–6.
8. Chadwick, D.L. (2006) *The evidence base in child protection litigation. Medical expert witnesses need legal protection too, to use the evidence effectively. [Editorial]* Br. Med. J. 333: 160–1.
9. Pringle, P. (1998) *Dirty Business. Big Tobacco at the Bar of Justice.* Aurum Press, London.

10. Daubert et al. v. Merrell Dow Pharmaceuticals 92-102. June 28, 1993. [113 S Ctr 2768 (1993)].

11. Hulka, B.S., Kerkvliet, N.L. and Tugwell, P. (2000) *Experience of a scientific panel formed to advise the Federal Judiciary on silicone breast implants ...* N. Engl. J. Med. 342: 812–15.

12. Dixon, L. and Gill, B. (2002) *Changes in the Standards for Admitting Expert Evidence in Federal Civil Cases since the Daubert Decision.* RAND Institute for Civil Justice, Santa Monica, California.

13. Hyams, A.L., Shapiro, D.W. and Brennan, T.A. (1996) *Medical practice guidelines in malpractice litigation: an early retrospective.* J. Health Polit. Policy Law 21: 289–313.

14. Hurwitz, B. (1998) *Clinical Guidelines and the Law: Negligence, Discretion and Judgement.* Radcliffe Medical Press, Oxford.

15. Chalmers, I. (1998) *Patients should sue when available research isn't put into practice. [Letter]* Health Serv. J. 108: 18.

Gentle Reader,

Empathise with the public health physician who had just put down Dickens' Bleak House with a strong sense of déjà vu. He had been readingChapter 4 in which the young heroine pays her first visit to the Jellybys to find Mrs Jellyby in great form, busily sorting out the problems of Africa.

> *'You find me, my dears,' said Mrs Jellyby, snuffing the two great office candles in tin candlesticks which made the room taste strongly of hot tallow (the fire had gone out, and there was nothing in the grate but ashes, a bundle of wood, and a poker), 'you find me, my dears, as usual, very busy; but that you will excuse. The African project at present employs my whole time. It involves me in correspondence with public bodies, and with private individuals anxious for the welfare of their species all over the country. I am happy to say it is advancing. We hope by this time next year to have from a hundred and fifty to two hundred healthy families cultivating coffee and educating the natives of Borrioboola-Gha, on the left bank of the Niger.'*

Commentary

Mrs Jellyby was engaged in a great public health initiative; unfortunately she spent so much of her effort on Africa that her own house was in great disorder: the dinner was delayed 'in consequence of such accidents as the dish of potatoes being mislaid in the coal scuttle, and the handle of the corkscrew coming off, and striking the young woman in the chin'. Throughout dinner, Mrs Jellyby had continued to discuss her good works with a reforming zeal that was excellent. However, the dinner itself was not quite of the same standard, as Miss Summerson recorded: 'We had a fine codfish, a piece of roast beef, a dish of cutlets, and a pudding; an excellent dinner, if it had had any cooking to speak of, but it was almost raw'.

Public health professionals have been prominent in the promotion of evidence-based decision-making in healthcare but the evidence base of public health itself is not particularly well established. It would be appropriate if some of the energy of the public health establishment directed at encouraging others to be more evidence-based were used to strengthen the evidence base of public health itself.

Evidence-based public health

The term 'public health' is a source of confusion because it has two meanings, being both:

- a type of professional activity, and
- the objective of that activity.

It is easier and clearer to distinguish between public health practice, a professional activity, and the improved health of populations, the objectives of that activity. Clinical practice focuses on the individual patient, whereas public health practice is concerned with both the individual and the population in which individuals live (Fig. 8.1).

The individuals and the population in which they live interact. The beliefs, values, attitudes and behaviour of individuals influence the determinants of health of a population, for example, by determining whether members of the population are willing to accept the wearing of seat belts or the taxation of cigarettes for health purposes. In return, the population influences the decisions and behaviour of individuals. A population in which binge drinking is tolerated is likely to have more individuals with alcohol problems than one in which such behaviour is not tolerated.

The term 'population', however, requires a more detailed consideration because within any population other groups can be identified, notably:

- communities – that is, groups of people who live in the same geographical area but one which does not necessarily represent a specific political jurisdiction
- subgroups of the population who share an attribute such as age or ethnicity – for example, children, older people or people of South Asian origin
- subgroups of the population who share a common interest – for example, service users or passengers.

Subgroups designated within a population are largely artificial constructs of the epidemiologist. For instance,

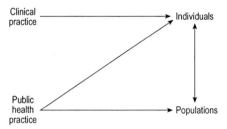

Fig. 8.1
The nature of public health practice in relation to that of clinical practice

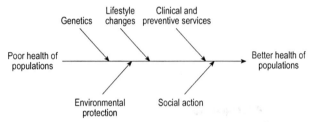

Fig. 8.2
Fishtail diagram to show the factors involved in health improvement

individual older people do not feel they are part of an 'elderly' subgroup. By contrast, communities and societies are real to the individuals who belong to them. The distinction between communities and societies, between Gemeinschaft and Gesellschaft, first described by the sociologist Ferdinand Tonnies in 1887, is powerful, but both provide a platform for public health practice.

The contribution of public health to improving the health of populations and individuals can best be depicted using a fishtail diagram (Fig. 8.2).

Although a fishtail diagram is useful for identifying causes, it does not have the capacity to depict the inter-relationship between activities which is better shown using a Venn diagram (Fig. 8.3).

8.1   The development of public health and the evolution of an evidence base

8.1.1   Public health practice and service development 1850–1950

There is no doubt that the decline in adult mortality that took place in England in the middle of the 19th century,

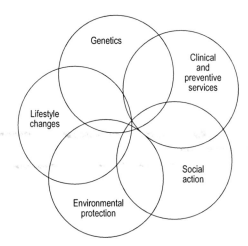

Fig. 8.3
Venn diagram to show the interrelationship of factors involved in
health improvement

similar to the declines observed in other developed
countries, was due primarily to environmental change
prompted by social action through legislation. The diseases
that declined were principally infectious diseases, and
the main reason for their decline was an improvement in
housing conditions and, more importantly, the provision of
clean drinking water and the effective disposal of sewage.
Vaccination, a health service, made a small contribution
to the decline in mortality, perhaps 5%, but most of the
change took place as a result of the transformation of society
in the 19th century. It is important to note that the basic
science was not understood before any control measures
were introduced. What was important was the belief that
infectious disease epidemics had natural, rather than
supernatural, causes and, in the case of cholera epidemic,
an agreement that the causal mechanism was related to the
water supply and not to smells in the air (the removal of the
Broad Street pump handle was important both practically
and symbolically).

The evidence base for 19th century public health
brought together an interesting combination of aesthetics
and science. Several 'nuisance' removal Acts were passed.
Although the term 'nuisance' as used today refers to a
trivial irritation, the word derives from the Old French
verb *nuire*, to harm, and in the middle of the 19th century a
nuisance was defined as anything that was offensive to the
senses and taken *ipso facto* to be injurious to health. Thus,
although a smell did not cause disease, the cause of a smell,

for example, raw sewage, was a cause of disease, and so by doing away with the untidiness and disorder that created the smell, disease was prevented and health improved.

The nuisance removal Acts provide interesting analogies for the patient safety movement in the 21st century, where it is clear that much harm to patients derives from disorder which can be observed in many aspects of clinical practice. By developing systems of care, care pathways or standard operating procedures, in which actions are determined by guidelines based on evidence, errors can be prevented and health improved. The ambitious project launched by the Institute of Healthcare Improvement in 2002 to save 100 000 lives by the introduction of relatively simple system changes can be regarded as analogous to the removal of the Broad Street pump handle. Donald Berwick and his colleagues did not need to understand all the reasons for system disorder; they simply took steps to ensure that it was dealt with appropriately and effectively (see Casebook 7.2).

The main factor that led to increased life expectancy in the 20th century, at least in England, was the improvement in child health and infant mortality which resulted from the introduction of health services at the turn of the 20th century. For instance, the Midwives Act of 1902 transformed a heterogeneous and disorderly workforce into a profession. School meals and a school health service were introduced in 1906 and 1908, respectively. The evidence on which these services were based was taken from Bismarck's 'Practical Christianity', in which were described changes introduced from 1870 onwards in the newly founded nation state of Germany.

It is essential to distinguish between the emotional drivers for change and the evidence base upon which a decision is made about what change should take place. In the middle of the 19th century, the emotional driver for change was enlightened self-interest, namely, rich and powerful people could contract cholera as well as poor people and so the rich were motivated to press for change that would benefit both rich and poor. Looking back at events in the early 20th century, it could be argued that the German Naval Act of 1902, which gave the Kaiser the authority to create a navy as powerful as any in the world, led to the establishment of the British 'Inter-Departmental Commission on Physical Degeneration'. In turn, the Commission's damning report on the health status of British children led to the Education Acts of 1906 and 1908, which introduced school meals and school health services.

In improving child health, the emotional driver for change was fear, a fear of Germany. This fear had arisen as a result of events ranging from the Agadir gunboat incident to the publication of the novel *The Riddle of the Sands*, in which a German invasion plan for England was described. These events led the British government, stimulated largely by the War Office and the Admiralty, to seek to improve child health through legislation, passing a series of Acts to do so.

8.1.2 Public health practice and health service development since 1950

Although health services have been trenchantly criticised by a wide range of commentators, most notably Ivan Illich, the impact of organised universal healthcare on the health of the population has been enormous, and at least half of the extra years of life gained since 1950 can be attributed to healthcare. Furthermore, there has been an increase in the number of disability-free years of life. Thus, well-organised universal healthcare has been responsible not only for improving the quantity but also the quality of life.

Health services can be classified into two different types:

1. services in which the main focus is the individual patient, e.g. orthopaedic or psychiatric services – these clinical services need to be organised on a population basis if the whole population is to benefit and not just those who are most wealthy
2. services in which the main focus is the population, e.g. occupational health, immunisation and screening – sometimes referred to as preventive services.

Traditionally, public health professionals have organised preventive services whereas their involvement in the delivery of clinical services varies from country to country. In some countries, public health professionals are part of the system that manages clinical services; in others, they are not directly involved but have a contribution of increasing importance in funding or commissioning healthcare, and making decisions about the most appropriate use of resources to maximise the value of healthcare.

8.1.2.1 The evidence base for preventive services

Whether directly managing or commissioning clinical services, or managing preventive services, the evidence base on which the public health professional is able to draw is one with which a clinician or someone who manages hospital services would be familiar. The systematic review of randomised controlled trials remains the single best source of evidence to demonstrate the benefits and harms of a health service, whether clinical or preventive. In the UK, the government based its decision not to introduce screening for prostate cancer on the results of two systematic reviews of the evidence (see Box 2.5), neither of which demonstrated any reduction in mortality from screening.[1,2] As screening always does some harm (see Section 3.4.1.1), policy-makers were able to conclude that screening would do more harm than good and therefore should not be introduced. It could be argued that this decision represented the values inherent in British decision-making which many people, particularly in the USA, see as over-cautious and timid (see Prologue, 'The USA and the rest of the developed world'). A further example of this can be found in Section 3.4 , where screening is described as an example of evidence-based public health in the context of service delivery.

A similar approach is necessary for other public health services, but the particular problems involved in constructing an evidence base for immunisation should not be underestimated as events in Britain have shown regarding the evidence about the relationship between autism and the measles, mumps and rubella vaccine (MMR). In general, a higher standard of safety and of evidence about safety are required when preventive services are being evaluated because preventive services are offered to a healthy population.

8.1.3   Public health practice and health education

In the second half of the 20th century, resources were invested in health education, that is, education about the body and risks to health. Much of the earlier work on controlled trials and meta-analysis was done by psychologists working within education and, therefore, there is a strong evidence base for education. The problems that health educators have had, however, derive not so much from the weakness of the evidence base as from a failure to agree on the objectives of health education.

In a linear theory of preventive medicine, there is a series of links from health education to increased knowledge to a change in attitude to changes in behaviour to better health (Fig. 8.4). In this theory, the

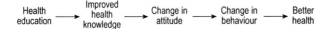

Fig. 8.4
The potential series of links in a linear chain from health education
to improved health

assumption is that, by stimulating change at any point in
the chain, change will take place further along the chain.
However, the relationship is not so simple. It is essential,
therefore, to design studies that have the capacity to
measure the impact of health education on health status,
if that is the objective of health education.

Because increased knowledge about health does not
necessarily lead to a change in behaviour, it is possible
to be confident only of the relationship between health
education and increased knowledge. This has led to a value
conflict within public health. Some practitioners believe
that a change in knowledge is sufficient justification for the
investment of resources, even if it does not lead to a change
in behaviour. Others argue that the objective is to change
behaviour, and they support the use of social marketing
techniques to achieve this end. Practitioners who champion
the strategy of increasing knowledge have questioned
the ethics of social marketing. Should public health
professionals use the techniques of the advertising agencies
to influence behaviour or is the role of health educators
to ensure that people are well informed about the risks to
health, leaving it to the citizen to decide whether they wish
to take action?

However, the implications of such a debate change when
the health of young people is involved. The relationship
between sex education and teenage pregnancy rates
demonstrates both the difficulty of relying on health
education alone to change behaviour and the need to define
outcomes clearly when investing resources in public health.
In a cluster randomised trial, Henderson et al.[3] investigated
the impact of a theoretically based sex education
programme (SHARE) delivered by teachers (intervention
group) on both conceptions and termination (as registered
by the NHS) compared with that of conventional education
(control group). Follow-up was 4.5 years after intervention
at age 20 years for the 4196 women in the study. No
significant differences were found between the two groups
and the lack of effect in the intervention group was not due
to quality of delivery of the SHARE programme.

In an accompanying editorial, Stammers[4] signals an urgent need for a change in approaches to school sex education, highlighting the evidence that unfortunately increased knowledge is a necessary but insufficient cause of change in sexual behaviour. Indeed, Henderson et al.[3] recommended that to reduce unwanted pregnancies there is a need to develop longer-term interventions that are complementary to high-quality sex education but address:

- socio-economic inequalities
- parental influences.

Stammers[4] also recommends that the wider sociocultural aspects influencing sexual behaviour require greater attention. One sociocultural factor that has potential to influence health risk behaviour in children is the ethos of the school itself, and Bonell et al.[5] recommend that interventions to improve school ethos which are complementary to classroom-based interventions need to be developed. Although it is important that any such interventions are tailored to the sociocultural context of the country in which they are implemented.

8.1.4 Public health practice and health promotion

In the last two decades of the 20th century, a significant shift took place from health education to health promotion, in which educational interventions aimed at individuals, communities or societies were complemented by other interventions in which individuals were educated not only about what they could do to change their own behaviour but also about how they could press for social action through legislation, such as the control of advertising.

Thus, health promotion is a term used to describe a wide range of activities. It was initially developed as part of a tripartite approach to public health, as shown in the Venn diagram in Fig. 8.5.

8.1.4.1 The evidence base for health promotion

The use of an evidence-based approach in public health practice and health promotion is the subject of much debate. Some practitioners hold the view that 'evidence-based' is synonymous with using evidence from randomised controlled trials. Others are against the approach believing it to be inappropriate for public health because it is

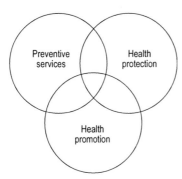

Fig. 8.5
The range of activities included under the term 'health promotion'

'positivist' or 'decisionist'. However, to deny that public
health decisions should be based on evidence from research
that is amplified, if possible, by evidence from experience
is unrealistic. Furthermore, evidence about the costs
and benefits of any public health or health promotion
intervention must be related to the other needs of the
population or community and the values that will also
influence a decision (Fig. 8.6).

In an editorial, Nutbeam puts inverted commas round
the terms 'evidence-based' and 'evidence', and concludes
that: 'the move towards evidence-based health promotion
should not be perceived as a threat'.[6]

It is rather an opportunity to engage in debate about
means and ends in health promotion interventions, and the
fit between intervention and evaluation methods. Indeed,
many practitioners are engaging in finding out what an
evidence-based approach means when applied to public
health practice and health promotion, including the nature
of evidence that needs to be applied for various types of
intervention.

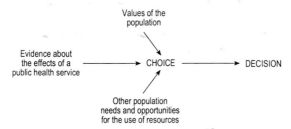

Fig. 8.6
Factors influencing decision-taking in public health

Rychetnik and Wise[7] propose an 'evidence-agenda map' to help advocates of evidence-based policy and practice identify the health promotion goals they want to influence against the available evidence. Rada et al.[8] have developed a framework to help prioritise health promotion interventions using different kinds of evidence in four domains. McQueen[9] highlights the need to develop appropriate standards for evidence-based evaluation of health promotion interventions in which the complex nature of such interventions is recognised. Green and Tones[10] advocate the use of a 'judicial principle' to assess the evidence for use in health promotion, and McMichael et al.[11] state that the public health evidence base is in urgent need of strengthening, including evidence of intervention effectiveness. Kemm[12] concludes that, although the concept of an evidence-based approach has been transferred from clinical medicine, for public health interventions, the RCT may not be wholly appropriate as a method of evaluation for complex interventions in communities where context is also important.

8.1.5   Public health practice and legislation

The traditional role of law is to protect the individual from harm by third parties rather than to protect the public health. However, legislation (including regulation if a change in the law is not required) is an intervention frequently used in public health practice. As such, it is vital for public health practitioners to gather evidence about the potential effects of proposed legislation on the health of the populations for which they are responsible. While this is necessary, it is important to remember that legislation does not affect people's 'health' directly. Instead, legislation is used to influence the social or socio-economic determinants of health.

There is an inverse relationship between the magnitude of a health problem and the strength of opposition to legislation framed to prevent it (Fig. 8.7). When public concern about a problem exceeds public opposition to legislation, a threshold is crossed and it is possible to legislate for the implementation of a policy.

However, the level of that threshold can be influenced by many factors other than the magnitude of the health problem; some of these factors raise the threshold while others lower it. Strong evidence is now a prerequisite before any public health policy can be introduced through

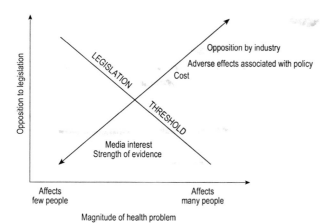

Fig. 8.7
Factors affecting the legislation threshold: those at the right-hand
end of the double-headed arrow will raise the threshold whereas
those on the left will lower it

legislation, but the converse is not true: the existence of
strong evidence indicating the need for a public health
policy does not necessarily result in legislation being
introduced.

Greater obstacles are faced when using the law to
implement a public health policy with the aim of protecting
individuals from their own inclinations – the paternalistic
role of law. Powerful evidence is needed to show that
such legislation is not only effective but also safe. When
legislation was being drafted to make the wearing of seat
belts compulsory, a law that now seems uncontroversial, it
was argued that the State should not introduce paternalistic
legislation for the benefit of a large number of people if it
resulted in the unnecessary harm of even one person. It was
considered tantamount to sacrificing one person for the
benefit of other people who did not wish to take protective
action of their own volition.

It is perhaps when pressing for legislation to improve
the public health that the public health professional has to
be most pragmatic about the influence of evidence during
the decision-making process (see also Section 7.8). The job
of the public health professional is to improve the health
of populations, in which task the use of evidence is
pre-requisite. In contrast, the job of the politician is to
introduce legislative power for the public good, in which
task values may be more influential than evidence.

Although some healthcare professionals may feel
indignant about the influence that politicians, and indeed the

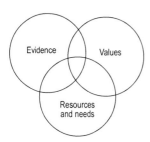

Margin Fig. 8.1

media, can have in public health decision-making, it is wholly appropriate for politicians and the public to take decisions in situations where values are dominant. In such cases, it is the role of the scientist to be clear about the evidence, and what it shows, including the balance of good to harm of an intervention for the population. However, this is the limit of the scientist's responsibility; it is the responsibility of those individuals who represent society to clarify the values of relevance in particular situations and make the appropriate decisions using those values (see Margin Fig. 8.1 for the factors affecting choice during decision-making).

8.1.6   Public health practice and policy-making

For public health policy-making, there is a greater body of research evidence available on which to base decisions, and as such there is a greater tradition of using evidence in decision-making (see Section 3.5), although values-based decision-making still occurs. For some decisions, in which resources are not a major determining factor and the values are relatively straightforward, policy-making can be based on evidence alone.

8.1.6.1 The evidence base in policy-making

The evidence base for public health practitioners working in policy-making is the literature of health and social policy, and of health economics, fields in which there are relatively few systematic reviews.

The Director General of the World Health Organization set up a Global Commission on the Social Determinants of Health in 2005. The objective of the Commission was to achieve policy change by learning from existing knowledge about the social determinants of health, and converting that learning into political and economic action on those social determinants.

A discussion paper was developed, entitled *Towards a Conceptual Framework for Analysis and Action on the Social Determinants of Health*,[13] in which was proposed a framework for the social determinants of health. In this paper, three key issues are identified, each of which would have a different evidence base, if effective action is to be taken to address the social determinants of health:

- the need to distinguish between structural issues (e.g. income and education) and 'intermediate' issues (e.g. behaviour) as determinants of health

- the need to understand and make explicit what is meant by the 'socio-political context' (aspects of the social system that impact on individuals)
- the need to take account of the actions that should be taken at different levels not only to improve health but also to reduce inequalities in health.

A working party produced a second paper entitled *The Development of the Evidence Base about the Social Determinants of Health;*[14] in it are set out eight principles to help tackle the three issues identified above:

1. A commitment to the value of equity – health inequity between and within societies is unfair and unjust (a political position).
2. Taking an evidence-based approach – finding the best possible evidence about social determinants in addition to developing an understanding of local context and tacit knowledge, and flexible use of evidence hierarchies.
3. Methods and epistemology – the need to develop multiple criteria to determine fitness for purpose, to judge thresholds of acceptability and to appraise critically the different forms of knowledge relevant to the social determinants of health.
4. Gradients and gaps – the importance of addressing health inequalities in the population by considering both health gaps and health gradients.
5. Causes: determinants and outcomes – a basis for developing the evidence as a causal model which crosses from the social to the biological.
6. Social structure – the need to make more explicit the range of dimensions of inequalities in the evidence base.
7. Social dynamics – the influence of changing social systems and sub-systems on health inequalities.
8. Explicating bias – the need to make sources of bias (political and ideological) explicit in the selection and interpretation of evidence.

Using this approach, every change in society could have an impact on health.

8.1.6.2 Using the public health evidence base to achieve health gain from non-health and health-related proposals

During the last decade, a methodology known as health impact assessment (HIA) has been used to increase the

Margin Note 8.1
HIA Gateway website

The Association of Public Health
Observatories hosts an HIA Gateway
website which includes information on
the following topics:

- Quick Guide
- Reports
- Guides and Evidence
- Networks and Events
- Links

The website is available online at:
http://www.apho.org.uk
Click on HIA

potential health gain from both non-health and health-related proposals. HIA has been defined by the WHO as:

a combination of procedures, methods and tools by which a policy, program or project may be judged as to its potential effects on the health of a population and the distribution of effects within the population.[15]

Thus, HIA is a way of modelling or predicting changes to health and well-being as a result of proposal implementation. Proposals for appraisal using HIA can range from national policies to projects at a local level, and any topic or subject can be covered from urban planning and spatial development to the introduction of a credit union, from the building of a new runway at an airport to the introduction of a minimum wage.

However, the main purpose of undertaking HIA is to give decision-makers information about the effects on health and well-being of a specific proposal. This information about the potential or predicted effects of a proposal is supported by suggestions about how the proposal could be changed or modified to achieve or optimise health gain. The methodology was developed partly in response to the inadequacy of other impact assessments (e.g. environmental impact assessment – EIA – and social impact assessment – SIA) which in the past have largely failed to address the effects of proposals on the health and well-being of a population or a community.

Potential effects on health and well-being are identified using a combination of both the main models of health:

1. the biomedical model of illness and disease
2. the social or socio-economic model of health and well-being.

Using a balance of both models, it is possible to identify potential health outcomes and trends in health as a result of proposal implementation. In this way, the impacts on the socio-economic determinants of health as well as the biophysical and/or environmental determinants of health are taken into consideration.

Suggestions to change or enhance the proposal cover the three main functions of public health:

- health protection – minimising or avoiding any negative or harmful effects
- health improvement – maximising or enhancing any positive or beneficial effects

- reducing health inequalities by addressing any differential impacts predicted to affect vulnerable, marginalised or disadvantaged groups in the population or community.

When implementing any complex intervention in a population or community, an eclectic approach needs to be taken to the collection of evidence. In HIA, the main sources of information are:

- the research literature covering different research methods
- the grey literature, including other HIA case-studies on similar types of proposal
- the analysis of routine and non-routine data about the population or community affected, and, if available, the effects of the intervention(s) in the proposal on similar communities elsewhere
- the knowledge and experience of people living and working in the population or community affected by proposal implementation.

These different types of information need to be collated and brought together in a report for decision-makers, who decide, on the basis of the health impacts in relation to other priorities, what, if any, changes they wish to make to the proposal to increase health gain.

8.1.7   Public health practice and humanitarianism

Accurate and unbiased information about health effects of policies, tactics, and weapons are rarely available, but act as an antidote to war propaganda and is essential to efforts to achieve a just peace.

MacQueen and Santa-Barbara, 2000[16]

Few public health interventions are as complex as those designed to tackle the major emergencies faced by populations, whether they result from civil war or natural disaster. However, the commitment to evidence-based public health in this most difficult of arenas was highlighted in an article by Banatvala and Zwi in the *British Medical Journal* entitled 'Conflict and health: Public health and humanitarian interventions: developing the evidence base'.[17] The authors make the following points:

- It is necessary to base policies and practice on the best available evidence to maximise the value of available resources.

- The evidence base must comprise not only evidence of effectiveness and efficiency, but also evidence related to other dimensions of health interventions such as their humanity, equity, local ownership, and political and financial feasibility.
- It is difficult to promote the uptake of good practice in the emergency aid sector due to rapid staff turnover, the perception that there is little time to learn lessons, and the scarcity of resources available for encouraging evidence-based practice.
- Humanitarian organisations need to meet the challenges of institutionalising a sensitive and inclusive culture informed by evidence and of building sustainable mechanisms through which policy advice is crystallised from the vast and valuable foundation of field experience.

The authors of this bold and visionary paper demonstrate how evidence from experience, i.e. tacit knowledge, can be integrated with evidence from scientific studies, i.e. explicit knowledge, to create evidence-based public health and humanitarian aid. This integration of the two types of knowledge requires that public health practitioners record their experience in a casebook, and make that experience widely available through publication.

Evidence about outcome can also be complemented by evidence about the effectiveness of the process of humanitarian aid. In a study of war-related fatality rates among the Kosovar Albanian population in Kosovo during 1998–99, it was found that men aged 50 years and older had a relative risk of dying from war-related trauma 3.2 times greater than that experienced by men of military age (15–49 years).[18] This finding indicates that it was safer for a man to be in the army than to be a civilian in an era of ethnic cleansing. Of greater importance, however, is the indication this study provides of the violation of international standards of conduct during warfare. It has led to the hypothesis that evacuation programmes to assist older people find refuge 'may prevent loss of life'. Although this hypothesis needs to be tested, on the basis of the evidence available from routine data the case for action is strong.

References

1. Selley, S., Donovan, J., Faulkner, A. et al. (1997) *Diagnosis, management and screening of early localised prostate cancer.* Health Technol. Assess. 1(2).

2. Chamberlain, J., Melia, J., Moss, S. et al. (1997) *The diagnosis, management, treatment and costs of prostate cancer in England and Wales.* Health Technol. Assess. 1(3).

3. Henderson, M., Wight, D., Raab, G.M. et al. (2007) *Impact of a theoretically based sex education programme (SHARE) delivered by teachers on NHS registered conceptions and terminations: final results of cluster randomised controlled trial.* Br. Med. J. 334: 133.

4. Stammers, T. (2007) *Sexual health in adolescents. [Editorial]* Br. Med. J. 334: 103–4.

5. Bonell, C., Fletcher, A. and McCambridge, J. (2007) *Improving school ethos may reduce substance misuse and teenage pregnancy.* Br. Med. J. 334: 614–16.

6. Nutbeam, D. (1999) *The challenge to provide 'evidence' in health promotion. [Editorial]* Health Promotion International 14: 99–101.

7. Rychetnik, L. and Wise, M. (2004) *Advocating evidence-based health promotion: reflections and a way forward.* Health Promot. Int. 19: 247–57.

8. Rada, J., Ratima, M. and Howden-Chapman, P. (1999) *Evidence-based purchasing of health promotion: methodology for reviewing evidence.* Health Promot. Int. 14: 177–87.

9. McQueen, D.V. (2001) *Strengthening the evidence base for health promotion.* Health Promot. Int. 16: 261–8.

10. Green, J. and Tones, K. (1999) *Towards a secure evidence base for health promotion.* J. Public Health Med. 21: 133–9.

11. McMichael, C., Waters, E. and Volmink, J. (2005) *Evidence-based public health: what does it offer developing countries?* J. Public Health (Oxf.), 27: 215–21.

12. Kemm, J. (2006) *The limitations of 'evidence-based' public health.* J. Eval. Clin. Pract. 12: 319–24.

13. Solar, O. and Irwin, A. (2005) *Towards a conceptual framework for analysis and action on the social determinants of health.* Discussion paper for the World Health Organization Commission on the Social Determinants of Health.

14. Kelly, M., Bonnefoy, J., Morgan, A. et al. (2006) *The Development of Evidence Base about the Social Determinants of Health.* World Health Organization Commission on Social Determinants of Health, Measurement and Evidence Knowledge Network.

15. World Health Organization (WHO) European Centre for Health Policy (1999) *Health Impact Assessment: main concepts and suggested approach. Gothenburg Consensus Paper.* WHO, Copenhagen.

16. MacQueen, G. and Santa-Barbara, J. (2000) *Peace building through health initiatives.* Br. Med. J. 321: 1293–6.

17. Banatvala, N. and Zwi, A.B. (2000) *Public health and humanitarian interventions: developing the evidence base.* Br. Med. J. 321: 101–5.

18. Spiegel, P.B. and Salama, P. (2000) *War and mortality in Kosovo, 1998–99: an epidemiological testimony.* Lancet 355: 2204–9.

8.2   Developing systematic reviews for the evidence base in public health

8.2.1   The Campbell Collaboration

The Campbell Collaboration was set up following a meeting of 80 people from four countries at University College, London, in July 1999. The aim is to synthesise the best research evidence about the effects of social and educational policies and practices. As such, the Campbell Collaboration is a social policy analogue of the Cochrane Collaboration and adopts the same principles towards research synthesis, namely:

- clarifying the question
- searching for and finding all the relevant evidence
- using specific criteria to distinguish the evidence that should be included in the synthesis from that which should be excluded
- synthesising the evidence
- keeping the synthesis up to date.

Work at the Campbell Collaboration has been focused on several topics, notably education and criminal justice. Although public health practitioners are acutely aware of and highlight the complexity of public health interventions, many of the topics considered by the Campbell Collaboration in the field of education and criminal justice are at least as complex.

The development of the Campbell Collaboration offers a firm platform on which to construct the evidence base for public health. The work undertaken so far demonstrates that it is possible to undertake a systematic review of different types of evidence.

8.2.2   The use of systematic reviews in public health decision-making

It is possible to use the methods that have transformed decision-making in clinical practice to improve public health. The results of randomised controlled trials and systematic reviews can make a valuable contribution to informing decision-making about public health interventions particularly those targeted at lifestyle determinants of health, for example, the results or outputs from:

- a randomised trial of the effects of two Mediterranean-style diets vs a low-fat diet on cardiovascular risk factors[1]
- a systematic review of the cost-effectiveness of healthcare-based interventions aimed at improving physical activity[2]
- guidance on four commonly used methods (exercise referral schemes, pedometers and community-based exercise programmes for walking and cycling) to increase physical activity based on a systematic review of the evidence[3]

- a systematic review of the cost-effectiveness of health promotion programmes.[4]

Indeed, more systematic reviews are needed, not fewer.[5] As it is likely that systematic reviews will be used increasingly in the future to make decisions about limited public health resources,[6] it is important for public health practitioners to understand and use them if they are to engage in the debate about setting public health priorities. One of the weaknesses in the argument of those who criticise the evidence-based approach is that they assume that systematic reviews comprise reviews of RCTs as the sole research methodology whereas this is not the case.

It will need a detached dispassionate historian to write an objective account of the debate between the different protagonists. As is usually the case, the arguments sometimes focus on marginal rather than central issues, and often have political or personal dimensions as well as the scientific issues. The author of an article in *Evidence and Policy* made a personal attack on the director of the UK Cochrane Centre under the title: 'Is the evidence-based practice movement doing more good than harm?'[7] The riposte of the person attacked had the wonderful title: 'If evidence-informed policy works in practice, does it matter if it doesn't work in theory?'[8] The abstract of this paper is worth quoting in full.

> *Professionals and policy makers sometimes do more harm than good when they intervene in the lives of other people. This should prompt humility and efforts to ensure that policies and practices are informed by rigorous, transparent, up-to-date evaluations of relevant empirical evidence. Systematic reviews of relevant evidence must be designed to minimise the likelihood of confusing the effects of interventions with the effects of biases and chance. Systematic reviews are essential, although insufficient, for informing policies and practice. Critiques of this approach based solely on theory are unhelpful in efforts to protect the public from harmful and useless interventions.[8]*

References

1. Estruch, R., Martinez-Gonzalez, M.A., Corella, D. et al. (2006) *Effects of Mediterranean-style diet on cardiovascular risk factors. A randomized trial.* Ann. Intern. Med. 145: 1–11.
2. Hagberg, L.A. and Lindholm, L. (2006) *Cost-effectiveness of healthcare-based interventions aimed at improving physical activity.* Scand. J. Public Health 34: 641–53.

3. National Institute for Health and Clinical Excellence (NICE) (2006) *Four commonly used methods to increase physical activity: brief interventions in primary care, exercise referral schemes, pedometers and community-based exercise programmes for walking and cycling.* Public Health Intervention Guidance no. 2. NICE, London.

4. Aldana, S.A.G. (2001) *Financial impact of health promotion programs: a comprehensive review of the literature.* Am. J. Health Promot. 15: 296–320.

5. Swingler, G.H., Volmink, J. and Ioannidis, J.P.A. (2003) *Number of published systematic reviews and global burden of disease: database analysis.* Br. Med. J. 327: 1083–4.

6. Brownson, R.C., Baker, E.A., Leet, T.L. et al. (2003) *Evidence-based Public Health.* Oxford University Press, Oxford.

7. Hammersley, M. (2005) *Is the evidence-based practice movement doing more good than harm? Reflections on Iain Chalmers' case for research-based policy making and practice.* Evidence and Policy 1: 85–100.

8. Chalmers, I. (2005) *If evidence-informed policy works in practice, does it matter if it doesn't work in theory?* Evidence and Policy 1: 227–42.

8.3   The need for an eclectic approach towards the evidence base for public health

The main differences between the nature and role of the evidence base in clinical practice and public health practice are shown in Matrix 8.1.

When implementing a highly complex intervention in a community, an eclectic approach has to be taken to the collection of evidence. The need for such an approach to the public health evidence base is outlined in a paper entitled

Matrix 8.1

	Clinical practice	Public health practice and health promotion
Nature of intervention	Mainly single or simple interventions	Mainly complex or multiple interventions
Nature of evidence to show effectiveness	• Systematic review • RCT	• Systematic review • RCT • Cohort study • Case-control study • Controlled before and after study • Interrupted time series
Sources of evidence	Published literature	• Published literature • Grey literature
Need for other types of knowledge	Tacit knowledge from clinicians' experience	Tacit knowledge of practitioners and end-users
Contextual factors	Emotional context of the decision	• Socio-political context of intervention • Local context

'Evidence, hierarchies and typologies: horses for courses'.[1]
Petticrew and Roberts identify an emerging consensus that
the 'hierarchy of evidence' used in clinical decision-making
may be difficult to apply in other settings. However, it may
not be appropriate to abandon the hierarchy without having
a framework or guide to replace it. Petticrew and Roberts
suggest a framework based around a matrix (Matrix 8.2), and
emphasise the need to match research questions to specific
types of research. The framework devised by Petticrew and
Roberts is based on the typology of evidence presented in
this book. They suggest that an emphasis on methodological

Matrix 8.2   An example of a typology of evidence: social interventions in children (Source: Petticrew and Roberts[1])

Research question	Qualitative research	Survey	Case-control studies	Cohort studies	RCTs	Quasi-experimental studies	Non-experimental evaluations	Systematic reviews
Effectiveness Does this work? Does doing this work better than doing that?				+	++	+		+++
Process of service delivery How does it work?	++	+					+	+++
Salience Does it matter?	++	++						+++
Safety Will it do more good than harm?	+		+	+	++	+	+	+++
Acceptability Will children/ parents be willing to or want to take up the service offered?	++	+			+	+	+	+++
Cost-effectiveness Is it worth buying this service?					++			+++
Appropriateness Is this the right service for these children?	++	++						++
Satisfaction with the service Are users, providers, and other stakeholders satisfied with the service?	++	++	+	+				+

appropriateness, and on typologies rather than hierarchies of evidence, may be helpful when organising and appraising public health evidence.

The prevention of death from fire by the installation of smoke alarms is an example of a public health activity that has been evaluated rigorously using a combination of different research methods. Rowland et al.[2] used a randomised controlled trial methodology to investigate smoke alarm installation in local authority housing in central London. To complement the trial, semi-structured group and individual interviews were conducted with some of the adult participants in the study to explore the barriers and levers to the use of this intervention.[3] This qualitative component of the study was important especially as mortality from fires is higher in lower socio-economic groups.

The importance of evaluating public health or social interventions in real-life situations as well as in research studies is highlighted in a paper by Roberts et al.,[4] who discuss mentoring to reduce antisocial behaviour in children. Although one meta-analysis had shown that mentoring schemes have benefits when assessed using self-reports and non-blinded reports of behaviour change (benefits were experienced for some young people for some programmes in some circumstances), an examination of existing reviews did not provide evidence of measurable gains in such outcomes as truanting and other antisocial behaviours. There is also evidence that some mentoring programmes can have a negative effect. Thus, to obtain evidence of effectiveness it is necessary to show that a public health intervention works, as well as to show that it works in real life. As social or public health interventions are complex, they need to be evaluated both before and after implementation. Roberts et al. conclude that for practitioners and members of the public, seeking research on programmes of intervention for common problems will be disappointed by the relative lack of good evidence.

References

1. Petticrew, M. and Roberts, H. (2003) *Evidence, hierarchies, and typologies: horses for courses.* J. Epidemiol. Community Health 57: 527–9.
2. Rowland, D., Di Guiseppi, C., Roberts, I. et al. (2005) *Prevalence of working smoke alarms in local authority inner city housing: randomised controlled trial.* Br. Med. J. 325: 998–1001.
3. Roberts, H., Curtis, K., Liabo, K. et al. (2004) *Putting public health evidence into practice: increasing the prevalence of working smoke alarms in disadvantaged inner city housing.* J. Epidemiol. Community Health 58: 280–5.
4. Roberts, H., Liabo, K., Lucas, P. et al. (2004) *Mentoring to reduce antisocial behaviour in childhood. [Education and debate]* Br. Med. J. 328: 512–14.

8.4   The basis for public health decision-making

As for decision-making in clinical practice, there are three types of input in public health decision-making:

- evidence
- values
- population needs and resources.

However, decision-making about population interventions affecting different categories of the determinants of health – physical, socio-economic, health services and genetic – involves a different balance of the three types of input. These relationships are best demonstrated using a Venn diagram, and the balance of inputs in decision-making about four different types of public health intervention is shown in Fig. 8.8 (a–d). As can be seen, some public health decisions can be value-based (see also Casebook 8.1) and often have difficult ethical implications. However, even when public health decisions are evidence-based, it is important to emphasise that values must always be taken into account.

8.4.1   The need for judgement

In order to make decisions about public health interventions, apart from the three types of input shown in Fig. 8.8, it is also necessary to apply judgement, as when making decisions about clinical services. The need for judgement during decision-taking was well analysed by Herbert Simon, who emphasised the need to distinguish:

> the element of judgement in decision-making is the ethical element ... in making administrative decisions it is continually necessary to choose factual premises whose truth or falsehood is not definitely known and cannot be determined with certainty with the information and time available for reaching the decision.[1]

The situation described by Simon is familiar to all public health practitioners.

Reference

1. Simon, H.A. (1997) *Administrative Behaviour: a study of decision-making processes in administrative organisations.* 4th edn. The Free Press New York.

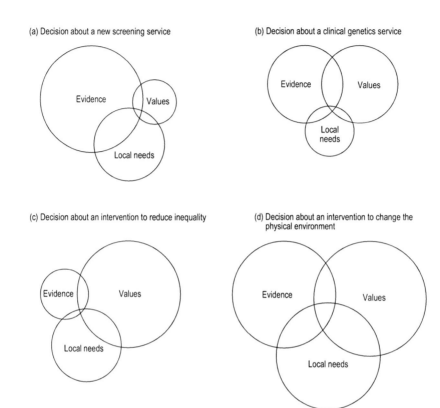

Fig. 8.8
The relative balance of the three main inputs – evidence, values and local needs – during decision-making about (a) a new screening service, (b) a clinical genetics service, (c) an intervention to reduce inequality, and (d) an intervention to change the physical environment

---

Casebook 8.1 Value-based policy-making

During 1999, there were frequent battles between the French government on the one hand and both the European Union (EU) and the United Kingdom on the other over the issue of the contamination of British beef with BSE. Although a panel of experts convened by the EU reviewed the evidence about the infectivity of British beef and recommended that it was safe for consumption, the French politicians declared British beef to be unsafe. The principal reason for this, as they openly stated, was the French general public's lack of faith in the capacity of the political system to protect the public health following the scandal surrounding the use of blood contaminated with HIV for transfusion. As a consequence, the politicians deemed any risk, however slight, to be unacceptable. Thus, in this particular decision, values were dominant.

8.5   Public health practice in the 21st century: knowledge-based public health

What does the future hold for public health practitioners? Some have said that the 21st century will be one in which genetics will dominate the health agenda, and it is important for public health practitioners to recognise this driver and the controversy it may generate. Some practitioners are already developing the concept of, and the evidence base for, public health genetics, i.e. the application of advances in genetic science to improve health and prevent disease.[1] It is important for politicians and policy-makers to learn about genetics and health so that they can respond to new technologies and any surrounding controversies on the basis of the evidence.[2]

However, it could be argued that the impact of the Internet and the influence it has on knowledge management will increase the importance of knowledge as a driver equal to that of genetics for improving the health of individuals and populations. Thus, to update the fishtail diagram of factors relevant to health improvement in the 20th century, knowledge can be added as a new driver for the 21st century (Fig. 8.9).

Knowledge-based public health will include not only evidence-based public health but also the traditional public health skills of data collection and analysis and the ability of public health practitioners to record and use the experience of communities and societies. Knowledge-based public health creates new opportunities for public health practice.

As discussed in Section 4.3, knowledge is like water, and knowledge has the potential to have a greater impact on health than any drug or technology likely to be introduced

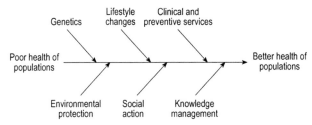

Fig. 8.9
Drivers in 21st century public health practice

during the next decade. Just as the 19th century epidemics of cholera, typhoid, typhus and smallpox were controlled by the provision of clean clear water, so 21st century epidemics will be controlled by the delivery of clean, clear knowledge. Just as public health services are responsible for monitoring and reporting on the quality and safety of water for their populations, they should also be responsible for monitoring, reporting on, and, if necessary, taking action to improve the quality and safety of the knowledge provided to their populations, including both professionals and members of the public.

In England, public health practitioners are ideally placed to be chief knowledge officers. Indeed, the plan is for the directors of public health to be the Chief Knowledge Officer for their local populations (see Section 2.5.1.1 and Box 2.4, and Section 7.4 and Box 7.6). Thus, the director of public health in the 21st century should ask questions not only about pollution and water quality but also about the quality of knowledge available to the whole population, and, in particular, to the least advantaged members of that population. If knowledge is regarded as a form of wealth, it is likely there will be an inequality in knowledge gain for different socio-economic groups just as there is an inequality in all other aspects of wealth. Given this, it will be necessary for the director of public health to provide a knowledge service to certain subgroups of the population who are unable to access knowledge on their own.

8.5.1 Knowledge-based health improvement

The World Health Organization (WHO) has recognised the importance of knowledge to health improvement, and, following the WHO summit in Mexico in 2005, produced a report entitled *World Report on Knowledge for Better Health*.[3] In addition to chapters on the need to improve health through health systems and health systems research and for better systems of health research, it contains a chapter called 'Linking research to action', in which the need to improve the use of evidence in decision-making, particularly by 'public policy-makers and health system managers', is emphasised. The WHO proposed that public policy-making and health system managers could support users of research knowledge in three ways:

- by developing their own or their representatives' capacity to use research knowledge

- by commissioning research or research syntheses when none exist
- by combining research knowledge with other types of knowledge to bring about change in health systems to achieve health equity.

Finally, WHO called for 'long-term relationships involving the producers and users of research', and identified knowledge exchange as the new frontier for bringing research into policy and practice. This commitment was reinforced by the newly elected Director General of WHO, Margaret Chan, who, in her inaugural speech, identified information and knowledge as one of six key issues on which she wants to focus. Public health practitioners are ideally trained and positioned to act as knowledge brokers, and knowledge management should be a core public health skill for the 21st century.

8.5.2 Supporting an evidence-based approach in healthcare systems

There are many challenges that practitioners of an evidence-based approach will have to face in the 21st century, and public health professionals are in a position to support them. Public health skills can be used to facilitate and mediate appropriate responses to three of these challenges.

The first challenge is to broaden the concept of effectiveness using criteria and standards that have been developed by people other than doctors and researchers. What do we mean when we use the word 'effective' and whose definition are we using?

The second challenge is to extend the culture of critical appraisal. Key criteria are likely to be equity, efficiency, and affordability, without all three of which the concept of effectiveness has little meaning.

The third challenge is to supplement and complement the use of evidence from quantitative research, especially that derived from RCTs, with that from good-quality qualitative research. As the primary determinant of the effective management of a healthcare system is the competence and behaviour of the professionals within it, there needs to be an increase in the amount of behavioural research conducted. A starting point for this strategy is to provide good-quality training in various research methodologies and their appropriate usage.

References

1. Marteau, T.M. and Lerman, C. (2001) *Genetic risk and behavioural change.* Br. Med. J. 322: 1056–9.

2. Zimmern, R., Emery, J. and Richards, T. (2001) *Putting genetics in perspective: requires better understanding and more rational debate.* Br. Med. J. 322: 1005–6.

3. World Health Organization (WHO) (2004) *World Report on Knowledge for Better Health. Strengthening Health Systems.* WHO, Geneva.

Gentle Reader,

Empathise with Dr John Hall, son-in-law of William Shakespeare, a man of good intentions. He wrote a treatise entitled Select Observations on English Bodies of Eminent Persons in Desperate Diseases. *In the preface, he reflects, 'we must study all ways possible to find out and appoint medicines of cheap rate and effectual for money is scarce and country people poor ...'.*

Commentary

Dr Hall's treatise provides an example of an early text on effectiveness.

Despite the worthiness of his objectives, his observational epidemiology was weak – most of his observations are of single cases. By today's standards, his level of skill was inadequate to the task, but in the 17th century he would have been considered highly skilled. Can this be said of all healthcare professionals practising today?

CHAPTER 9

Developing the skills of individuals

Developing skills for evidence-based practice

Evidence-based practice is not a one-off activity; it requires integration of the key concepts, and use of the key evidence-based practice skills, into everyday work. There is evidence to suggest that the following factors can support the development and use of evidence-based practice skills:[1]

- a degree of social exchange during which professionals work together to interpret evidence and reflect upon its significance for the context in which they are working
- the use of highly context-specific evidence
- sustained problem-solving to deal with the number of variables at work.

The benefit of integrating teaching and learning into routine practice is that, over time, self-directed and lifelong learning skills will become embedded.[2] The way evidence-based practice skills are learned can also determine success. A systematic review of postgraduate teaching in evidence-based medicine found that an integrated approach, rather than a stand-alone course, is more likely to lead to gains in appraisal skills.[3] Although stand-alone teaching improves knowledge, clinically integrated learning improves knowledge, skills, attitudes and behaviours in postgraduate learners. The authors of this review conclude that teaching and learning evidence-based practice should be moved from the classroom to clinical practice. This further supports the need for the entire organisation to focus on learning and suggests an organisational shift is required to sustain a culture of enquiry and explicit application of evidence (see Section 7.1.2).

The quality of teaching and learning cannot be viewed as an activity isolated from the rest of the organisation.[4] The environment will determine the extent to which the learner is able to engage with evidence-based practice. A climate of continually changing organisational structures cannot be ignored if teaching and learning are to contribute to solutions and reduce fragmentation. If these organisational issues are ignored, there is a danger that learning will be bolted on to existing activities and lack any educational coherence.

Although any health service will undergo numerous system changes, it is wise to remember that management, although supported by systems, is a human activity, and it is the competence of individuals within any system that is a major determinant of system performance.

References

1. Cordingly, P. (2004) *Teachers using evidence: using what we know about teaching and learning to reconceptualise evidence based practice.* In: Thomas, G. and Pring, R. (eds) *Evidence Based Practice in Education.* Open University Press, New York, pp. 77–87.
2. Mennin Stewart, P. (2003) *Position paper on problem based learning.* Educ. Health 16: 98–113.
3. Coomarasamy, A. and Khan, K.S. (2004) *What is the evidence that postgraduate teaching in evidence based medicine changes anything? A systematic review.* Br. Med. J. 329: 1017–19.
4. Ramsden, P. (2003) *Learning to Teach in Higher Education.* 2nd edn. RoutledgeFalmer, London.

9.2 Approaches to learning

A study of what is known as 'approaches to learning' can:

- help to identify factors that can facilitate the understanding and application of knowledge
- provide a way of identifying how learning can be supported in different situations.

There is evidence that learners take different approaches to learning depending on how they perceive their learning environment.[1]

A deep, surface or strategic approach to learning describes the relationship between the learner and the learning task.[2,3] The critical variation in approaches to learning is between a 'surface' approach, characterised by the student intending to fulfil a set of requirements without engaging with the material or the learning process, and a 'deep' approach, characterised by the learner being intent on making personal meaning of subject matter. It is important to be aware that students vary their approach according to their perceptions. For example, if a student, practitioner, healthcare manager or policy-maker perceives their workload to be overwhelming, they are likely to take a surface approach to learning.[1,2]

Students' prior experience of learning may also determine their approach to learning. A learner who has previously adopted a surface approach to learning may find it difficult to develop a more complete conceptual understanding. This can occur when the previous emphasis has been on learning a lot of facts, and may inhibit a critical approach and active learning.

9.2.1 Problem-based learning

Problem-based learning (PBL) is an educational strategy in which learning is organised around problems, with an emphasis on integrating knowledge and using cognitive skills to deepen understanding. Problem-based learning encourages active learning and independent study with a focus on lifelong learning skills. As an approach to learning, problem-based learning is implemented in various forms, often being modified to suit local policy, but the key focus is always on a problem rather than on a discipline.

The starting point when undertaking problem-based learning is problems of immediate interest that require learners to explore prior knowledge and to formulate questions.[4,5] By seeking the active engagement of the learner through contextualising and situating knowledge in real work activity, reflective learning is encouraged, as students are asked to interpret and understand cases or situations. The process of turning problems into questions facilitates the application of evidence and helps the learner to adopt a position towards the problem with which they have been presented in relation to both their prior experience and the new knowledge they have retrieved.[6] Developing this independence of enquiry can help learners understand and manage the ambiguities that exist in professional life, and build leadership skills through the development of learning strategies for critical enquiry in order to deal with different sources of information and interpretations of the evidence.[7]

The method of problem-based learning originated at McMaster University Medical School in Canada in the mid-1960s, and has been adopted and adapted by many schools world-wide. Problem-based learning cuts across disciplines by integrating learning across subjects. Problem-based learning starts with a problem or brief case presentation that is ill defined in order to prompt students to identify the questions they need to answer. As students discuss the problem, they generate knowledge within the group. For problem-based learning to be successful:

- realistic problems should be selected
- tutor facilitation should support reflection and cooperation
- sufficient time should be scheduled for independent study
- any assessment should be aligned with the learning issues, problem packages and other teaching sessions.[8,9]

9.2.1.1   Problem-based learning and continuing professional development

Problem-based learning can be used as a technique to motivate active and deep learning by engaging the learner with the problem. A high degree of engagement in which students search for understanding and meaning can help promote intellectual growth,[10] which is essential for meaningful continuing professional development. This level of 'realisation' is achieved by students interacting with the domains of knowledge for the discipline.[11] Thinking beyond a problem, and the accompanying set of solutions, to the application of the solutions can result in an analysis of the respective strengths and weaknesses of each solution for different contexts. This level of engagement with learning generates an environment that supports a deep approach to learning. Problem-based learning, by encouraging learners to identify and use information from a wide range of sources to solve a problem, requires students to make an effort to integrate information. As a result, problem-based learning is more likely to result in deep learning and facilitate long-term retention.[3,12]

9.2.2   Self-directed and reflective learning

Reflective learning is a deliberative process of interpreting and understanding cases or situations[6] and therefore can facilitate the application of evidence. This is sometimes referred to as reflective observation, in which the learner evaluates their own work critically by reflecting on the range and depth of evidence used to enhance professional development.

John Dewey, the American philosopher and psychologist, emphasised learning as a dialectic process, integrating experiences and concepts, observations and action. He was one of the first proponents to advocate that education should engage with experience by focusing on problem-solving and critical analysis.

However, Dewey recognised that a major educational problem was the 'postponement of immediate action' in order to allow 'observation and judgment to intervene'.[13]

9.2.2.1 Meeting appraised learning needs

What people want they do not need.
What people need they do not want.

Traditional knowledge proved

The evidence is accumulating, and has been summarised in a systematic review,[14] that self-directed learning has its limitations as well as its strengths. The team at the University of Toronto with a particular interest in continuing professional development has carried out a review of the literature relating to the identification of learning needs, both self-directed and directed during the process of appraisal. The following conclusions can be drawn from the systematic review:

- the learning priorities identified by the individual do not relate to the weaknesses in their clinical practice
- those people whose clinical practice is worst are also worst at identifying their learning needs
- people who are most confident about the identification of their learning needs are no more accurate at identification than those who are not.

From this evidence, it is apparent that self-directed learning cannot be relied on as a sole means of identifying the learning needs of individuals. It is likely that these findings will be applicable to people who manage or pay for healthcare, and to public health practitioners, as well as to clinicians.

In the light of this evidence, it is essential that all individuals undergo external appraisal of their performance, and the learning implications that flow from a study of their performance. This has been introduced in some healthcare systems, for example, the UK National Health Service, but needs to become a standard feature in all healthcare systems.

9.2.3   e-Learning

e-Learning provides an alternative way for learners to gain knowledge, and virtual-learning communities may provide high-quality learning environments. However, in the light of experience, the initial enthusiasm for, and wholesale move towards, e-learning has been tempered by the recognition that the inclusion of some face-to-face contact facilitates learning. Face-to-face sessions provide individualised support and help the learner to develop ways in which they can engage with online resources, thereby ensuring that accessing information becomes more than just a simple retrieval exercise. This blended approach[15] utilises the advantages of online learning by providing students with access to a wide range of information to appraise critically, and an online forum that can facilitate communication and collaboration through peer learning. It can also provide a means for enhancing the learners' interaction with content through simulated exercises, which students can undertake at their own pace. The barriers to a successful online learning experience include:

- a low level of interaction
- inadequate induction
- a seemingly haphazard delivery of online resources, which do not appear to be integrated with the curriculum.

9.2.4   Learning by doing

Formal training has certain connotations for people: seminar rooms, overhead projectors, one person being active, many people being passive. In fact, formal training in which only one person is active while the learners are passive is relatively ineffective. Although some formal training is necessary, for example, to introduce people to critical appraisal, the best way to learn is to learn by doing. Learning by doing involves using skills on the job to face practical decisions and then reflect upon the theory and/or training received. The 'learning by doing' cycle is shown in Fig. 9.1.

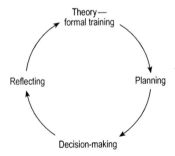

Fig. 9.1
The learning-by-doing cycle

9.2.4.1 Informatics support for staff who are learning by doing

Often, the need for evidence arises in meetings or on a ward round, during a debate, discussion or difference of opinion. However, in these situations, it is almost always impossible to resolve the matter by going to the library to carry out a search, appraising the articles found, and assembling the evidence on which a decision could be based. Although this strategy may sometimes be necessary, particularly when clinicians are making decisions in a life-or-death situation, a more realistic scenario is for staff to have ready access to a computer – at a clinical work station, or in a meeting – at which a search could be performed. At present, this is not a common occurrence in many countries. New developments in technology, such as the personal digital assistant (PDA), are facilitating the uptake of such a strategy.

9.2.4.2 Support for staff learning by doing: the educational prescription

As certain developments in informatics are not widely available at present, it is necessary to find viable alternatives. Questions raised during debate, discussion or differences of opinion in meetings or on the ward round can be used as a starting point to drive the learning process. In the absence of a mechanism to capture such questions, and monitor progress toward finding the answers, it is more than likely that these opportunities to learn will be lost due to pressure of work.

One low-technology alternative that can be used to capture questions that arise during learning by doing is the educational prescription (Fig. 9.2). Educational prescriptions were originally devised by Dave Sackett and co-workers at the Centre for Evidence-Based Medicine, Oxford, in order to keep track of a learner's progress from the formulation of an appropriate (or 'right') question about a patient's needs to a clinically useful answer.[16] The use of an educational prescription helps both learners and teachers in five ways:

1. it specifies the clinical problem that generated the questions
2. it states the question in all of its key elements
3. it specifies who is responsible for answering it
4. it provides a reminder of the deadline pertinent to answering the question (taking into account the urgency

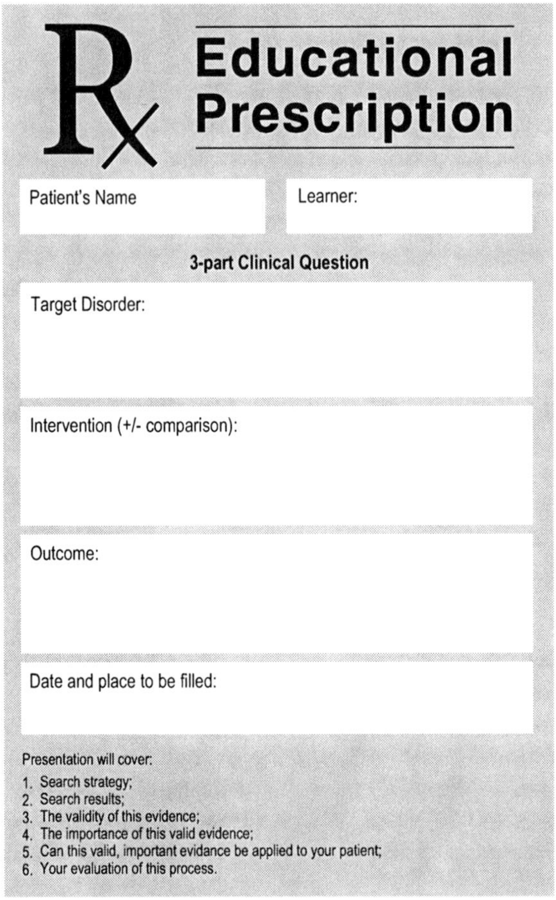

R x **Educational Prescription**

Patient's Name	Learner:

3-part Clinical Question

Target Disorder:

Intervention (+/- comparison):

Outcome:

Date and place to be filled:

Presentation will cover:
1. Search strategy;
2. Search results;
3. The validity of this evidence;
4. The importance of this valid evidence;
5. Can this valid, important evidance be applied to your patient;
6. Your evaluation of this process.

Fig. 9.2
Proforma for an educational prescription (Source: Straus et al.[16])

of the clinical problem from which the question was generated)

5. it furnishes an aide-mémoire of the steps necessary for searching, critically appraising, and relating the answer back to the patient.

One outcome of the educational prescription was the PECO(T)/PICO(T) formulation, described in Section 9.4.1.

References

1. Prosser, M. and Trigwell, K. (1999) *Understanding Learning and Teaching.* Society for Research into Higher Education and Open University Press: The Experience in Higher Education, Buckingham.
2. Ramsden, P. (2003) *Learning to Teach in Higher Education.* 2nd edn. RoutledgeFalmer, London.

3. Biggs, J. (1993) *What do inventories of students' learning processes really measure? A theoretical review and clarification.* Br. J. Educ. Psychol. 63: 3–19.

4. Davies, P. (2005) *Approaches to evidence based teaching.* Med. Teach. 22: 14–21.

5. Mennin Stewart, P. (2003) *Position paper on problem based learning.* Educ. Health 16: 98–113.

6. Eraut, M. (1994) *Theories of professional expertise.* In: Eraut, M. (ed.) *Developing Professional Knowledge and Competence.* Falmer Press, London, pp. 123–57.

7. Savin-Baden, M. (2000) *Problem-based Learning in Higher Education: Untold Stories.* The Society for Reasearch into Higher Education and Open University Press, Buckingham.

8. Biggs, J. (1996) *Enhancing teaching through constructive alignment.* Higher Education 32: 347–64.

9. Hendry, G.D., Frommer, M. and Walker, R.A. (1999) *Constructivism and problem based learning.* Journal of Further and Higher Education 23: 359–71.

10. McLean, M. (2006) *Pedagogy and the University.* Continuum, London.

11. Perry, W.G. (2006) *Different worlds in the same classroom.* In Ramsden, P. (ed.) *Improving Learning: New Perspectives.* Kogan Page, London, p. 158.

12. Dent, J.A. and Harden, R.M. (2005) *A Practical Guide for Medical Teachers.* Churchill Livingstone, Edinburgh.

13. Dewey, J. (1938) *Experience and Education.* Collier Books, New York.

14. Davis, D.A., Mazmanian, P.E., Fordis, M. et al. (2006) *Accuracy of physician self-assessment compared with observed measures of competence: a systematic review.* JAMA 296: 1094–102.

15. Donnelly, R. (2004) *Investigating the effectiveness of teaching 'on line learning' in a problem based learning on-line environment.* In: Savin Baden, M. and Wilkie, K. (eds) *Challenging Research in Problem Based Learning.* Society for Research into Higher Education and Open University Press, New York, pp. 50–64.

16. Straus, S.E., Richardson, W.S., Glasziou, P. et al. (2005) *Evidence-based Medicine: How to Practice and Teach EBM,* 3rd edn. Churchill Livingstone, Edinburgh.

9.3 Teaching and learning evidence-based practice

Teaching and learning evidence-based practice integrates the principles of problem-based and reflective learning by using questions and problems arising from work to engage the learner actively. Over time, as the evidence-based practitioner becomes competent in applying the skills of evidence-based practice, it becomes easier to deal with uncertainty while at the same time making a commitment to an explicit interpretation of the evidence.

However, a high level of competence does not of itself guarantee good performance; performance is also directly related to an individual's motivation and inversely related to the barriers that individual has to overcome:

$$P = \frac{M \times C}{B}$$

Table 9.1 Paradigms in learning

Old	New
Knowledge-based	Problem-based
Knowing what one should know	Knowing what one does not know
Intuition very powerful	Ability to generate and refine a question, and to search for, appraise and act on the evidence to find the answer
Learning from received wisdom	Ability to question received wisdom
Learning almost 'complete' at end of formal training – only a finite amount of knowledge to be absorbed	Life-long learning – there is always new knowledge to be absorbed
Learning dominated by knowledge from experience	Learning involves complementing experience with knowledge from research

where:

P=performance

C=competence

M=motivation

B=barriers

In order to practise an evidence-based approach, individuals need to develop their competence in the core skills of evidence management – searching, appraisal and storage. The development of these skills requires training, but with the advent of an evidence-based approach there has evolved a new paradigm in learning (Table 9.1) in which some of the methods of conventional training, in which learners are passive, are eschewed.

9.4 The five steps to evidence-based practice

The key skills for evidence-based practice are described in the following five steps:[1]

1. converting a problem or 'information need' into an answerable question
2. searching for and retrieving the best sources of evidence to answer the question
3. critically appraising the evidence for validity (closeness to truth), impact (size of the effect) and applicability (usefulness)
4. integrating and applying the best evidence with patient, client or population values as appropriate, and with professional judgement and costs; and applying the evidence to practice
5. evaluating and reflecting on the practice and learning of evidence-based practice.

9.4.1   Asking the right question

Real education begins with a question in the life of the learner.
Leo Tolstoy

The key to learning and teaching evidence-based practice
is recognising opportunities for asking questions and
formulating these into a question that can be answered,
and then searching, appraising and applying the evidence
to the question.[2] This helps to ensure relevance and equips
users with a framework that can be easily employed in
decision-making, in addition to providing a mechanism for
making decisions under conditions of uncertainty. Although
this statement might appear to be self-evident, many
people hasten to find the evidence and appraise it *before*
defining precisely the question they wish to answer. Careful
consideration of the question that needs answering is the
foundation for evidence-based decision-making.

Recognising a healthcare problem is relatively easy;
translating the problem into an answerable question is
not always straightforward. This may be because the
healthcare problem is broad, for example, it is concerned
with a programme, policy or the organisational structure of
a healthcare facility, or it may require general information
about a health condition.

Broad questions encompass the general aspect of a topic
and include a who, what, when, where, how or why type of
question.[1] However, broad questions may provide a context
for a narrow, more focused question. Narrow questions
are inevitably more specific, for example, enquiring about
a particular intervention, risk factor, test, aetiology or
phenomenon.

A well-constructed question, whether broad or narrow,
will usually have four parts:[3]

- the patient or population (P)
- the intervention (I) or exposure (E)
- the comparison intervention (C)
- the outcome (O), including the time at which it was
  measured (T).

The acronym PICO or PECO (PICOT or PECOT if a
timeline is included) is used to describe this structure. The
PECO(T)/PICO(T) formulation for questions provides
precision and focus, and can be used to unpick the elements
of a healthcare problem such that an answerable question
can be formulated. It can also be used to strengthen
decision-making because a poorly focused question can lead

to unclear decisions. If time (T) is used as an extra searching category, it should be noted that it will restrict the search, and it is difficult to search for.

An example of a broad problem is exploring the impact of a quality improvement programme. Using the PECO(T)/PICO(T) formulation, this problem can be broken down into the specific elements of the programme in such a way that a series of answerable questions can be constructed. Quality improvement includes a range of activities, for example, audit, benchmarking, guidelines, utilisation review and quality indicators. Defining these different activities provides a key to formulating a series of answerable questions. As an alternative, it may be more helpful to focus on the management of a particular patient group, such as patients with a hip fracture who have a high risk of thrombo-embolic complications following surgical management.[4]

Imposing too many limits on a question may limit the generalisability of the answer, that is, the extent to which the answer can be extrapolated to the setting in which the practitioner is working. A more useful approach to a broad problem is to develop a series of related questions. In the above example, this took the form of identifying the separate elements of a quality improvement programme. Alternatively, the healthcare problem may relate to the organisation and delivery of services, for example, case management or discharge planning. In the case of discharge planning, defining what is and is not discharge planning is not immediately obvious, but breaking down the possible components into a series of discrete interventions can help articulate the policy that is being examined. For example, pre-admission assessment, case-finding on admission, in-patient assessment and preparation of a discharge plan based on individual patient needs, pre-discharge home visits, implementation, and monitoring.[5]

9.4.1.1 Competencies

Everyone who makes decisions about groups of patients or populations should be able to identify the clinical question they are seeking to answer, for example, using the PECO(T)/PICO(T) formulation.

9.4.2 Searching for evidence

The issues about which decisions must be made usually arise without warning or at inconvenient times. In an ideal world, a manager would request a search for evidence from a librarian; however, in reality, managers often have to find the evidence for themselves.

Using a structured question following the PECO(T)/ PICO(T) formulation will provide precision and focus to the search terms you use to identify evidence from the electronic databases, such as Medline (or PubMed), EMBASE, and CINAHL (see Section 9.7 for a list of resources).

If time (T) is used as an extra searching category, not only will it restrict the search but also it is difficult to search for. Time factors, however, might be useful when a clinician is considering an individual patient.

When defining the intervention, it is possible to list the different synonyms relating to the intervention and identify which are Medical Subject Headings (MeSH) and which are free text terms. Using the example of quality assurance, the synonyms will include:

- Utilisation Review/
- Program Evaluation/
- Guidelines/
- Benchmarking/
- Total Quality Management/
- Medical Audit/
- Management Audit/
- Quality Indicators, Health Care/
- "audit" (text word)
- "guideline" (text word).

Combining these terms with Boolean operators will create a more powerful search strategy. The term 'AND' is used to combine words with different meanings where both words will appear in the same article, for example 'children AND mental health'; 'AND' will narrow the search. The term 'OR' is used to broaden a search and to combine words with the same or similar meaning, for example 'total quality management OR audit'.

Sources of high-quality evidence are shown in Margin Note 9.1.

9.4.2.1 Retrieval

My storage system? I've got a foot and a half of papers torn out of the BMJ in a pile on my dining-room table.
A physician, 2 years after graduation

Storing paper is easy, at least for the short term. However, the young doctor quoted above could have storage

Margin Note 9.1
Sources of high-quality evidence

- TRIP database
  http://www.tripdatabase.com/
- National Library for Health
  http://www.library.nhs.uk/
- Cochrane Library
  http://www.cochrane.org/

Aphorisms on storage and retrieval

Filing cabinets will always be full to capacity.

A photocopier is a machine for creating storage problems.

Only highly obsessional healthcare professionals can store paper in a system that will enable them to find what they need when they need it by themselves.

One of the few ways in which computers have made life easier for healthcare professionals is the development of bibliographic management software.

problems in 20 years' time if his rate of acquisition continues at 9 inches (22.86 cm) per year. It is highly likely that he could maintain a storage system of three four-drawer filing cabinets, filing papers alphabetically by surname of the first author, for example. The drawback with such a system, however, is the difficulty of retrieval unless the user has a good memory or the author of the paper has a memorable name. Retrieval from an alphabetically or chronologically ordered paper storage system is compounded when the user wants to retrieve all the papers on a particular subject. Although it is possible to store papers or reference cards by disease grouping, concepts or patient groups, it is impossible to combine any of these, e.g. to retrieve all the papers describing trials of coronary heart disease prevention on one occasion and all the papers investigating coronary heart disease in women on another. Only computer-based storage systems have the potential to store useful information in a form that will allow retrieval from several different 'entry' points.

9.4.2.2 Competencies

Everyone who makes decisions about groups of patients or populations should be able:

1. to define and identify the sources of evidence appropriate to a particular decision that must be made
2. to construct simple search strategies in Medline, using Boolean operators ('AND', 'OR') for:

   (a) the following types of healthcare intervention:
   - therapy
   - test
   - screening programme
   - health policy or policy-making

   (b) the following service characteristics:
   - effectiveness
   - safety
   - acceptability
   - cost-effectiveness
   - quality
   - appropriateness.

Ideally, a manager should be able to carry out a search without the help of a librarian, but obtaining assistance and feedback from a librarian is encouraged.

3. to download the citations retrieved from a search into bibliographic management software such as Reference Manager or Endnote
4. to use bibliographic management software in the following ways:
    - to enter references and abstracts using self-selected keywords
    - to search for references
    - to download sets of references from an electronic database.

As there are several different types of bibliographic management software available and healthcare professionals are highly 'mobile', it is important that librarians are able to support staff who use any of the common bibliographic management software packages, irrespective of that used in the library. After a short period of induction training, anyone who is intelligent enough to be a decision-maker in a health service should be able to use bibliographic management software.

9.4.3   Appraising evidence

Appraisal is the explicit assessment of evidence for:

- validity, i.e. closeness to the truth
- usefulness, i.e. applicability.

The assessment process is a series of steps to determine:

- if the evidence from research is biased
- the type of bias present
- in what way the bias undermines the validity of the evidence.

In addition, appraisal involves an assessment of the usefulness of that evidence when applying it in practice.

Librarians are being trained to appraise evidence as well as to search for it, and to teach both skills. At present, the main source of appraisal skills when making decisions about groups of patients or populations is in departments of public health. However, all those who make decisions about populations or groups of patients must have the skills to appraise research articles on healthcare, that is, to take a scientific approach to health service management.

9.4.3.1 The GATE frame

The GATE frame is: 'a visual framework that illustrates the generic design of all epidemiological studies'.[6]

(GATE stands for a Graphic Appraisal Tool for Epidemiological Studies.) Jackson and colleagues have developed the GATE frame to teach critical appraisal skills that will enable users not only to answer individual appraisal questions but also to assess overall study quality. The GATE frame is a simple diagram (Fig. 9.3) that helps the user to organise information and re-frame a problem. Thus, it is possible to superimpose the PECO(T)/PICO(T) formulation onto the GATE frame to guide the user to organise the elements of a structured question, which can then be used to structure a search of electronic databases for evidence. The GATE frame can also be used to identify and describe the different study designs.

In the GATE frame there is:

- a triangle labelled P, which represents the population studied or participants
- a circle labelled E or I and C, which represents the exposure or intervention group and the comparison group, respectively
- a square labelled O, which represents outcomes
- a set of two arrows labelled T, which represents time.

This labelling corresponds to the acronym PECOT/PICOT.

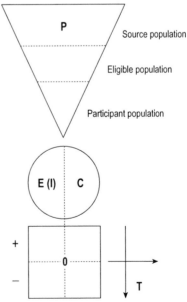

Fig. 9.3
The GATE frame (Source: Jackson et al.[6])

The triangle P is inverted and split into three overlapping levels:

- the source population, from which participants were selected, represented by the whole triangle
- the lower two levels marked in the triangle represent the eligible population, that is, participants who met the eligibility criteria
- the lowest level marked in the triangle represents the people who agreed to take part, that is, the study participants. Thus the study participants are funnelled into the exposure.

This structure enables a judgement to be made about how representative the study population is.

The circle is divided in two to represent:

- the exposure group (E), often referred to as the intervention group (I) in a trial
- the comparison group (C) who receive a placebo, usual care or another comparator.

The square labelled O is usually divided into four using the 2 × 2 table from epidemiological studies representing two exposures (either E and C or I and C) and two outcomes (yes and no). The top two squares represent participants from E or I and C who experienced the specified study outcome. The bottom two squares represent the participants from E or I and C who did not experience the specified study outcome. In the full form of the GATE frame, it is possible for the user to identify whether the measurement of outcomes was blinded or subjective.

The set of two arrows represents time, the horizontal arrow being used for study outcomes at one point in time (prevalence of cross-sectional measures) and the vertical arrow being used for outcomes measured over a period of time (incidence or longitudinal measures).

The GATE frame allows users to become familiar with some of the core epidemiological concepts that underpin evidence-based practice, and it helps to combine intuitive and quantitative analysis that facilitates effective reasoning.[7]

9.4.3.2 Competencies

Everyone who makes decisions about groups of patients or populations should be able to appraise:

1. the evidence presented in a review article on the following types of intervention:
   - a therapy (see Section 3.2.3)

- a test (see Section 3.3.3)
- a screening programme (see Section 3.4.3)
- a health policy (see Section 3.5.3)
2. the quality of the following research methodologies:
   - systematic review (see Section 5.3.3)
   - RCT (see Section 5.4.3)
   - case-control study (see Section 5.5.3)
   - cohort study (see Section 5.6.3)
   - controlled before and after studies (see Section 5.7.3)
   - interrupted time series (see Section 5.8.3)
   - survey (see Section 5.9.3)
   - qualitative research (see Section 5.10.3)
   - decision analysis (Section 5.11.3).

Margin Note 9.3
Courses in critical appraisal

In the UK, courses in critical appraisal are organised by several organisations:

- Centre for Evidence-Based Medicine (CEBM) http://www.cebm.net/
- Public Health Resource Unit (PHRU) Critical Appraisal Skills Programme (CASP) and Evidence-Based Practice http://www.phru.nhs.uk/casp/casp.htm

In New Zealand, courses in critical appraisal are organised by EPIQ – Effective Practice, Informatics & Quality Improvement. Available online at: http://www.health.auckland.ac.nz/populatioon-health/epidemiology-iostats/epiq.index.html

The skills of appraisal should be developed during the basic training of all healthcare professionals. At present, these skills are virtually ignored; very few decision-makers have been taught how to be systematic in their appraisal of a report or a research project. Indeed, a critical appraisal skills programme is necessary to the development of any healthcare organisation (Margin Note 9.3).

9.4.4 Integrating and applying the evidence

Decisions on if and how to integrate evidence into practice can be complex, as the realities of the workplace, organisational climate and health systems have to be considered. Often the population or setting will differ from that reported in the primary research or systematic review, making the transfer of results less than straightforward. However, rather than starting off from a position of 'the evidence cannot be applied', it is more helpful to list the important differences and ask if any of these differences undermine the validity of the results across different settings and populations. The next stage is to identify barriers and constraints that may limit the application of evidence (see Sections 6.1.5 and 6.4.1, and Box 6.3).

It is vital to appraise the evidence found in the context of local circumstances: a decision-maker must consider not only the applicability of the findings to a particular population, but also the local factors that may affect the outcomes of applying those findings.

9.4.4.1 Competencies

Everyone who makes decisions about groups of patients or populations should be able to:

1. assess the population outcomes of an intervention against the following criteria:
   - acceptability (see Section 6.6.1.1)
   - equity (see Section 6.3)
   - effectiveness (see Section 6.4)
   - safety (see Section 6.5)
   - patient satisfaction and patients' experience of care (see Section 6.6)
   - cost-effectiveness (see Section 6.7)
   - quality (see Section 6.8)
   - appropriateness (see Section 6.9)

2. assess the population outcomes of an intervention against the following biological and cultural factors:
   - variations in settings
   - variation in compliance
   - variation in baseline risk.

3. evaluate and reflect on their performance and practice of evidence-based healthcare.

References

1. Straus, S.E., Richardson, W.D., Glasziou, P. et al. (2005) *Evidence Based Medicine: how to Practice and Teach EBM*, 3rd edn. Churchill Livingstone, Edinburgh.
2. Sackett, D.L., Rosenberg, W.M., Gray, J.A. et al. (1996) *Evidence based medicine: what it is and what it isn't*. Br. Med. J. 312: 71–2.
3. Richardson, W.S., Wilson, M.C., Nishikawa, J. et al. (1995) *The well-built clinical question: a key to evidence-based decisions*. ACP J. Club 123; A12–13.
4. Handoll, H.H.G., Farrar, M.J., McBirnie, J. et al. (2007) *Heparin, low molecular weight heparin and physical methods for preventing deep vein thrombosis and pulmonary embolsim following surgery for hip fractures.* Cochrane Database of Systematic Reviews 2007, Issue 1. Abstract available online at: http://www.cochrane.org/reviews/en/ab000305.html
5. Shepperd, S., Parkes, J., McClaren, J. et al. (2007) *Discharge planning from hospital to home*. Cochrane Database of Systematic Reviews 2007, Issue 1. Abstract available at: http://www.cochrane.org/reviews/en/ab000313.html
6. Jackson, R., Ameratunga, S., Broad, J. et al. (2006) *The GATE frame: critical appraisal with pictures*. Evid. Based Med. 11: 35–8.
7. Schon, D. (1986) *Educating the Reflective Practitioner*. Jossey-Bass, San Francisco.

9.5   Developing capacity as well as skills

A focus on developing skills is better than a focus on developing knowledge, because there are many examples of people who have knowledge but lack skill. It is, however, important to recognise that some people have a greater capacity for learning than others. Managers or public health professionals have certain characteristics that can probably be enhanced by offering training; however, the outcome of professional development is a function not only of the effectiveness of the training provided but also of the capacity of the individual to learn.

Leadership is much talked about, and many consultants are trainers who have made the leap from 'developing leadership skills'. Although it would be unwise to cling to the old adage 'Leaders are born and not made', it is important to appreciate that some people have a greater capacity for leadership than others. The same probably applies to evidence-based decision-making skills. Some people may be less able to tolerate uncertainty than others. Some people find it more difficult than others to accept that their opinion, based on experience, should be complemented by evidence, or that when a young colleague describes evidence that does not conform to their opinions, the colleague is simply stating propositions and not questioning their bureaucratic authority or their credibility.

The converse is that some people have a much greater capacity for both learning and teaching than others, and these people need to be identified and supported, not only by the type of simple techniques described in this book but also by the opportunity to carry out research in evidence-based decision-making as part of a programme of study for a higher degree.

9.6 Case-studies of applying evidence-based practice skills

The following learning examples are from students who graduated from the MSc programme in Evidence-Based Health Care at Oxford University. This is a modular course that encourages students to integrate the skills of finding and appraising evidence by formulating and exploring a healthcare question that has arisen at their workplace. If there is insufficient evidence, students learn the practices and principles of research design to generate new evidence. The students come from a range of healthcare backgrounds, which reflects the variety of problems they identify from their workplace. During the MSc course, students examine these problems by converting them into an answerable question, identifying and utilising evidence to answer the question, and in some cases generating evidence from primary research.

9.6.1   Diagnosis

An emergency room physician was unsure about the accuracy of measuring ischaemia-modified albumin (IMA), in addition to cardiac troponin, in patients presenting to the emergency department with chest pain. This was a new test being introduced as a means of identifying low-risk patients with chest pain and could potentially reduce the time these patients spent in emergency departments.

A systematic search of the literature revealed little evidence for the accuracy of IMA with troponin, compared with the current gold standard of delayed measurement of cardiac troponin 8 hours after the onset of pain. Therefore, a prospective, observational, two-centre research study was designed and implemented, into which 399 patients with features of possible ischaemic cardiac chest pain and a normal electrocardiogram were recruited. The results of the study showed that measuring IMA at presentation was not an effective method of assessing risk in this patient population. The sensitivity of the test was 97.6% (95% confidence interval (CI) 87.4 to 99.9), the specificity was 13.6% (95% CI 9.5 to 18.7) and negative predictive value 97% (95% CI 84.2 to 99.9). Further analysis showed that the cut-off level used did not alter the accuracy of the test.[1]

Specificity indicates how good the test is at identifying people who do not have the disease. The low specificity of 13.6% reported in this research study meant that there were many false-positive results, which limits the use of the test because these patients would go on to have further investigation, even though they did not have the condition. Using the new test, only 32 out of a total 235 people who tested negative were classified as not having the disease. The negative predictive value refers to the proportion of people with a negative test who are free of the condition being investigated (see Section 3.3.1.2).

9.6.2   Decision analysis

9.6.2.1 Introduction

The need to analyse decisions is now accepted widely, and the science of decision analysis is developing.[2] Indeed, the recognition of the way in which clinicians use heuristics and what is known as bounded rationality to complete the work demanded of them is now well described both in theoretical[3] and practical terms.[4]

Decision analysis provides a structure for the consideration of how an action or incident will lead to an outcome. It is a technique that exposes assumptions for discussion and requires a critical reading of research. A premise of decision analysis is that the success of a desired outcome is uncertain and that the decision-maker has specific preferences for each individual outcome. This is based on the assumption that both the probability of each outcome and its perceived benefit (i.e. utility) to the decision-maker are measurable,[2] while being explicit about the level of uncertainty surrounding the different options. A decision tree is a graphic representation of the alternative strategies for intervention or decision-taking and the possible outcomes associated with each (see, for example, Fig. 5.7). In Fig. 9.4, the decision tree shows the evidence of probabilities for a situation in which a doctor has suffered a needlestick injury while treating a patient with a heroin overdose.

9.6.2.2 Case-study

A dentist was concerned by the number of adults with large dental restoration who complained of toothache. He looked at the evidence for the different management options, which included:

- saving the tooth using root canal therapy, post and core build-up (P&C), crown lengthening periodontal surgery and convention crown restoration (CC)

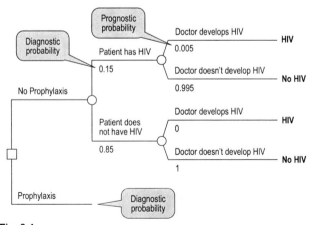

Fig. 9.4
A decision tree showing the evidence of probabilities when a doctor suffers a needlestick injury while treating a patient with a heroin overdose (With permission from Paul Glasziou)

- extracting the tooth and replacing it with a partial denture, a conventional dental bridge or a single tooth implant.

Recognising the role of the patient in decision-making, he collected data on the way patients value the different treatment options and used this data to complete a decision analysis.

The amount of out-of-pocket expense influenced the decisions people made. The expected utility value for a 5-year prosthetic survival was highest for a conventional dental bridge in the case of an abscessed mandibular molar, and highest for a single-tooth implant if the maxillary incisor, which is more visible, was affected. This remained constant if the success of the root canal therapy and the risk of damage to the adjacent tooth were varied.[5]

9.6.3   Treatment

A doctor training as an ophthalmologist observed that eye patches are often recommended for treating the common eye problem of corneal abrasion despite a lack of evidence of effect. He conducted a systematic review to determine if patching an eye following a corneal abrasion improves healing or reduces pain. From a systematic search of the published and unpublished literature, he identified 11 trials in which patching the eye was compared with no patch for treating a simple corneal abrasion. Data from seven trials were combined, and the results showed that if a patch is used:

- initial healing is at a slower rate
- pain is not reduced
- there is a loss of binocular vision.[6]

References

1. Keating, L., Benger, J., Beetham, R. et al. (2006) *The PRIMA study: presentation ischaemia modified albumin in the emergency department.* Emerg. Med. J. 23: 764–8.
2. Hunink, M., Glasziou, P. et al. (2001) *Decision Making in Health and Medicine. Integrating Evidence and Values.* Cambridge University Press, Cambridge.
3. Gigerenzer, G. and Todd, P.M. (1999) *Simple Heuristics That Make Us Smart.* Oxford University Press, New York.
4. Del Mar, C., Doust, J. and Glasziou, P. (2006) *Clinical Thinking: Evidence, Communication and Decision Making.* BMJ Publishing, London.

5. Balevi, B. and Shepperd, S. (2007) *The Management of an Endodontically Abscessed Tooth: Patient Health State Utility, Decision-tree and Economic Analysis.* BMC Oral Health 7:17 doi: 10.1186/1472-6831-7-17.
6. Turner, A. and Rabiu, M. (2007) *Patching for corneal abrasion.* Cochrane Database of Systematic Reviews 2007, Issue 1. Abstract available online at: http://www.cochrane.org/reviews/en/ab004764.html.

9.7   Resources

There are many resources to support the teaching and learning of evidence-based practice, including user guides, checklists, reference books and guidelines to improve the clarity of reporting research.

9.7.1   Resources for critical appraisal

- The Evidence-Based Medicine Working Group (2002) *Users' Guides to the Medical Literature: Essentials of Evidence-Based Clinical Practice.* Guyatt, G. and Rennie D. (eds) JAMA & Archives Journals, American Medical Association. Available online at:

    http://pubs.ama-assn.org/misc/usersguides.dtl
    http://www.cche.net/usersguides/why.asp

- Users' Guides Interactive (UGI) for individuals with a personal subscription to JAMA and/or Archives Journals or who register their Users' Guides textbooks, available online at:

    http://www.usersguides.org/

- CASP appraisal checklists, available online at:

    http://www.phru.nhs.uk/casp/critical_appraisal_tools.htm

- Resources from the Centre of Evidence-Based Medicine, Oxford, UK, available online at:

    http://www.cebm.net

9.7.2   Guidelines to improve the standard of reporting published research

- The CONSORT Statement is aimed at improving the quality of reports of randomised controlled trials. Available online at:

    http://www.consort-statement.org/Statement/revisedstatement.htm

- The STARD statement is aimed at improving the accuracy of reporting studies of diagnostic accuracy. Available online at:

  http://www.consort-statement.org/
  stardstatement.htm

- The TREND statement is aimed at improving the reporting of non-randomised evaluations of behavioural and public health interventions. Available online at:

  http://www.trend-statement.org/asp/documents/
  statements/AJPH_Mar2004_Trendstatement.pdf

9.7.3 Educational resources

- The Sheffield Centre for Health Related Research in the UK (ScHARR) provides an online list of evidence-based practice resources and sites.

  Netting the Evidence: A ScHARR introduction to Evidence Based Practice on the Internet

- The TRIP database in the UK supports evidence-based practice by providing evidence-based answers to clinical questions within a clinically relevant time-frame. Available online at:

  http://www.tripdatabase.com/index.html

- Cochrane e-Learning provides short modules, taking just a few minutes' time to complete, including: an Introduction (8 minutes)

  http://www.brainshark.com/wiley/cochrane1

  Tips on Advanced and MESH searching (7 minutes)

  http://www.brainshark.com/wiley/cochrane2

- The Perinatal Education Programme (PEP) is produced and distributed by the Perinatal Education Trust, a non-profit organisation, which aims to improve the care of pregnant women and their newborn infants, especially in poor, rural communities. Available online at:

  http://www.pepcourse.co.za

- Searching PubMed® is a web-based learning programme that will show you how to search PubMed®, the National Library of Medicine's (NLM®) journal literature search system. Available online at:

  http://www.nlm.nih.gov/bsd/pubmed_tutorial/
  m1001.html

- DISCERN provides online tools for information providers and users (including patients, carers and their representatives) to judge the quality of information available to the public on treatments and genetic tests. Each resource is accompanied by a free training resource for self-directed learning. Available online at:

  http://www.discern.org.uk
  http://www.discern-genetics.org.uk

- A practical and interactive workbook that will help to develop practitioners' skills in evidence-based medicine is available, based on workshops developed by Professors Glasziou and Del Mar. The workbook helps users to increase their competencies in:

  - asking clinical questions
  - searching for answers
  - using the answers to make clinical decisions.

  Glasziou, P., Del Mar, C. and Salisbury, J. (2003) *Evidence-based Medicine Workbook*. BMJ Publishing, London.

- EBM Teaching Tips Online is a companion resource to Users' Guides Interactive for those interested in teaching or learning about evidence-based practice. Available online at:

  http://meta.cche.net/clint/hirex.asp?
  FOLDER=1414@scriptshirex&HEAD=SCRIPTS

Gentle Reader,

Empathise with the late Stephen Jay Gould.

In July 1982, I learned that I was suffering from abdominal mesothelioma, a rare and serious cancer usually associated with exposure to asbestos. When I revived after surgery, I asked my first question of my doctor and chemotherapist: 'What is the best technical literature about mesothelioma?'. She replied, with a touch of diplomacy (the only departure she has ever made from direct frankness), that the medical literature contained nothing really worth reading.

Of course, trying to keep an intellectual away from literature works about as well as recommending chastity to Homo sapiens, *the sexiest primate of all. As soon as I could walk, I made a beeline for Harvard's Countway medical library and punched* mesothelioma *into the computer's graphic search program. An hour later, surrounded by the latest literature on abdominal mesothelioma, I realised with a gulp why my doctor had offered that humane advice. The literature couldn't have been more brutally clear: mesothelioma is incurable, with a median mortality of only 8 months after discovery. I sat stunned for about 15 minutes, then smiled and said to myself: so that's why they didn't give me anything to read.*

Then my mind started to work again, thank goodness.

The problem may be briefly stated: what does 'median mortality of 8 months' signify in our vernacular? I suspect that most people, without training in statistics, would read such a statement as 'I will probably be dead in 8 months' – the very conclusion that must be avoided, both because this formulation is false and because attitude matters so much.'

Stephen Jay Gould, 'The median isn't the message' in Adam's Navel, 1995

Commentary

Stephen Jay Gould, world-class palaeontologist, baseball fan and beautiful writer, was not perhaps the average patient, but neither should his experience, attitude and skills be disregarded. As the 21st century progresses, patients will become more literate, better organised and better educated, and many of them will be better at finding, but not necessarily appraising, knowledge using the World Wide Web. The relationship between clinician and patient will continue to evolve, and in the future clinicians should be prepared to encounter more patients like Stephen Jay Gould.

Coda

After an experimental treatment of radiation, chemotherapy and surgery, Gould lived for almost another 20 years after his initial diagnosis.[1]

Reference

1. http://en.wikipedia.org/wiki/Stephen-Jay-Gould

Evidence-based clinical practice

Every year, for every million population receiving health services, many decisions are made, including:

- hundreds of resource allocation decisions
- thousands of managerial decisions
- millions of clinical decisions.

Clinical decisions are of direct and immediate importance to patients. They are also of importance to those who manage or pay for health services because one of the outcomes of clinical decision-making is expenditure on health services. In a system in which resources are finite, changes in the volume and intensity of clinical practice are the major factors driving the increase in healthcare costs that can be controlled,[1] and over which managers can exert considerable influence (see Section 2.5).

In order to exercise this influence, it is essential for those who make decisions about groups of patients or populations to understand how clinicians, in consultation with their patients, make and take decisions.

Reference

1. Eddy, D.M. (1993) *Three battles to watch in the 1990s.* JAMA 270: 520–6.

10.1   Clinical decision-making

There are two main types of clinical decision-making:

- 'faceless'
- face-to-face.

10.1.1   'Faceless' decision-making

'Faceless' decisions are those in which the decision is based on either a specimen taken from, or an image taken of, the patient. Such decisions are the clinician's interpretation of

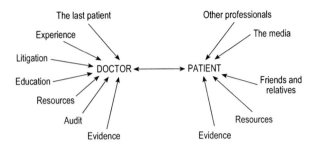

Fig. 10.1
The decision drivers in a clinical consultation

a test result, sample or image; there is no discussion with either the patient or the patient's relatives. As the clinician is a human being and not a mechanical instrument, the decision will be influenced not only by what can be seen or measured but also by other variables (see left-hand side of Fig. 10.1).

Owing to the influence of these other variables, 'faceless' decisions are always characterised by:

- inter-observer variability, in which different clinicians interpret the same image or test results in different ways
- intra-observer variability, in which the same clinician interprets the same image or test results differently on separate occasions.

These characteristics of 'faceless' decision-making can be observed among even the best clinicians; moreover, the level of variability increases as the image or test result approaches 'borderline'. Although certain levels of inter- and intra-observer variability are unacceptable and must be eradicated through clinical audit, inter- and intra-observer variability are inevitable consequences of using human beings as measuring and decision-taking instruments (see Section 3.3.1.3, 'Words').

10.1.2   Face-to-face decision-making

The principal characteristic of face-to-face decision-making is the dialogue between clinician and patient, to which the patient will bring his/her own set of beliefs, attitudes and values. Consequently, there are many more variables involved when face-to-face decisions are made (see right-hand side of Fig. 10.1).

The numerous interactions that take place during face-to-face decision-making may be classified as either non-verbal or verbal communication. Although non-verbal communication is important, the focus in this book is on verbal communication because it is upon words and numbers that evidence-based clinical decisions are made.

10.2   Communicating with patients

You have an exorbitant auditory impediment, replied the doctor, ever conscious of the necessity for maintaining a certain iatric mystique, and fully aware that 'a pea in the ear' was unlikely to earn him any kudos. 'I can remove it with a fishhook and a small hammer; it's the ideal way of overcoming un embarras de petit pois.' He spoke the French words in a mincingly Parisian accent, even though his irony was apparent only to himself.

Louis de Bernières, *Captain Corelli's Mandolin*, 1994

Failures in communication with respect to providing information about illness and treatment are the most frequently cited source of patient dissatisfaction.[1] However, communication with patients is a complicated topic that has many aspects, some of which are contentious, such as the issue of disclosure, that is, how much should be revealed to patients, especially to those who are terminally ill?[2] In this chapter, part of the focus is on verbal communication in face-to-face decision-making, which comprises three elements (Fig. 10.2):

1. the provision of evidence-based information to the patient by the clinician after a diagnosis has been made
2. interpretation of that information by the patient
3. discussion between clinician and patient.

10.2.1   The provision of evidence-based information

For the clinician, steps in the provision of evidence-based information to a patient include:

- finding all the available research evidence using the best possible searching techniques

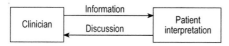

Fig. 10.2
The interaction between patient and clinician during face-to-face decision-making

- appraising that research evidence systematically to identify the best evidence available
- determining whether the best evidence available is relevant to the individual patient currently under care.

Determining the relevance of the best evidence available to an individual patient includes the following calculations:

- the probability that the patient will benefit
- the magnitude of any benefit
- the probability that the patient will suffer from any adverse effects of treatment
- the magnitude of any adverse effects.

When giving evidence-based information to a patient, the clinician must present it in a form that patients will find useful. For example, in one study in which patients chose the therapy for lung cancer, it was found that patients would prefer the results to be expressed in terms of life-expectancy rather than in terms of the probability of surviving.[3]

It is also important to tailor the information to individual patients' needs. In a study of 1012 women who had a confirmed diagnosis of breast cancer,[4] one of the objectives was to identify the women's priorities for information. It was found that:

- for women over 70 years of age, their priority was to have information about the chance of cure, and the spread of the disease
- for women less than 50 years of age, their priority was for information about the effect of treatment on their sexuality
- for women who had positive family histories, their priority was for information about family risk.

10.2.1.1 Other sources of information for patients

Clinicians are not the only source of information for patients. Other sources of information include:

- relatives, friends, and acquaintances
- the World Wide Web
- the pharmaceutical industry.

Many patients now access medical information from the World Wide Web. However, as there is no control over the content of material put up on the Web, the information that patients are able to find can vary widely in quality. It is important, therefore, that healthcare professionals contribute to providing good-quality information on the Web, i.e. information that is easy to find, easy to read, and free from bias.

10.2.2   Interpretation

Once a patient has been given the information, s/he has to interpret it, and may require time for reflection (Margin Fig. 10.1).

A patient will seek to interpret the information in two ways.

1. how the evidence provided applies to his/her particular case: this is difficult for a patient, who may need guidance; it is the responsibility of the clinician to assess the relevance of the evidence to the particular patient who is consulting
2. how the outcomes, good and bad, sit within the context of his/her values; for example, a patient who has deep vein thrombosis and is offered treatment has to weigh up two risks:
   - that of complications or death as a result of treatment
   - that of experiencing complications or death if treatment is refused.

It is possible to delineate these values using decision analysis techniques. In one study, all patients suspected of having venous thrombosis preferred to follow a course in which the risk of an early death from treatment was reduced rather than a course in which the risk of long-term complications from the disease was reduced.[5]

The provision of written information (patient leaflets) can be used to support the verbal communication, and aid the process of interpretation. Such leaflets can be used to give a clear indication of the strength of the evidence, for instance, by highlighting which statements are supported by research and which by opinion or anecdote. Tools, such as DISCERN, have been developed to enable those who produce information for patients to ensure that the information provided is based on the best current knowledge, and takes into account the needs of patients and carers.[6]

10.2.3   Discussion

The quality of a discussion between clinician and patient is determined not by the quality of the evidence or the

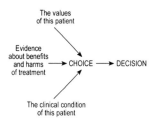

Margin Fig. 10.1

Margin Note 10.1
DISCERN

DISCERN provides online tools for information providers and users to judge the quality of information available to the public on treatments and genetics tests, respectively:
http://www.discern.org.uk/
http://wwww.discern-genetics.org/

patient's knowledge of medical terms but primarily by the relationship between clinician and patient. If a patient feels powerless, the discussion will be stilted, inconclusive and unsatisfactory. If a patient feels empowered to participate with the clinician in decision-making, a satisfactory discussion will take place.

Skelton and Hobbs[7] have taken a novel approach to analysing the language used during the doctor–patient consultation. They applied the technique of computer concordancing, a methodology established in linguistic research but rarely applied to professional language, which enables both a quantitative and qualitative study of language. Skelton and Hobbs investigated the language of 40 doctors (native English speakers) and their patients during 373 primary care consultations, to determine:

- the use of jargon by doctors
- the use of the language of power, and that of the absence of power
- the ways in which language was used to diminish the potential threat of the presenting disorder.

The authors found that doctors did not use jargon, which suggests that they are aware of the need to avoid it. However, some doctors did use language associated with social power, and some patients used language associated with absence of power, which could imply that consultations may be less democratic than is appropriate. Finally, there was substantial evidence that doctors used language to express emotions, to diminish threats, and to reassure patients, which Skelton and Hobbs feel denotes a therapeutic use of language.

References

1. Coulter, A. and Cleary, P.D. (2001) *Patients' experiences with hospital care in five countries.* Health Aff. 20(3): 244–52.
2. Annas, G.J. (1994) *Informed consent, cancer and truth in prognosis.* N. Engl. J. Med. 330: 223–5.
3. McNeil, B.J., Pauker, S.G., Sox, H.C. et al. (1982) *On the elicitation of preferences for alternative therapies.* N. Engl. J. Med. 306: 1259–62.
4. Degner, L.F., Kristjanson, L.J., Bowman, D. et al. (1997) *Information needs and decisional preferences in women with breast cancer.* JAMA 277: 1485–92.
5. O'Meara, J.J., McNutt, R.A., Evans, A.T. et al. (1994) *A decision analysis of streptokinase plus heparin as compared with heparin alone for deep-vein thrombosis.* N. Engl. J. Med. 330: 1864–9.
6. Coulter, A. (1998) *Evidence based patient information.* Br. Med. J. 317: 225–6.
7. Skelton, J.R. and Hobbs, F.D.R. (1999) *Concordancing: use of language-based research in medical communication.* Lancet 353: 108–11.

10.3   Facilitating evidence-based patient choice

For a patient to exercise choice based on the available evidence, all three elements of patient communication must occur.

When patients are given information, their preferences for treatment may change. In one study of people aged between 60 and 99 years, who were asked if they wished to receive cardiopulmonary resuscitation (CPR), 41% said 'yes' initially; when they were apprised of the evidence and realised that survival after CPR was lower than their expectations, the proportion of those wishing to receive it dropped to 22%.[1] However, the nature of the information provided may also affect patient preference. Mazur and Hickam[2] compared the preference for intubation and ventilatory support (IVS) in two groups of patients randomly assigned to alternative explanations of the purpose of the intervention. One group considered IVS in an unspecified medical condition (general explanation); the other considered IVS in the context of severe pneumonia. They found that those patients who had been given a general explanation were willing to accept significantly fewer days of intubation (65 days vs 96 days; $P = 0.009$), and significantly fewer of them wanted to continue IVS when the probability of a successful outcome was less than 50% (30% vs 64%; $P < 0.0001$).

The provision of information to patients about new interventions can vary in difficulty depending on the treatment. The introduction of a new drug is usually easy; the means of administration will probably not be different to those of established drugs and therefore it is more likely to be acceptable to patients. In contrast, the introduction of a new operation is much more difficult; patients may want evidence about both the operation and the skill of the operator. In this case, there are two inter-related questions the patient may ask:

- 'Should I have this operation?'
- if the answer is in the affirmative, 'Whom should I ask to perform this operation?'

A patient's decision about whether to have an operation is usually determined by the level of confidence the patient has in a particular operator. This is wise because the evidence on which any clinician's advice is based has been

> **Box 10.1** Questions a patient contemplating laparoscopic cholecystectomy should ask about the operator (Source: Nenner et al.[3])
>
> - Is the surgeon board-certified?
> - Does the surgeon have hospital privileges to do open cholecystectomy?
> - Was the surgeon formally trained in a recognized programme in laparoscopic cholecystectomy?
> - How many laparoscopic cholecystectomies did he or she do and what were the frequency and types of complications?

derived from trials in which high-quality professionals work within stringent criteria on a carefully defined and often relatively healthy subset of patients.

To resolve this situation, a patient can ask for evidence about those characteristics of the process of care that have been demonstrated as leading to good outcomes. For example, any American patient considering laparoscopic cholecystectomy is advised by Nenner et al.[3] to ask the questions shown in Box 10.1.

10.3.1   Factors inhibiting evidence-based patient choice

There are several factors that may prevent a patient exercising evidence-based choice about treatment options:
- clinical ignorance
- the emphasis clinicians place on the beneficial effects of intervention
- lack of full disclosure by clinicians
- withholding information about relevant organisational policies.

10.3.1.1 Clinical ignorance

Clinical ignorance will limit patient choice and might impede the delivery of effective care. The causes of clinical ignorance are shown in Box 10.2. As can be seen,

> **Box 10.2** Causes of clinical ignorance
>
> - There may be no knowledge to know
> - There may be knowledge not known to the clinician
> - There may be knowledge known to the clinician, but that knowledge does not allow the clinician to assess the probabilities of the outcomes of the different options available to the clinician and the patient

clinicians are not always aware of the best evidence available. For instance, in a study in which doctors' beliefs about the treatment of high blood pressure were compared with the treatment known to be effective based on the best evidence available,[4] it was found that doctors thought treatment should be commenced at a level of blood pressure that increased with the age of the patient, whereas the evidence shows that treatment is indicated at lower levels of blood pressure as a patient grows older.

10.3.1.2 Emphasising the benefits of intervention

Clinicians tend to emphasise the beneficial rather than the adverse effects of intervention, as this harrowing account of a person treated for myeloid leukaemia illustrates:

> We were told that the condition was serious, but in 50% of cases people were cured. When it was discovered there were sideroblasts the success rate was reduced to 25%. It was not until the second course of chemotherapy that the head of the department, B, saw Jeffrey and said that only 15% of patients can be treated successfully and for someone of Jeffrey's age a remission was impossible.[5]

10.3.1.3 Disclosure

It can be argued that any patient should have full disclosure of the evidence from a clinician, much as they would expect to be fully informed by a lawyer or television engineer who was working for them. Indeed, one speaker at a conference on bioethics in the USA said, 'I trust my lawyer more than I trust my doctor', meaning that she trusted the lawyer to tell her all the options available and execute the one she chose, whereas she would not have this confidence in her doctors if she were terminally ill.

In a survey in the USA in 1982,[6] it was found that:

- 85% of Americans wanted a realistic estimate of 'how long they had to live if their type of cancer' usually leads to death in less than 1 year
- only 41% of physicians if, or when, asked by a patient with 'a fully confirmed diagnosis of lung cancer at an advanced stage' would give either a straight statistical prognosis (13%) or 'say that you can't tell how long the patient might live but stress that in most cases people lived no longer than a year' (28%).

Owing in part to the fear of litigation, clinicians are now more open and frank, particularly with patients who have a severe illness where a decision to proceed with treatment may expose the patient to interventions that have major side-effects but carry little prospect of cure. It is most common for this type of decision to be faced when there is a choice between further treatment for a malignancy or palliative care.

10.3.1.4 Withholding information about organisational policies

Clinical care is provided in the context of a set of policies at every level from the local to the national, and it is these policies that define the limits of healthcare provision. Policies, therefore, can have an influence on the care a patient receives, and Williamson argues that patients should be told about specific policies that might concern them.[7] Of course, disclosure of such policies will probably expose the fact that policy is often influenced by the level of resources available.

References

1. Murphy, D.J., Burrows, D., Santilli, S. et al. (1994) *The influence of the probability of survival on patients' preferences regarding cardiopulmonary resuscitation.* N. Engl. J. Med. 330: 565–9.
2. Mazur, D.J. and Hickam, D.H. (1997) *The influence of physician explanations on patient preferences about future health-care states.* Med. Decis. Making 17: 56–60.
3. Nenner, R.P., Imperato, P.J. and Will, T.O. (1994) *Questions patients should ask about laparoscopic cholecystectomy. [Letter]* Ann. Intern. Med. 120: 443.
4. Dickerson, J.E.C. and Brown, M.J. (1995) *Influence of age on general practitioners' definition and treatment of hypertension.* Br. Med. J. 310: 574.
5. Anonymous (1994) *Dying for palliative care.* Br. Med. J. 309: 1696–9.
6. Annas, G.J. (1994) *Informed consent, cancer and truth in prognosis.* N. Engl. J. Med. 330: 223–5.
7. Williamson, C. (2005) *Withholding policies from patients restricts their autonomy. [Education and debate]* Br. Med. J. 331: 1078–80.

10.4   Understanding evidence-based clinical practice

10.4.1   Definitions and dimensions

Evidence-based clinical practice or evidence-based medicine is:

> *... the conscientious, explicit and judicious use of current best evidence in making decisions about the care of individual patients. The practice of evidence-based medicine means integrating individual clinical expertise with the best available external clinical evidence from systematic research. By individual clinical expertise we mean the*

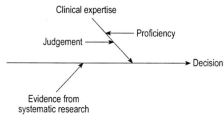

Fig. 10.3
Evidence-based decision-making

> *proficiency and judgement that individual clinicians*
> *acquire through clinical experience and clinical practice.[1]*

This process of evidence-based decision-making described above can be represented diagrammatically, as shown in Fig. 10.3.

The use of the adjective 'judicious' signifies that the clinician must take into account a patient's condition, baseline risk, values, and circumstances when making a decision (Fig. 10.4); evidence-based clinical practice is not cookbook medicine.[1] In itself, the possession and provision of the current best evidence does not constitute a decision; the evidence must be interpreted in the context of the individual patient's needs, which requires clinical judgement, good communication skills, and humanity.[2]

In evidence-based clinical practice, a clinician must also link the evidence to the other activities that promote the exercise of evidence-based patient choice (Fig. 10.5).

Contrary to the widely held belief that only 15–20% of clinical practice is based on good research evidence, it has been found that in several specialties and sub-specialties, the majority of patients are treated on the basis of good evidence, i.e. on evidence from good-quality RCTs and convincing non-experimental evidence (Margin Note 10.2).[3–14] From Table 10.1, it can be seen that the specialty and sub-specialties of surgery appear to be more dependent

Margin Note 10.2
What proportion of healthcare is evidence-based?

For a resource guide on the proportion of healthcare that is evidence based, visit: http://www.shef.ac.uk/~scharr/ir/percent.html

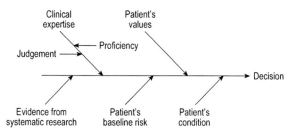

Fig. 10.4
The 'judicious' use of evidence in relation to a patient's baseline risk, condition and values during decision-making

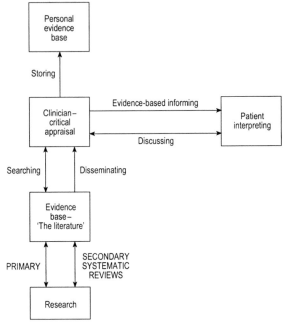

Fig. 10.5
Factors in the promotion of evidence-based patient choice

Table 10.1   The nature of the evidence supporting the use of interventions in various specialties and sub-specialties (Sources: Refs.[3–14])

Specialty	No. interventions/ patients	Nature of supporting evidence for intervention		
		Evidence from good-quality RCTs	Convincing evidence from non-RCT study designs	No convincing evidence
General medicine[3]	108/108	53%	29%	18%
General surgery[4]	100/100	24%	71%	5%
Haematology, UK[5]	?/83		70%	30%
Haematology/oncology, USA[6]	154/?	24%	21%	55%
Dermatology outpatients, Denmark[7]	?/115	38%	33%	23%
Psychiatry, UK[8]	40/40	65%		
Psychiatry, UK[9]	160/158	53%	10%	37%
Community paediatrics, UK[10]	1149/247	39.9%	7%	
Paediatric surgery, UK (regional unit)[11]	281/281	11%	66%	23%
Paediatric surgery, UK (tertiary referral unit)[12]	70/49	26%	71%	3%
Laparoscopic surgery, France[13]	428/?	50%	28%	
General thoracic surgery, USA (tertiary cancer care unit)[14]	50/?	14%	64%	22%

on convincing evidence from studies with designs that are not RCTs. For non-surgical specialties, there is a greater tendency for interventions to be based on evidence from RCTs (see Table 7.5 for the evidence base of consultations in general practice).

10.4.1.1 Failures in clinical decision-making

When evidence is not used during clinical practice, important failures in clinical decision-making occur:

- ineffective interventions are introduced
- interventions that do more harm than good are introduced
- interventions that do more good than harm are not introduced
- interventions that are ineffective or do more harm than good are not discontinued.

When considering the reasons why these failures happen, it is helpful to remember the three factors that influence clinical performance (see Section 9.3):

- a professional's competence
- a professional's motivation
- the barriers a professional has to overcome.

There is no evidence that clinicians lack motivation, but some skills (competence) do need to be improved (see Chapter 9) and many barriers need to be removed.

Barriers to using evidence during clinical practice
Of those factors contributing to the presence of barriers, some are external (Table 10.2), over which clinicians have

Table 10.2 External factors contributing to the barriers that impair a healthcare professional's performance, and their solutions

External causes	Solutions outwith the power of clinicians
Poor quality of research producing biased evidence	Better training of research workers and more stringent ethics committees
Studies too small to produce unequivocal results	Promotion of systematic reviews
Unpublished research unavailable to clinicians	Publication of all research findings by pharmaceutical companies
Publication bias towards positive findings	Prevention of publication bias
Failure of research workers to present evidence in forms useful to clinicians	Tougher action by journal editors
Inaccessible libraries	Extension of access to the World Wide Web to all clinicians

Table 10.3 Internal factors contributing to barriers that impair a healthcare professional's performance, and their solutions

Internal causes even a busy clinician can modify	Solutions for the busy clinician
Out-of-date textbooks	Don't read textbooks for guidance on therapy
Biased editorials and reviews	Don't read editorials and reviews for guidance on therapy except Cochrane Collaboration reviews and reviews in DARE
Too much primary research (the average clinician needs to read 19 articles a day to keep up)	Read good-quality reviews rather than primary research
Reviews difficult to find	Improve searching skills (Sections 4.2.2 and 9.4.2)
Inability to spot flaws in research	Improve appraisal skills (Sections 4.2.3 and 9.4.3)
Difficulty in retrieving evidence identified as useful	Develop skills to use reference management software (Section 9.4.2)
Translating the data about groups of patients in research papers into information relevant to an individual patient	Develop/improve understanding of baseline risk and NNT (Section 6.4.3.1) and ability to explain how research results apply to an individual patient (Section 10.2.1)[15-17]
Insufficient time	Be more discerning about what to read by developing a good scanning strategy (Box 4.1)

very little control, and others are internal (Table 10.3), over which clinicians can take action.[15-17]

Owing to the small number of studies, in a Cochrane Review of interventions tailored to overcome identified barriers to change, whether in healthcare professionals or organisations,[18] it is not clear whether tailored strategies are more effective than those that are not. The reviewers conclude that more research is needed about how to identify and overcome barriers.

10.4.2 The clinician's dilemma

10.4.2.1 Treating individual patients

Gentle Reader,

Empathise with Mr B.
'What do you think, doctor?' asked Mr B., who had been found to have narrowing of the arteries to his brain after investigation for a transient ischaemic attack. His GP had put him on aspirin and referred him to hospital. Mr B. knew the aspirin was safe and effective, and he had no trouble taking it. However, after numerous tests, the hospital doctor had advised him to have an operation

on his carotid arteries – an endarterectomy – not unlike, he was cheerily told, rodding out pipes that had become furred up. So here he was, back in the surgery of his GP, whom he trusted, asking: 'What do you think, doctor?'

Gentle Reader,

Empathise with the GP. On being asked what she thought by Mr B., she was assailed by so many different thoughts. Why didn't consultants make the decisions? Isn't it great to be a GP, trusted by both the patient and the consultant to whom the referral had been made! She thought of Mrs B., who had Alzheimer's disease: if Mr B. has a stroke, she's had it. But there again, he might not: not everyone with carotid artery stenosis does. What if he dies on the table? Some people do. What are the risks and benefits for Mr B.? Where do I find the evidence? Why are these bloody difficult decisions always booked into a routine slot in morning surgery?

Commentary

Carotid endarterectomy is classified as effective, i.e. it does more good than harm on a population level, but some people are harmed by the operation.[19] In fact, some of those who suffer harm would not have had a stroke even if they had not had the operation. It is essential for any clinician to know how to target treatment to individual patients who are at high risk of a poor outcome without treatment but who are also at a low risk of a poor outcome with treatment. In making this particular decision, the GP and Mr B. were fortunate because an epidemiologist had completed and published the necessary research.[20] Only 20% of people at risk of carotid stenosis becoming stroke will have a stroke on medical treatment alone. Thus, 80% will not. If everyone at risk of stroke had a carotid endarterectomy, some of the 80% would be harmed. Fortunately, a risk factor can be calculated that indicates which of those with carotid stenosis are most likely to benefit from an operation, and would therefore have a higher than average probability of being helped rather than harmed.[21]

The clinician's dilemma is:

'How relevant is this research to this particular patient?' In order to answer this question, the clinician must consider the 'baseline risk of the patient', that is, the degree of risk of a particular individual who shares the same characteristics as the patients in the trial.[16] Although this issue does not have to be addressed by health service decision-makers directly, they should be cognisant of the dilemma faced by the clinician and the patient, both of whom have to weigh up not only the probability of good and harmful outcomes occurring but also the magnitude of any beneficial and of any adverse effects (Fig. 10.6).

One approach that can be taken to help clinicians and patients resolve this dilemma is the use of a decision support system. A computer-based decision support system (CDSS) has been defined as any software designed to aid the clinician directly in clinical decision-making, in which the

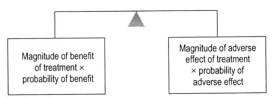

Fig. 10.6
The balance between the magnitude of beneficial effects and that of harmful or adverse effects

characteristics of individual patients are matched to a computerised knowledge base for the purpose of generating patient-specific assessment or recommendations that are then presented to the clinician for consideration.[22] For advice on how to use an article evaluating the clinical impact of a computer-based clinical decision support system, see Randolph et al.[23]

10.4.2.2 Clinical freedom

> *Everything is what it is: liberty is liberty, not equality or fairness or justice or culture, or human happiness or a quiet conscience.*
>
> Isaiah Berlin, *Two Concepts of Liberty*, 1958

Isaiah Berlin's ebullient personality dominated Oxford, and much of the London intelligentsia, in the second half of the 20th century. From a brilliant career in Intelligence during the Second World War to his death in 1997, Berlin's irresistible flow of ideas enlivened many a dull academic and establishment meeting. In one of his most interesting essays, *Two Concepts of Liberty*, Berlin distinguished between what he called 'negative liberty', the freedom to do what we want without constraint (wear a seat belt or not, smoke cannabis or not), and 'positive liberty', the freedom to decide how much negative liberty we have.

Very often healthcare professionals, particularly doctors, will fight for negative liberty, namely the freedom for individual clinicians to do anything they see fit. However, it is of equal, if not greater, importance to maintain the positive liberty of the profession, i.e. the freedom to decide how much negative liberty each individual member of the profession has. Unfortunately, in fighting to preserve negative liberty, clinicians have failed to recognise not only the change in public attitudes to the profession, reflected in a change in political attitudes, but also the growing concern about variations in the quality of professional

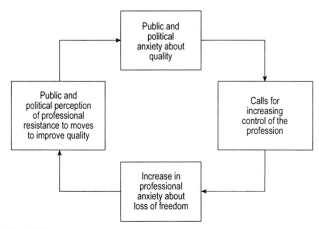

Fig. 10.7
The interaction of public anxiety about the quality of healthcare and
professional anxiety about the loss of freedom

practice (Fig. 10.7). A desire now exists among the public
and politicians, usually supported by the media, to
introduce controls on the behaviour of the profession as a
whole but particularly on that of its worst members.
It is ironic that the clinicians who call for the retention of
negative liberty are often the most responsible members
of the profession who base their clinical decisions on good
evidence and best practice. However, by emphasising
the need to maintain negative liberty, the profession is in
danger of losing the trust of the public and politicians,
which may lead to greater controls on the profession.
In this situation, healthcare professionals need to embrace
the concept of evidence-based decision-making and, where
systems of care can be developed, the introduction of
guidelines and audit (see Fig. 1.4).

In the UK, the establishment of the National Institute
for Health and Clinical Excellence (NICE) and the
Healthcare Commission probably represents the best
balance between positive and negative liberty that
could be obtained. The overall aim for NICE is to
provide national guidance on promoting good health
and preventing and treating ill health, whereas the
Healthcare Commission is empowered to identify failures
in the quality of care and to take action to remedy
them. The initial response of healthcare professionals to
this development has been positive: it is viewed as an

important opportunity for the professions to maintain positive liberty even though it will mean some diminution of negative liberty.

10.4.2.3 Clinical governance

The debate about the nature of liberty acceded to the professions is not new. In his book *The Death of the Guilds*, Elliott Krause[24] analyses the steady decline in prestige of the medical and several other professions in five countries – Italy, Germany, France, the UK and the USA. Krause discusses how the influence of the Guilds, precursors of the professions, waned, sometimes as a result of capitalism, sometimes as a result of state action, but usually as the result of combined action by the two forces. He also emphasises that there is now a third force affecting the status of the professions – consumerism. Throughout this process, the professions seem to have been relatively unaware of what was happening or unable to take a strategic view.

In the UK, the concept of clinical governance has been introduced. Clinical governance, which could have been termed 'clinical self-governance', gives clinicians the responsibility to monitor and manage their performance as part of the general management of healthcare organisations; this concept is central to preserving positive liberty. However, in clinical governance, chief executives have been given the responsibility for the quality of clinical care, which could be seen as a loss of negative liberty, except for the understanding that this responsibility can be fulfilled only with the full involvement of clinicians.

The range of views about clinical governance can be represented on a spectrum, as shown in Fig. 10.8. At one end are those who believe that clinical freedom has been abused and professionals need to be policed; at the other are those who believe that education is the key to improved performance. However, it is necessary to

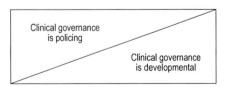

Fig. 10.8
The spectrum of views about the function of clinical governance

reconcile these two views because both approaches are complementary. For any professional activity, performance can be measured and categorised according to quality standards. The policing function is necessary to identify those individuals who fall below the minimal acceptable standard, but quality assurance is not simply a matter of identifying poor performance. The aim is to help all professionals improve their performance, which can be achieved through continuing professional development. As performance improves, it is important to re-set standards to ensure that healthcare professionals do not become complacent but are motivated to seek further improvement.

10.4.2.4 To whom should the clinician be loyal: patient or State?

The concepts of clinical freedom and clinical governance beg the question of how the individual clinician relates to the State on the one hand and to the patient on the other.

Patients want to trust that clinicians will give them the best possible care, but it is often not feasible for clinicians to do this because the majority of them work in health systems in which resources are finite and limited. Some people believe that clinicians should play no part in resource allocation or rationing; some, however, argue that the definition of evidence-based medicine is misguided to absolve clinicians of concerns about the resource consequences of each and every decision.

The approach taken in the development of the concepts of evidence-based medicine and evidence-based healthcare was that decision-making for groups of patients or populations was qualitatively different to that in clinical practice, even though the evidence used for both would be the same. This distinction enables the clinician and the patient to focus on assessing the best current evidence in the context of the patient's values and baseline condition without worrying about cost.

As an example, consider the ethical problems that might be raised when considering the use of either tissue plasminogen activator (tPA) or streptokinase for patients who have suffered an acute myocardial infarction (AMI). One possible approach in this situation is to let the clinician be responsible for deciding whether to administer tPA or streptokinase on a case-by-case basis: if tPA is the drug of choice in the majority of cases because it may be slightly more effective, as the financial year progresses the budget will be under increasing pressure because tPA is almost ten times more costly than streptokinase. In this scenario, the clinician's decision-making becomes dominated by the availability of resources. A better approach is for those who pay for or commission health services to decide whether tPA or streptokinase should be used. Although there are some minor additional benefits with the use of tPA, the population as a whole would be better served if the additional money necessary to fund the use of tPA were spent on improving the quality of care within the service, for example, the introduction of programmes to reduce the door-to-needle time for the administration of streptokinase, known to be a key factor influencing survival after AMI.

In the USA, Ubel has recommended that physicians need to relax their advocacy duties towards patients in order to control healthcare costs[25] to the extent of being willing to forego small benefits for patients by acceding to 'reasonable' rationing mechanisms introduced by those who pay for healthcare.[26] This means that each physician must decide what constitutes:

- a small benefit
- reasonable rationing mechanisms.

In the UK, if a clinician disagrees with any decisions made by those who pay for healthcare, she or he can lobby the relevant member of parliament for more money to be allocated to the health service to fund the use of specific interventions. However, it is better to make decisions about money, and marginal differences in effectiveness of interventions, at a population level to reduce:

- the number of factors that a clinician has to take into account
- the part that emotion can play in the process.

The example of which clot-busting agent to choose highlights the nature of the ethical problems that clinicians practising evidence-based medicine in organisations promoting evidence-based healthcare might encounter. Thus, there can be conflict between the patient and the clinician, with the consultation as the focal point of that conflict, in which clinicians must balance the needs of the individual and the needs of society at large. If society has to limit the resources expended on healthcare, and ensure those resources are used to best

Casebook 10.1 The book that was nearly the death of the man (Source: Koller[27])

Clinicians are able to see the need for wisdom and discretion most clearly when they become patients, as Chad Koller described in the *Annals of Internal Medicine* series entitled 'On being a patient'. He had had major surgery and wanted analgesics for postoperative pain. The surgical intern and senior resident prescribed famotidine, 'according to the book', but the pain was worsening. Two and a half hours later, when Koller was told by the nurse his blood pressure was normal, he thought, 'Normal unless you consider my history of hypertension and my current pain. Mildly worrisome, actually'.

He then asked what his last haemoglobin level was, to which the nurse replied, 'It was 7.1 mg/dL this morning, I think. I told the surgical intern, but he said that the book says you don't need a transfusion'.

However, Koller knew his preoperative haemoglobin level had been 13.6 mg/dL, and was concerned that it had dropped from the postoperative level measured that morning.

The pain continued to worsen, and when the anaesthesia resident arrived, she discovered that owing to a kink in the line the epidural had not been administered by the pump, even though the readout indicated that it had. When Koller informed the anaesthesia resident of his last-measured haemoglobin level and she wondered why he had not been given any blood, the surgical intern said, 'Not unless the hemoglobin level is less than 7.0 mg/dL'.

The patient then outlined his concerns, giving the entire clinical picture and strongly recommending that the intern consider giving a blood transfusion immediately. The intern paused and 'chanted', 'The book says your hemoglobin level has to be less than 7.0 mg/dL before we give you blood'.

However, the intern did agree to consult the senior resident, who responded that 'the book says no transfusion'. Koller then pleaded to have his haemoglobin level re-checked. At this point, his blood pressure had dropped to 72/50 mmHg, and he felt very weak and everything 'looked dark and fuzzy'. The next thing he was aware of was the arrival of 2 units of blood. His last haemoglobin level had dropped to 6.6 mg/dL, and as the surgical intern said, 'The book said to give you blood'.

In this case, the book was nearly the death of the man.

effect, rules and controls are essential, but so too are clinicians who can interpret those rules with wisdom and discretion (Casebook 10.1).[27]

10.4.2.5 Remember the multiple goals of therapy: applying wisdom and discretion

Gentle Reader,

Empathise with the clinician facing this dilemma: it is 11.30 p.m. and he is responsible for the care of a woman who is bleeding and near to death. However, she cannot accept she is dying and is desperate to see her son, who is 5 hours away but coming as quickly as he can to her bedside. Blood is scarce; the clinician knows that; he also knows that blood given to this woman will merely postpone the inevitable. There is no evidence that it will make her feel any better or increase her life-expectancy, it will simply use up blood that could have been transfused into patients undergoing surgical interventions for which there is good evidence of effectiveness. However, the clinician chooses to give the woman six units of blood over a period of 5 hours. The woman is reconciled with her son and dies peacefully when the transfusion stops.

Commentary

The clinician involved in this case was accused of acting unethically by a health economist who thought he had wasted society's resources on a patient who was clearly close to death. A jury would probably have found for the clinician on the grounds of humanity.

As resource constraints increase, conflicts between the professional primarily concerned with the care of the whole population and the professional primarily concerned with the care of individual patients will become more common. In fact, the clinician who made the decision to transfuse was one of the healthcare professionals most active not only in his hospital but also in the UK in the promotion of an evidence-based approach to decision-making, and had championed the need for the profession to take a much more systematic, explicit and judicious approach to the use of evidence in the care of patients, whatever the goals of therapy might be.

The goals of therapy can include:

- to treat a person's illness
- to control a person's symptoms
- to extend a person's life.

In many cases, there will be a principal goal of therapy.

One of the problems faced by people suffering from cancer is that the clinicians caring for them can be confused about whether the principal goal of therapy is life extension or control of symptoms. When a decision has been made jointly with the patient that the principal goal of therapy is control of symptoms, a different pattern of care can be instituted which may be just as active and equally as, or even more, expensive than life-extension therapy.

Finally, although evidence-based decision-making requires the application of evidence, it may be appropriate on occasion for values to trump evidence through the application of wisdom and discretion.

10.4.3   Shared decision-making

Patients want the opportunity to make choices in relation to their health care, but choosing a provider is only one of the choices they can make. Knowing about the various treatment options available and having a say in these is more important to most patients than having a choice of where to be treated.

Angela Coulter, 2005[28]

One of the aims of the provision of healthcare in the 21st century should be to promote shared decision-making. In shared decision-making, it is recognised that:

- the evidence-based clinician's contribution to the decision must take into account the patient's preferences and values
- the consultation is no longer the only source of information – for example, patients can download information from the World Wide Web and relate that to their own preferences and values (Margin Fig. 10.2).

Margin Fig. 10.2

The results of a poll run in 1999 by the *British Medical Journal* to coincide with a theme issue on 'Embracing Patient Partnership' are shown in Matrix 10.1.[29] Visitors ($n = >850$) to the website from 17 September to 4 October were asked who should make treatment decisions. As can be seen, the majority of patients preferred shared decision-making. When asked which consulting style would predominate in 10 years' time, 65% of visitors responded that it would be shared decision-making, and 26% of visitors thought that the patient would be making the decision. In 2004, in the National Patient Survey Programme for England,[30] the

	Doctor decides	Doctor and patient decide together	Patient decides
As a patient, which consulting style do you prefer?	56	737	54
Which consulting style predominates today?	503	298	43
Which consulting style do you think will predominate in 10 years' time?	75	546	223

Matrix 10.1
'Embracing Patient Partnership' (Source: e-BMJ[29])

following types of patient reported that they definitely had a say in decisions about their treatment:

Margin Note 10.3
Shared decision-making

A website devoted to the promotion of shared decision-making is available online at: http://www.shared-decision-making.org/

- 53% of inpatients
- 70% of outpatients
- 64% of A&E patients
- 61% of coronary heart disease patients.

From these figures, it would seem that there is a developing trend towards shared decision-making, although there is still room for improvement. The use of patient decision aids (see Section 10.4.3.1) to facilitate shared decision-making and ensure that patient choice is informed is a trend that in 2007 reached a tipping point.[31,32]

However, it is important to be aware that different patients may want different levels of control and participation in decision-making. In the study of 1012 women who had a confirmed diagnosis of breast cancer (discussed also in Section 10.2.1), Degner et al.[33] investigated the level of control and participation the women desired in decision-making about their treatment, and the degree to which their desired level of control had been achieved. They found that:

- 22% wanted to select their own treatment
- 44% preferred a collaborative approach
- 34% wished to delegate the responsibility to the clinician.

The best single predictor of preference was a woman's educational status.

It can be seen that the majority of women (78%) did want to participate in the decision-making about their treatment, however, only 42% of the women felt that they had achieved their preferred level of control. From this study, it would appear that clinicians should not make assumptions but actively determine each individual patient's preferred level of control and participation in decision-making about treatment options, and tailor their approach accordingly. It is possible also that a patient's preference about participation may change during the course of an illness, and it is advisable to review this at suitable points during treatment.

10.4.3.1 Decision aids

In the UK, there are about 2 million consultations between healthcare professionals and patients in the NHS every day. These 2 million consultations are the drivers for about 10 million decisions relating to the diagnosis and treatment of individual patients. During the consultation, some of these decisions will be made by the patient and clinician together, and within such clinician–patient decision-making there is a spectrum of patient participation.

Decision aids have been developed to support the process of decision-making about patients' diagnosis and treatment. There are two main types of decision aid:

- knowledge support and computer-based clinical decision support systems for professionals, which help to identify the options available
- patient decision aids or support technologies, which help patients come to a decision about which treatment option to choose – there is strong evidence to show that patient decision aids can improve decision quality and prevent the over-use of options that informed patients do not value.[32]

The Cochrane Collaboration has set up a registry of patient decision aids as part of an ongoing systematic review of such aids (Margin Note 10.4). As at mid-2006, over 400 aids were included in the registry. In addition to the Cochrane Collaboration cataloguing patient decision aids and their development, the quality of available decision aids is appraised using the CREDIBLE criteria.[34]

Building on the work of the Cochrane Collaboration, a framework of quality criteria for patient decision aids has been designed using an online Delphi consensus process[35] involving people from 14 countries in four stakeholder groups:

- researchers
- practitioners
- patients
- policy-makers.

This framework is the basis of a checklist for appraising the quality of patient decision aids (see Box 10.3 for the main question categories in the checklist).[35]

Margin Note 10.4
The Cochrane Collaboration Decision Aids Registry

The Cochrane Decision Aids Registry comprises:

- The Cochrane Inventory, a resource for researchers, is a registry of *all* decision aids identified to date by the Cochrane Systematic Review Group
- The A to Z Inventory, a resource for patients, is a registry of decision aids that meet a set of five minimal inclusion criteria, i.e. satisfy the Cochrane definition of a patient decision aid, have a development process that includes expert review, have an update policy, support statements with scientific evidence, and disclose funding sources and/or conflicts of interest.

Access to the Cochrane Collaboration's Decision Aids Registry is available online at: http://www.ohri.ca/decisionaid/cochinvent.php

---

Box 10.3 IPDAS patient decision aid user checklist (Source: Elwyn et al.[35])

1. Content: does the patient decision aid:
   - provide information about options in sufficient detail for decision-making?
   - present probabilities of outcomes in an unbiased and understandable way?
   - include methods for clarifying and expressing patients' values?
   - include structured guidance in deliberation and communication?

2. Development process: does the patient decision aid:
   - present information in a balanced manner?
   - have a systematic development process?
   - use up-to-date scientific evidence that is cited in a reference section or technical document?
   - disclose conflicts of interest?
   - use plain language?
   - meet additional criteria *if* the patient decision aid is Internet based?
   - meet additional criteria *if* stories are used in the patient decision aid?

3. Effectiveness: does the patient decision aid ensure decision-making is informed and values-based?
   - decision processes leading to decision quality. The patient decision aid helps patients to:
     - recognise a decision needs to be made
     - know options and their features
     - understand that values affect decision
     - be clear about option features that matter most
     - discuss values with their practitioner
     - become involved in preferred ways
   - decision quality: the patient decision aid improves the match between the chosen option and the features that matter most to the patient.

References

1. Sackett, D.L., Rosenberg, W.M.C., Gray, J.A.M. et al. (1996) *Evidence-based medicine: what it is and what it isn't. [Editorial]* Br. Med. J. 312: 71–2.
2. McAlister, F.A., Straus, S.E., Guyatt, G.D. et al. (2000) *Users' guides to the medical literature: XX. Integrating research evidence with the care of the individual patient.* JAMA 283: 2829–36.
3. Ellis, J., Mulligan, I., Rowe, J. et al. (1995) *In-patient general medicine is evidence based.* Lancet 346: 407–10.
4. Howes, N., Chagla, L., Thorpe, M. et al. (1997) *Surgical practice is evidence based.* Br. J. Surg. 84: 1220–3.
5. Galloway, M., Baird, G. and Lennard, A. (1997) *Haematologists in district general hospitals practise evidence-based medicine.* Clin. Lab. Haematol. 19: 243–8.
6. Djulbegovic, B., Loughran, T.P.Jnr, Hornung, C.A. et al. (1999) *The quality of medical evidence in haematology-oncology.* Am. J. Med. 106: 198–205.
7. Jemec, G.B.E., Thorsteinsdottir, H. and Wulf, H.C. (1998) *Evidence-based dermatologic out-patient treatment.* Int. J. Dermatol. 37: 850–4.

8. Geddes, J.R., Game, D., Jenkins, N.E. et al. (1996) *What proportion of primary psychiatric interventions are based on randomised evidence?* Qual. Health Care 5: 215–17.

9. Summers, A. and Kehoe, R.F. (1996) *Is psychiatric treatment evidence-based? [Letter to the Editor]* Lancet 347: 409–10.

10. Rudolph, M.C.J., Lyth, N., Bundle, A. et al. (1999) *A search for the evidence supporting community paediatric practice.* Arch. Dis. Child. 80: 257–61.

11. Kenny, S.E., Shankar, K.R., Rintala, R. et al. (1997) *Evidence-based surgery: interventions in a regional paediatric surgical unit.* Arch. Dis. Child. 76: 50–3.

12. Baraldini, V., Spitz, L. and Pierro, A. (1998) *Evidence-based operations in pediatric surgery.* Pediatr. Surg. Int. 13: 331–5.

13. Slim, K., Lescure, E., Voitellier, M. et al. (1998) *Is laparoscopic surgery really evidence-based in everyday practice? Results of a prospective regional survey in France.* Presse Med. 27: 1829–33.

14. Lee, J.S., Urschel, D.M. and Urschel, J.D. (2000) *Is general thoracic surgical practice evidence-based?* Ann. Thorac. Surg. 70: 429–31.

15. Guyatt, G.H., Cook, D.J. and Jaeschke, R. (1995) *How should clinicians use the results of randomized trials?* ACP Journal Club Jan–Feb: 122(1): A12–13.

16. Guyatt, H.G., Cook, D.J. and Jaeschke, R. (1995) *Applying the findings of clinical trials to individual patients. [Editorial]* ACP J. Club Mar–Apr: 122(2): A12–13.

17. Glasziou, P.P. and Irwig, L.M. (1995) *An evidence based approach to individualising treatment.* Br. Med. J. 311: 1356–9.

18. Shaw, B., Cheater, F., Baker, R. (2007) *Tailored interventions to overcome identified barriers to change: effects on professional practice and health care outcomes.* Cochrane Database of Systematic Reviews 2007 Issue 2. Cochrane Collaboration. Abstract available online at: http://www.cochrane.org/reviews/en/ab005470.html.

19. European Carotid Surgery Trialists Collaborative Group (1991) *MRC European Carotid Surgery Trial: interim results for symptomatic patients with severe (70–99%) or with mild (0–29%) carotid stenosis.* Lancet 337: 1235–43.

20. Rothwell, P.M. (1995) *Can overall results of clinical trials be applied to all patients?* Lancet 345: 1616–19.

21. Rothwell, P.M. and Warlow, C.P. (1999) *Prediction of benefit from carotid endarterectomy in individual patients: a risk modelling study. European Carotid Surgery Trialists' Collaborative Group.* Lancet 353: 2105–10.

22. Hunt, D.L., Haynes, R.B., Hanna, S.G. et al. (1998) *Effects of computer-based clinical decision support systems on physician performance and patient outcome: a systematic review.* JAMA 280: 1339–46.

23. Randolph, A.G., Waynes, R.B., Wyatt, J.C. et al. (1999) *Users' guides to the medical literature: XVIII. How to use an article evaluating the clinical impact of a computer-based clinical support system.* JAMA 282: 67–74.

24. Krause, E.A. (1996) *The Death of the Guilds: Professions, States and the Advance of Capitalism, 1930 to the Present.* Yale University Press, New Haven and London.

25. Ubel, P.A. and Arnold, R.M. (1995) *The unbearable rightness of bedside rationing: physician duties in a climate of cost containment.* Arch. Int. Med. 155: 1837–42.

26. Ubel, P.A. (1999) *Physicians' duties in an era of cost containment: advocacy or betrayal?* JAMA 282: 1675.

27. Koller, C. (1997) *What the book says.* Ann. Intern. Med. 127: 238–9.

28. Coulter, A. (2005) *What do patients and the public want from primary care? [Education and debate]* Br. Med. J. 331: 1199–201.

29. e-BMJ (1999) *Poll results.* Br. Med. J. 319: 1026.

30. Coulter, A. (2005) *Opinion and experience: do they concur?* In: Coulter, A., Nye, R. and Pollard, S. (eds) *What Patients Really Want.* Populus, London, pp. 33–58.

31. Gladwell, M. (2000) *The Tipping Point.* Little Brown, London.

32. O'Connor, A.M., Wennberg, J.E., Legare, F. et al. (2007) *Toward the 'tipping point': decision aids and informed patient choice.* Health Aff. 26(3): 716–25.

33. Degner, L.F., Kristjanson, L.J., Bowman, D. et al. (1997) *Information needs and decisional preferences in women with breast cancer.* JAMA 277: 1485–92.

34. O'Connor, A.M., Stacey, D., Entwistle, V. et al. (2007) *Decision aids for people facing health treatment or screening decisions.* Cochrane Database of Systematic Reviews 2007 Issue 2. John Wiley and Sons. Abstract available online at: http://www.cochrane.org/reviews/en/ab001431.html

35. Elwyn, G., O'Connor, A., Stacey, D. et al. for the International Patient Decision Aids Standards (IPDAS) (2006) *Developing a quality criteria framework for patient decision aids: online international Delphi consensus process.* Br. Med. J. 333: 417.

10.5   Dealing with the patient's anxiety

Gentle Reader,

Empathise with the eminent American surgeon and his son, both of whom were prominent gastroenterologists. The surgeon was suffering from stomach cancer. Father and son searched and appraised the literature to determine what was the best course of action. They went to see expert after expert, each of whom gave different advice or behaved so cautiously that they merely re-stated the evidence, saying that it was inconclusive. Weary and dispirited, the son said to the last expert, 'What more do we need to get a good decision?'. To which the expert replied, 'You need a good doctor'.

Commentary

Throughout most of this book, it has been argued that there is a need for a scientific, evidence-based approach to decision-making. However, there are situations in which clinical decisions are not clear-cut, in fact only a small proportion ever are; as such, the relationship between clinician and patient is of central importance in decision-taking. Although evidence is influential in decision-making, in decision-taking, the fears, anxieties and values of the patient may predominate.

Although patients do want to be treated as rational beings, that is, offered evidence, helped to assess the various options and left to take the decision, this approach does not take account of the effect of an important aspect of any consultation, that of anxiety. Anxiety may be felt by both clinician and patient. Patients can be anxious about many aspects of illness and disease, such as the diagnosis, when it is unknown, or the treatment options and outcomes when it is; clinicians may feel anxious about the possibility of misdiagnosis.

Clinicians do use certain techniques to control patient anxiety, either consciously or unconsciously. One technique is to appear to be more certain, or to state or imply that the evidence of effectiveness is certain when, as is usually the case, it indicates only a probability of success. The clinician does this with the best of intentions, and some patients want the clinician to deal with their anxiety and actively seek reassurance and comfort. However, evidence-based clinical practice, while improving the quality of healthcare given to any patient, is not necessarily a way of minimising their anxiety.

Having to make a choice can expose a dilemma, and there is usually a dilemma associated with every clinical decision, not just those where there is a stark contrast between the options, e.g. a choice between palliative care and interventions with a low probability of success and a high risk of side-effects. Patients have to make decisions about which treatment option to choose, e.g. mastectomy or breast-conserving treatment (lumpectomy), or about whether to opt for preventive intervention or risk acceptance, e.g. treatment of high blood pressure or no action.

In one study of decisions made between two types of treatment, Fallowfield et al.[1] investigated the association between being offered a choice of treatment and a patient being anxious or depressed after treatment. No difference was found in the prevalence of anxiety and depression between the patients who had been offered a choice of treatment and those to whom a firm recommendation had been made about a treatment option, which suggests that offering choice does not increase anxiety or depression. What is striking about this result is that it is impossible to generalise about patients and their preferences. For example, of the 62 women offered choice, eight refused to choose, whereas a proportion of patients who were not offered choice expressed a wish for more autonomy. Thus, there may not be any relation between preference for a style of decision-making and anxiety but neither does this mean a patient's preference should be ignored.

Reference

1. Fallowfield, L.J., Hall, A., Maguire, P. et al. (1994) *Psychological effects of being offered choice of surgery for breast cancer.* Br. Med. J. 309: 448.

10.6 Dealing with conflict around limiting treatment

For many clinicians one of the most difficult and challenging situations they can face is handling conflict with relatives about decisions regarding treatment towards the end of a patient's life (Section 6.9.1.6). Goold et al.[1] propose a 'differential diagnosis' of such conflicts, distinguishing between and describing the various factors or characteristics contributing to the situation (Fig. 10.9) and providing strategies for 'diagnosing' the dominant factors. Several factors can be present in any one situation and interact. A checklist of questions to help clinicians understand and manage these situations has been developed, divided into:

- questions to ask the family
- questions to ask oneself as clinician
- questions to interrogate the social and organisational influences.

Goold et al. suggest the next step is to 'treat' or 'prevent' such conflicts occurring.[1]

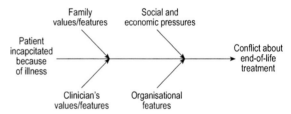

Fig. 10.9
The factors contributing to conflicts between clinicians and relatives about end-of-life treatment for incapacitated patients (Source: adapted from Goold et al.[1])

Reference

1. Goold, S.D., Williams, N. and Arnold, R.M. (2000) *Conflicts regarding decisions to limit treatment. A differential diagnosis.* JAMA 283: 909–14.

Evidence-based healthcare in the 21st century

Evidence, economics and ethics

If you want to learn people's values, present them a choice.
Roger Neighbour, *The Inner Apprentice*

People making decisions about health and healthcare policy face five great challenges:

- population ageing
- new technology and new knowledge
- rising expectations for both consumers and professionals, those of consumers being stimulated and driven by the explosion of information on the World Wide Web
- new diseases, such as SARS
- the prevalence of HIV/AIDS.

As a result of these challenges, the need and demand for healthcare are increasing at a rate that is greater than the rate at which resources are being made available. As a consequence, it is necessary for decision-making to be open, explicit, and evidence based.

The use of an evidence-based approach makes it possible to differentiate between a proposition that is supported by evidence and one made on unsubstantiated assertion or opinion (Fig. E.1). However, any evidence-based decision, whether being made in clinical practice or healthcare management or policy-making, is influenced by values. The clinician has to take into account the condition and values of the individual patient; the policy-maker has to take into account not only best current knowledge but also the needs of the population, the values of that population, the resources available, and the opportunity costs of any decision.

In evidence-based policy-making and management, it is important also to distinguish between decision-making and decision-taking. For effective decision-making in healthcare, scientists have a responsibility to ensure that the best current knowledge is available, but decisions need to

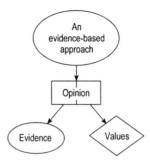

Fig. E.1
An evidence-based approach clarifies the basis of any proposition

be taken by the public or their representatives, because all healthcare decisions involve the allocation of finite resources and have significant opportunity costs. In general, the provision of information improves the quality of decision-making, but it is important to bear in mind Maynard Keynes' statement that there is nothing that a politician likes so little as to be well informed, because it makes decision-taking even more complicated and difficult.

Although it is sometimes possible to make a sharp distinction between evidence and values, it is important for the evidence-based decision-maker to bear in mind that values are all pervasive. The assumption made throughout this book that evidence and values can be distinguished, like oil and water, is a necessary convenience. The reality is that our values influence the way we ask questions, collect information, interpret data, and express the results.

Values trump evidence

The job of the decision-maker is to take the option that their judgement tells them is the best option. In the words of the English civil service: 'Officials advise, Ministers decide'.

The need for judgement and the difference between the capacity for good judgement and the skills of evidence appraisal have been well analysed, for example, in Mark Moore's book *Creating Public Value*[1] and in the fourth edition of the monumental *Administrative Behaviour* by Herbert Simon.[2]

Those who represent the public can take any decision they want on the basis of their values. If this decision goes against the evidence-based advice officials have given, the official can either accept the difference in the nature of their relative roles and responsibilities, or resign. Any person involved in decision-making who does not know their point of resignation is not thinking hard enough about the ethics of what they do.

References

1. Moore, M.H. (1997) *Creating Public Value. Strategic Management in Government*. Harvard University Press, Boston, Massachusetts.
2. Simon, H.A. (1997) *Administrative Behavior: A study of Decision-making Processes in Administrative Organizations*, 4th edn. Free Press, New York.

Doing better, feeling worse

Although *Doing Better and Feeling Worse*[1] is the title of a collection of essays about the American healthcare system, it also describes how many people felt about clinical practice and healthcare during the 1990s. This feeling of unease is experienced by those within the service, who feel criticised as never before, and those who use the service, who feel that health services are not as good as they were. The title is just as relevant at the time of writing in 2007, and this feeling may be ever with us. Yet never has the provision of healthcare been so effective or so efficient, never have clinicians been trained to communicate so well, nor has more attention been given to the needs and aspirations of patients and carers. New complaint systems have been introduced, and the clinical professions are open to scrutiny as never before. Finally, and most recently, clinicians are practising evidence-based decision-making, and managers are making open and explicit decisions about health services based on best current evidence.

As proponents of an evidence-based approach, we must ask ourselves two profound questions:

1. Why is it that as healthcare professionals, although we have become so effective and concerned with communication and the patient's experience, we have never been so unpopular?
2. Why is it that as healthcare professionals, although we have never been more self-critical, more scientific and more thoughtful, we have never been more insecure or less certain?

It may be that the phenomenon we are witnessing is simply a widening gap between consumer expectations and the delivery of a health service subject to increasing pressure exerted by the population ageing and the advent of new technology and new knowledge. However, there is the possibility that in clinical practice and healthcare management other more complex factors are at work, which may stem from the marked ambivalence that society has to the advances of science and technology.

Reference

1. Knowles, J.H. (ed.) (1977) *Doing Better and Feeling Worse: Health in the United States*. W.W. Norton, New York.

The modernisation of medicine

It is possible to divide the practice of medicine into three main eras:

First era: *pre-modern medicine*, in which the enthusiasm and conviction of the individual clinician, and of the profession as a whole, was sufficient to bring about change.

Second era: *modern medicine*, which was based on science and characterised by scepticism and uncertainty. This era began not with the technological developments after the Second World War but in the 1960s when the new breed of epidemiologists, epitomised by Archie Cochrane with his conceptualisation of effectiveness and efficiency, sowed the seeds of doubt in the minds of once-confident clinicians.

Third era: *post-modern medicine*, the current era, which, while retaining the characteristics of modern medicine, needs to take account of, and adapt to, the following social concerns and trends:

- for many patients, the process of care is as important as the outcome
- the process of care can influence the outcomes of care, not only with respect to patient satisfaction but also in terms of the patient's state of health and the effectiveness of treatment
- modern medicine and complementary medicine can be used together in what Dr Andrew Weil, the leading protagonist of this movement, has called 'integrative medicine'
- the involvement of patients as partners in clinical decision-making, although it is important to be aware that different patients will require different degrees of involvement (Section 10.4.3)

- the public are more concerned about the risks of modern medicine than the medical establishment which, until now, has emphasised the benefits.

Post-modern medicine

Die Risikogesellschaft

Ulrich Beck, Professor of Sociology at Munich, is one of the leading figures in his discipline. In his book *The Risk Society*, he proposed that:

> *the scientists are entirely incapable of reacting adequately to civilisational risks since they are prominently involved in the origin and growth of those very risks. Instead – sometimes with a clear conscience of 'pure scientific method', sometimes with increasing pangs of guilt – the science has become the legitimising patron of a global industrial pollution and contamination of air, water, foodstuff, etc.*[1]

Beck castigates the sciences as 'a branch office of politics, ethics, business and judicial practice in the garb of numbers' and the scientists have, in his opinion, 'squandered until further notice their historic reputation for rationality'. Beck's main concerns, and his arguments, derive from his study of risk and pollution. He points out that it would be more honest to replace the phrase 'permitted maximum levels' of a harmful substance with another – 'collective standardised poisoning'.

His arguments are powerful, both as an analysis of the public views of science and as a trenchant stimulus to those involved in the sciences to re-think their claim to objectivity and rationality. Medicine, in strengthening its scientific base, and through its claim to be a branch of science, exposes itself to the general public's distrust of science. It is also worth considering what medicine may have lost in moving away from a style of practice based on the personal opinion of the physician to one based on 'impersonal' scientific evidence.

Beck has one further important message for evidence-based decision-makers, whether clinicians or managers: the 21st century will be one dominated by concerns about risk and the adverse effects of intervention, whereas scientists, including clinical scientists and epidemiologists, have hitherto emphasised the positive aspects of science and the benefits to be gained from intervention.

Evidence-based risk management

As evidence accumulates about the prevalence of medical errors, public concern about the quality of healthcare provision will increase. This could lead to an exponential rise in the number of complaints and in the level of litigation. However, it is possible to adopt a pro-active approach to risk management.

In a review of the implementation of a 'humanistic risk management policy' at the Veterans Affairs Medical Center in Lexington, Kentucky, from 1990 to 1996,[2] Kraman and Hamm assessed the impact of introducing 'a policy that seems to be designed to maximize malpractice claims'. The policy included:

- early injury review
- steadfast maintenance of the relationship between the hospital and the patient
- pro-active full disclosure to patients who have been injured because of accidents or medical negligence
- fair compensation for injuries.

From their analysis, Kraman and Hamm judged the financial consequences of full disclosure to be 'moderate', and the liability payments were found to be comparable with those of similar facilities. They concluded that an honest and forthright policy in which the patient's interests come first may be relatively inexpensive, because it enables healthcare institutions to avoid lawsuit preparation, litigation, court judgement and settlements at trial. Important additional advantages of such a policy are goodwill and the maintenance of the care-giver role. In an accompanying editorial in the *Annals of Internal Medicine*, Wu states: 'only by changing the expectations of both patients and physicians can we achieve the solutions that will decrease medical errors and their devastating consequences.'[3]

References

1. Beck, U. (1986) *The Risk Society*. Sage, London.
2. Kraman, S.S. and Hamm, G.H. (1999) *Risk management: extreme honesty may be the best policy*. Ann. Intern. Med. 131: 963–7.
3. Wu, A.W. (1999) *Handling hospital errors: is disclosure the best defense?* [Editorial] Ann. Intern. Med. 131: 970–2.

Post-modern clinical practice

'… a primordial image', as Jacob Burckhardt once called
it – the figure of a physician or teacher of mankind.
The archetypal image of the wise man, the saviour or
redeemer, lies buried and dormant in man's unconscious
since the dawn of culture; it is awakened whenever the
times are out of joint and a human society is committed to
a serious error. When people go astray they feel the need
of a guide or teacher or even of the physician.

Carl Gustav Jung, *Modern Man in Search of a Soul*

It is likely that the 21st century will be one in which
there will be greater uncertainty – economic, social and
environmental. Against this background, it will be necessary
for the clinician to practise evidence-based medicine
(although the term may fall into disuse as evidence-based
medicine becomes part of the accepted paradigm).

Anxiety and disease

There are several interesting trends that should give the
proponents of evidence-based medicine cause to stop and think:

- the sector in healthcare undergoing the fastest growth is
  complementary medicine
- bookshops contain more books about alternative
  medicine than those about what might be termed
  scientific, evidence-based, or conventional medicine
- vitamins and nutritional supplements, for which there
  is no evidence of effectiveness, are two of the fastest
  growing retail lines – new 'health' shops are opening
  more rapidly than new healthcare facilities.

As proponents of an evidence-based approach, we must
ask ourselves what it is that people want that they are not
getting from conventional health services.

Perhaps it is certainty they need, and uncertainty is
undoubtedly the hallmark of evidence-based healthcare and
a critical approach to decision-making. In the past, a doctor
was always certain, always had a diagnosis, and always had a
treatment in which s/he believed, or at least appeared to believe.
The modern doctor is sceptical, uncertain, and participative.
Some patients welcome this development, but many do not.
More confusing for the clinician, some patients apparently
welcome the change but also want a doctor who is certain.

Thus, it is important to recognise that many patients want more than uncertainty from a consultation. People who are ill are anxious, and they want their anxiety assuaged as well as their disease treated. Many patients, however, do not have a disease that doctors can recognise; they simply bring to the doctor their feelings of unwellness and anxiety. Sometimes, reassurance that they do not have a disease is sufficient, but this is not always the case.

Dealing with uncertainty

Evidence-based medicine, although a very good way of dealing with disease, is not necessarily a good way of dealing with the anxiety that symptoms and/or a diagnosis may cause. In fact, for some people, it may increase the level of anxiety which is why they might seek complementary care. Complementary therapists are rarely as uncertain as practitioners of evidence-based clinical practice, and are sometimes absolutely certain, both about the theory on which they base their practice and about the advice they give an individual patient, even though they do not have what the author of this book would consider to be 'evidence'. Although some practitioners of evidence-based medicine are good at alleviating anxiety and some patients are not anxious, currently there is no mechanism through which the anxieties of individual patients can easily be identified and met by a busy clinician; moreover, a clinician's style of practice will stem not just from a learned skill but also from his/her personality.

However, the development of the DUET database has introduced a new paradigm: instead of clinicians telling patients only what is known, it is now possible to tell them what is not known (Section 1.5.1.1). There are two types of uncertainty:

- uncertain uncertainty, that is, we do not know if anyone knows
- certain uncertainty, that is, we know that no one knows, which is the type of uncertainty anatomised in the DUET database.

When given the information about any uncertainty relevant to their condition, many patients may welcome this honesty and be empowered to take steps to deal with it, for instance, by finding out if it is possible to participate in an RCT.[1]

Reference

1. Chalmers, I. (1995) *What do I want from health research and researchers when I am a patient? [Education and debate]* Br. Med. J. 310: 1315–18.

Back to the future: 21st century healthcare

The 21st century clinician

Three things which judgement demands:

- *wisdom*
- *penetration*
- *knowledge.*

Ninth Century Irish Triad

David Pencheon suggested that the three most important words in medical education are 'I don't know': learning is about knowing how to find out what you don't know.[1] For a clinician in the 21st century, openly admitting to patients that no one can keep abreast of all the information being generated and taking on the role of, and working as, a knowledge manager is the most appropriate strategy. It is a better strategy than trying to retain a status as the fount of all knowledge, which was how physicians were viewed (and sometimes portrayed themselves) in the past.

In his book *Business @ the Speed of Thought*,[2] Bill Gates identified one of the important debates for the digital age as the need to identify the function of the human being; nowhere will this be more important than in clinical practice. Indeed, the Joint Learning Initiative, an independent network of over 100 global health leaders, has identified that the role of human beings as the workforce in health services will be critical to building sustainable health systems in all countries.[3]

The 21st century patient

If the 20th century was the century of the clinician, with biographies such as that of Harvey Cushing describing how the rise of the great physician or surgeon paralleled the growing power and prestige of the medical profession,[4] in the 21st century, the power of the individual clinician and of the profession as a whole is waning.

If the 20th century was the century of the clinician, the 21st century will be the century of the patient. Which adjective is it most appropriate to apply to informed patients? Some people have suggested the 'expert' patient, but the opposite of 'expert' is 'inexpert', which is inaccurate. Another approach has been to talk about the 'resourceful' patient, namely, a patient who has the resources needed to make decisions about their own healthcare, for example, access to knowledge, skills to interpret information, access to their notes, and the confidence to challenge authority.[5]

Although, to state the obvious, the resourceful patient needs resources, they also need a change in attitude on the part of the medical profession, as the insights from a doctor as the parent of a patient vividly demonstrate (Box E.1).[6] However, as a change in professional attitude may take too long to evolve, the most appropriate course is to promote evidence-based clinical practice and ensure that the patient has access to good-quality evidence.

Does the 21st century patient want choice?

Choice is hell.

Isaiah Berlin, in a letter to Lord David Cecil, 8 November 1953

It is impossible to generalise about patients. As people, they possess a range of different types of knowledge and a wide range of literacy, including health literacy. Furthermore, in any group of individuals there will be a wide variation in their tolerance of anxiety.

As discussed in Chapter 10, Isaiah Berlin's essay *Two Concepts of Liberty* provides a helpful framework when thinking about the degree of freedom people might want. Berlin emphasised that there are two types of liberty:

Box E.1 'Our special girl': what was important for us? (Source: Dunkelberg[6])

- To be protected from specialists who propose more and more tests but cannot admit they do not know what is wrong.
- To accept that we don't have a diagnosis and will probably never have one.
- To have the opportunity to try a treatment, even though there is no evidence for its efficacy.
- To clarify my own role as doctor, co-therapist, or mother.
- To be taken seriously and treated with respect.
- To shift from the focus on pathology and abnormality to Mathilda's health and to the positive aspects of her life.

1. negative liberty – freedom from restraint, barriers or obstacles
2. positive liberty – freedom or ability/opportunity to take control to achieve certain purposes or ends.

Applying Berlin's concept of negative liberty to patient choice would mean that patients should be allowed to choose anything or everything. However, simply giving patients freedom to choose, i.e. maximising their negative liberty, is not the best course of action. Positive liberty is of much greater importance in this situation.

The individual patient wants to have control, namely, the positive liberty of deciding whether, in any particular situation, he or she has complete freedom:

- to make whatever decision they want
- to ask the clinician to make the decision
- to share the decision-making with the clinician.

The 21st century patient wants the positive liberty of controlling how much choice they as a patient will have.

Sharing knowledge from experience

In the 21st century, the individual patient will also be able to rely not only on the clinician facing them, but also on the collected wisdom of many clinicians and patients, available through the direct experience of patients provided in the Database of Individual Patient Experience (DIPEx) (Box E.2), and by the use of patient decision aids.

Patient decision aids are one of the clinical resources of greatest use to both patients and clinicians (see Section 10.4.3.1). Patient decision aids, whether as CDs or websites, offer easy access to unbiased information. This is important because clinicians may not be either unbiased or clear in the provision of information to patients.

In the 21st century, many patients will be able to use digital sources of information and then have the capacity to discuss the options with a trusted professional. The role of the appropriately trained clinician will be to help patients reflect on the evidence and relate it to their values when considering the options available. As such, patient decision aids will become clinical tools of central importance.

Rapport et al.[7] explored users' views and reactions to three patient decision aids (two CD-Roms and one paper-based aid) for genetic testing for breast cancer. One pilot and six extended focus groups were set up.

Box E.2 DIPEx

DIPEx provides access to a variety of personal experiences of health and illness. In addition to personal experiences on the website, there is information on treatment choices and where to find support. The following topics are covered:

- cancers
- heart disease
- HIV
- mental health
- neurological conditions
- screening programmes
- immunisation
- pregnancy
- chronic illness
- chronic pain
- rheumatoid arthritis
- intensive care
- living with dying
- teenage health (http://www.youthhealthtalk.org/).

DIPEx is available online at: http://dipex.org/.

The groups comprised women over the age of 18 years ($n = 39$) at high, moderate and population risk of familial breast cancer who had been referred to the Cancer Genetic Service for Wales. It was found that the women had different preferences for different types of decision aids, and there was no consensus over the most appropriate aid, and no systematic differences among the risk groups. The women reported that the aids did increase their knowledge, and that they wanted the aids designed within the context of the NHS and by an authoritative source.

The results of this study underline the need:

- to involve users in the development of patient decision aids
- to provide a range of formats
- to contextualise the information so that it is relevant to the health service in which it is used.

In the absence of the development of user-sensitive decision aids, patients will continue to access information from a variety of sources that will undoubtedly vary in quality.

References

1. Editor's Choice (1999)'*I don't know': the three most important words in education*. Available online at:
   http://www.bmj.com/cgi/content/full/318/7193/0
2. Gates, B. (2000) *Business @ the Speed of Thought*. Penguin, London.
3. Chen, L., Evans, T., Anand, S. et al. (2004) *Human resources for health: overcoming the crisis*. Lancet 364: 1984–90.
4. Bliss, M. (2005) *Harvey Cushing: A Life in Surgery*. Oxford University Press, New York.
5. Gray, J.A.M. (2002) *The Resourceful Patient*. eRosetta Press, Oxford.
6. Dunkelberg, S. (2006) *A patient's journey: our special girl*. Br. Med. J. 333: 430–1.
7. Rapport, F., Iredale, R., Jones, W. et al. (2006) *Decision aids for familial breast cancer: exploring women's views using focus groups*. Health Expect. 9: 232–44.

Conclusion

Providing patient-centred care is the simplest way to run health services. As healthcare becomes more complex – a greater number of networks, a greater number of staff working part-time and increasing use of the independent sector – the patient becomes the only constant. In this situation, it is the patient who should hold their own record, which is the simplest way to run a patient record system, and knowledge should be given to patients with the expectation that they will use that knowledge to make decisions about their own healthcare.

If evidence-based practice dominated the 20th century, it is likely that evidence-based patient choice will dominate the 21st.

Index

Page numbers in *italics* refer to boxes and tables, and those in **bold** type to figures.

D

W